# SERIOUS MENTAL HEALTH PROBLEMS IN THE COMMUNITY

# SERIOUS MENTAL HEALTH PROBLEMS IN THE COMMUNITY
## Policy, Practice and Research

*Edited by*

## Charlie Brooker

*PhD MSc BA(Hons) RMN RNT DipNEd*

*Professor of Nursing, School of Nursing,
Health Visiting and Midwifery, University of Manchester,
Manchester*

*and*

## Julie Repper

*MPhil BA(Hons) RMN RGN*

*Research Student, School of Nursing, Health Visiting and Midwifery,
University of Manchester, Manchester*

## Ballière Tindall

London   Philadelphia   Toronto   Sydney   Tokyo

Ballière Tindall  24–28 Oval Road
London NW1 7DX

The Curtis Center
Independence Square West
Philadelphia, PA 19106–3399, USA

Harcourt Brace & Company
55 Horner Avenue
Toronto, Ontario M8Z 4X6, Canada

Harcourt Brace & Company, Australia
30–52 Smidmore Street
Marrickville, NSW 2204, Australia

Harcourt Brace & Company, Japan
Ichibancho Central Building, 22–1 Ichibancho
Chiyoda-ku, Tokyo 102, Japan

A catalogue record of this book is available from the British Library

ISBN 0–7020–2127–X

Typeset by Paston Press Ltd, Loddon, Norfolk
Printed and bound in Great Britain by Bell & Bain Ltd, Glasgow

# CONTENTS

# CONTRIBUTORS

**Elizabeth Armstrong**   RGN RHV, Director, National Depression Care Training Centre, Nene College of Higher Education, Northampton

**Max Birchwood**   BSc MSc PhD FBPsS, Director, Early Intervention Service, Northern Birmingham Mental Health Trust, Birmingham

**Charlie Brooker**   PhD MSc BA(Hons) RMN RNT DipN Ed, Professor of Nursing, School of Nursing, Health Visiting and Midwifery, University of Manchester, Manchester

**Gráinne Fadden**   BA MPhil C.Psychol AFBPsS, Consultant Clinical Psychologist, Aylesbury Vale Healthcare, Aylesbury, Buckinghamshire

**Richard Ford**   BSc RMN MSc, Head of Service Evaluation, Sainsbury Centre for Mental Health, London

**Kevin Gournay**   MPhil PhD C.Psychol AFBPsS RN, Professor of Psychiatric Nursing, Institute of Psychiatry, London

**Andrew Healey**   BSc(Hons) MSc, Lecturer in Health Economics, Centre for the Economics of Mental Health, Institute of Psychiatry, London

**David G. Kingdon**   MD MRCPsych, Medical Director, Nottingham Healthcare Trust, Nottingham

**Martin Knapp**   BA MSc PhD, Professor of Health Economics, Centre for the Economics of Mental Health, Institute of Psychiatry, London, and Professorial Fellow, London School of Economics and Political Science, London

**Fiona Macmillan**   MD MRCPsych, Consultant Psychiatrist, St Edwards Hospital, Cheddleton, Staffordshire

**Dermot McGovern**   MPhil MBChB MRCPsych, Northern Birmingham Mental Health Trust Headquarters, Birmingham

**Edana Minghella**   BSc(Hons) RMN PGCEA, Senior Researcher, Sainsbury Centre for Mental Health, London

**Steve Morgan**   BA BPl (Town Planning), DipCOT, SROT, Training and Development Officer, Sainsbury Centre for Mental Health, London

**Steve Onyett**   MSc AFBPsS C.Clin Psychol, Senior Research Fellow, Tizard Centre, University of Kent at Canterbury and Head of Clinical Psychology Service, South Kent Community Healthcare NHS Trust

**Edward Peck**   BA(Hons) MA PhD, Director, Centre for Mental Health Services Development, Kings College, London

**Rachel E. Perkins**   BA(Hons) MPhil PhD, Clinical Director and Consultant Clinical Psychologist, Rehabilitation and Continuing Care Service, Pathfinder Mental Health Services NHS Trust, London

**Peter Pratt**   BSc(Pharm) MRPharmS, Chief Pharmacist, Community Health Sheffield, Sheffield

**Julie Repper**   MPhil BA(Hons) RMN RGN, Research Student, School of Nursing, Health Visiting and Midwifery, University of Manchester, Manchester

**Tom Sandford**   BSc DipN RMN RGN, Mental Health Advisor, Royal College of Nursing, London

**Helen Smith**   BA MSc (Clin Psychol), Strategic Commissioner for Mental Health, Lambeth, Southwark and Lewisham Health Authority

**Jo Smith**   BSc MSc PhD, Consultant Clinical Psychologist, Head of Rehabilitation, Department of Clinical Psychology, Newtown Hospital, Worcester

# PREFACE

Despite the recent emphasis which government policy has placed upon people with serious mental health problems, few texts provide an overview of current understanding about this client group, their needs and the provision of services to meet these needs. In this book we have endeavoured to draw together policy, research, practice and educational experts from a range of disciplines to provide a comprehensive and contemporary account of community services, approaches, interventions and teaching programmes for people who are disabled by serious and ongoing mental health problems.

This is not, however, a step-by-step guide. Local populations differ as do local services, community resources, personnel and visions of excellence: it is only through creativity and innovation that new ideas can be tried and tested and we do not advocate nor guarantee any single model of service provision. Nevertheless, each of the contributors does provide research evidence and practical illustrations of approaches and interventions which have been shown to be effective and they detail the problems and possibilities of implementing such practice within local services. It is for local commissioners, planners, practitioners and educational establishments to piece this evidence together and fit it into local services to meet the needs of the local people.

The book has been written with this broad mental health service constituency in mind. Theoretical models and research findings are presented alongside case studies and practical examples so that all those involved in the support of people with serious mental health problems will find it valuable and interesting – whether commissioning, planning, providing teaching or using services.

Although the book is launched onto a sea of political change, it is clear that the new administration will largely emphasise many aspects of good practice already highlighted by contributors working at the cutting edge. The clearest indication of the direction of forthcoming changes is the proposals to strengthen links between all agencies impacting on health: primary and secondary services, health and social care, housing and employment. Throughout this text, the importance of close collaboration between care agencies is all too evident, as are the deleterious effects of homelessness, poor housing, poverty and unemployment. As such, the book does not detail the problems and struggles of the last two decades but looks towards solutions, challenges and changes for the years ahead.

# SECTION I

# CONTEMPORARY ISSUES IN COMMUNITY MENTAL HEALTH SERVICES

# CHAPTER 1

# Serious Mental Health Problems in the Community

## The Significance of Policy, Practice and Research

## Julie Repper and Charlie Brooker

The 1990s mark a period of unprecedented attention on people who have serious mental health problems. Shifts in the location of mental health services have raised ongoing questions about what their function should now be and the increased visibility of people with mental health problems has led to paradoxical public views – with widespread concern and sympathy coexisting with fear and opposition to local mental health facilities. The growing voice of service users and their families has drawn attention to the rights of people with mental health problems and their potential role in planning, providing and evaluating services. A synthesis of biological explanations of mental illness with an increased understanding of psychological and social factors has given rise to new ways of working which are supported by increasingly rigorous research.

The broad policy context of health care has provided a backdrop to this activity, but has also been coloured by it. With the health service reforms, the introduction of the internal market is driving the development of adequate needs assessment tools for this population. Also, as the importance of collaboration between different purchasing bodies, and between purchasers and providers has become apparent, so specific policy for people with serious mental health problems has been introduced to ensure that mechanisms for monitoring and review are in place. The focus on this population is also reflected in the NHS Research and Development (R&D) policy: mental health was the first priority topic in the nationally commissioned R&D programme in 1993; serious mental illness was a key area in the subsequent regional R&D programmes; and in 1995 the Mental Health Research Initiative was part of the centrally commissioned Department of Health (DoH) programme.

Such intense activity in relation to people with serious mental health problems has not occurred without reason. Although the large-scale movement away from institutional to community-based care for people with mental illness began almost four decades ago, the full implications of this shift are only now becoming clear. Numerous reports, inquiries and media commentaries have drawn attention to the broad impact of de-institutionalisation, and more detailed research continues to describe the lives of people who would previously have spent long periods in psychiatric hospitals. Overall, it is apparent that community living is particularly difficult for people who have serious mental illness, many of whom experience frequent re-admissions in times of crisis and survive inadequately: in poverty and isolation, without work, with poor social supports and networks, and at risk of victimisation, exploitation, homelessness and imprisonment. Indeed the community tenure of this population is often dependent upon the support of informal carers who inevitably have problems and needs themselves.

Given rather more publicity in the general media, is the risk that people with serious mental health problems pose for the general public. Although newspaper articles proclaiming the success of community support projects are few and far between, maximum coverage is given to the relatively rare incidents of violence perpetrated by people with mental health problems. Indeed the Confidential Inquiry into Homicides and Suicides identified a total of 39 homicides by mentally ill people in a total period of three years. Undoubtedly negative media coverage has contributed to a popular association between madness and dangerousness and added to the reluctance of local communities to accommodate facilities for people with mental health problems. However, by raising public concern it has directly influenced the development of policy: Virginia Bottomley's '10 point plan' was announced in the aftermath of several widely publicised tragic incidents.

The complex, multiple and long-term needs of people with serious mental health problems cannot be met by the time-limited, unidisciplinary therapy provided for people with short-term problems. A number of interventions which take into account the effect and interaction of biological vulnerability with psychological, social and cultural influences demonstrate promising levels of effectiveness with this client group. However, these are clearly not sufficient in themselves. A comprehensive range of mental health services which are accessible and acceptable is also needed, but, since many people with serious mental health problems withdraw from services at times of crisis, may not wish to be associated with psychiatric services, or may find it difficult to organise themselves sufficiently to use community services, it is also necessary to provide support within clients' own homes. Service evaluation research demonstrates the benefits of assertive outreach working on a long-term, intensive, continuous but flexible basis. In those services found to be most effective, such principles are combined with skilled bio-psychosocial interventions from a supportive team, drawing on multidisciplinary and multi-agency resources. However, the implementation of this approach within local settings is fraught with difficulties, such as limited resources and skills, contradictory demands, poor communication and collaboration between services. To minimise the risks of neglect, self-harm and violence a series of policy initiatives have been introduced which offer explicit guidance for the support and prioritisation of 'people with severe or serious mental illness'. These are summarised in Box 1.1. Although this focus of attention on people with serious mental health problems demonstrates a commitment to protecting the public and service users alike – and might well be considered long overdue – in itself, such policy has not guaranteed effective change within local services.

The planning of this book arose out of our concern that despite the intense policy and research focus upon people with serious mental health problems, the provision of adequate services remains problematic. With the help of the contributors, we therefore set out with the clear aim of examining the relationship between policy, research and practice. We have endeavoured to achieve this by organising the book in two sections. The first traces the effect of policy on the functions of purchasing and providing services, the second examines, in some detail, specific ways in which broad categories of interventions might be tailored to meet the needs of people with serious mental health problems.

A text such as this cannot do justice to all the work that has been going on in recent years and might be noted as much for its omissions as for its inclusions, but in selecting topics for inclusion, we were guided by two principles. First, the book is primarily intended to provide a practical guide to issues that are of day to day relevance to those planning, providing and evaluating services for people who have serious mental health problems. Thus, priority has been given to those areas in which a substantial body of knowledge and understanding has accrued, rather than the many new aspects of treatment and service delivery that are at an early stage of development and remain relatively untried in practice. For example, although epidemiological research and neuropsychiatry are beginning to reveal new leads in the treatment and management of people with serious mental health problems, their implications for the delivery of local services remain, as yet, unclear.

**Box 1.1** Mental Health Policy Developments 1990–1997

1990 NHS and Community Care Act
       Community Care. House of Commons Social Services
       Committee report
1991 Care Programme Approach
       Mental Illness Specific Grant
1992 Health of the Nation White Paper – Mental Illness one of
       five key areas
       Review of services for mentally ill offenders (chair: J. Reed)
1993 Mental Illness Key Area Handbook (Health of the Nation)
       Mental Health Task Force set up
       Review of legal powers on the care of mentally ill people in
       the community
       Secretary of State's 10 point plan:
         1. Review of standards of care for people with
            schizophrenia (CSAG)
         2. Agreed programme of work for Mental Health Task
            Force
         3. Ensure Health Authority and GP fundholder plans cover
            mental health
         4. The London Implementation Group to improve services
            in the capital
         5. Better training for keyworkers under the Care
            Programme Approach
         6. Publication of the review of legal powers
         7. Seek legislation for supervised discharge, and
            extended leave under Section 3
         8. Publication of revised code of practice for Mental
            Health Act
         9. Guidance on the discharge of mentally disordered
            people
        10. Development of better information systems
1994 DoH guidance for introducing supervision registers from 1
       April 1994
       DoH guidance for discharge and continuing care
       Mental Health Nursing Review (chair: T. Butterworth)
       Inquiry into care of Christopher Clunis (chair: J. Ritchie)
       House of Commons Health Committee report – Better off in
       the community?
       Audit Commission report – Finding a place
       Mental Illness Key Area Handbook (2nd edition)
       Health of Nation thematic review – The prevention of
       suicide
       Mental Illness Specific Grant to target those most at risk
1995 Mental Health (Patients in the Community Bill) – Supervised
       Discharge
       Health of Nation guide to interagency working – Building
       Bridges
       Additional Mental Illness Specific Grant funding to target
       severely mentally ill
       CSAG report on schizophrenia
1997 Green Paper: Developing Partnerships in Mental Health

Second, neither the policy context, nor the delivery of services can be properly understood outside the context of the NHS policy for research and development. At the crux of this is Peckham's comment on the use and development of research in the NHS in 1991: 'Strongly held views based on belief rather than sound information still exert too much influence in health care. In some instances the relevant knowledge is available but is not being used; in other situations additional information needs to be generated from reliable sources' (Department of Health, 1995). Throughout the book, therefore, an emphasis has been placed on the research evidence that does exist in order to understand the effects of policy initiatives in areas as broad as 'the coordination of care' and 'purchasing', and to justify the use of specific interventions for particular groups of people with serious mental health problems.

These principles not only enabled us to select broad chapter headings for the book, they also informed the approach taken by authors. Case study material is included wherever possible to illustrate the use of the interventions and approaches discussed and make their application more accessible. Relevant research is cited throughout the text, and the need for further research is specifically indicated. Each chapter begins with a summary of key points – to give the reader a succinct insight into its content – and ends with questions for consideration and a list of key texts for further reading. These are intended to help the reader reflect on the broader implications of the chapter and enable him to access more detailed information in the area.

For a book entitled 'Serious mental health problems...', we had to be clear from the outset about the client group we were referring to. Although the term 'serious mental health problems' is commonly used, it clearly has different meanings for different people. For policy makers driven by the publicity given to high profile cases of violence and neglect, the term originally referred to those people who caused most problems if they were not carefully monitored and provided for. Policy guidance has not given precise definitions of the client group it refers to, but increasingly includes criteria used by local services in the prioritisation of people who have serious mental health problems. Research, on the other hand, has generally focused on those with a diagnosis of schizophrenia as a proxy for all people who experience serious mental health problems. Although a narrowly defined client group might be necessary in the rigorous evaluation of interventions, the question for local services is whether these interventions can and should be used with the whole population who have serious mental health problems, including people with a range of diagnoses, multiple diagnoses, multiple health and social problems, different wishes and aspirations, and various levels of social disability.

In the implementation of policy, local services have needed to develop clear criteria for prioritising those clients whom they consider to have the most severe mental health problems. This involves judgements of relative need: should greater priority be given to people with a diagnosis of schizophrenia than to those with a diagnosis of personality disorder or long-term, severe depression? Should people with alcohol or drug dependency be excluded? Who is responsible for supporting people who have pre-senile dementia or Huntington's chorea? It is this debate that brings us closest to defining serious mental health problems: in policy and practice terms, the prioritisation of people with serious mental health problems refers to those with greatest need. But if efforts and resources are to be focused on those with greatest need, how should need be defined? Rather than attempt to adjudicate between different interest groups (clients, the courts, professionals, relatives, neighbours) who adopt different definitions of a person's needs, it is perhaps more helpful to consider the dimensions generally used by services in the prioritisation of clients: diagnosis, disability and duration (Bachrach, 1988; Powell and Slade, 1995). Two further dimensions have been added in the recent policy document *Building Bridges*: safety, and the need for formal and informal care, which 'have secured widespread acceptance at a local level' (Department of Health, 1995, p. 11). Local services are advised to agree locally an operational definition which is consistent with this 'SIDDD' framework (Safety, Informal and formal care, Disability, Duration and Diagnosis).

However, these dimensions are not straightforward, and the manner in which the framework is used greatly influences the number and characteristics of clients prioritised in any local service (Perkins and Repper, 1998). The criterion of safety encompasses both the safety of the individual client from him/herself and others, and the safety of other people. It covers 'unintentional' harm such as self-neglect, more active self-harm, harm to other people and harm by other people. Although these issues are critical in providing adequate support, clinical judgements in this area are fraught with problems about what constitutes 'acceptable risk'.

The criterion of informal and formal care refers to the level of care a person requires to achieve a reasonable level of social functioning. As such, it includes help from informal carers and from formal services, including detention under the Mental Health Act. The problems with prioritising those who apparently need most formal and informal support include the risk of perceiving those who are compulsorily detained to be in greatest need. It follows that resources will be committed to this client group which may inadvertently lead to inadequate investment in ongoing support, respite and early preventative work - services which could reduce the need for compulsory admission.

*Building Bridges* (Department of Health, 1995) suggests that diagnostic dimensions of serious mental health problems *may* include psychotic illness, dementia, severe neurotic illness, personality disorder or developmental disorder. Given such broad criteria, local services must either prioritise people with specific diagnoses (usually schizophrenia and manic depressive psychosis) and exclude others (for example personality disorder), or they must use some other criteria to distinguish those with greatest need, for example level of disability. This refers to a person's ability to function in the community. From the perspective of people using services, social disability is perhaps the most meaningful criterion. In the second chapter of this book, Perkins and Repper argue that the aim of mental health services should be to minimise the socially disabling impact of mental health problems by ensuring that the person has access to ordinary roles, relationships, activities and opportunities. However, as a principle for prioritising those with greatest need, questions arise over whether resources should be directed towards those people whose social functioning has deteriorated most or towards the prevention of social disability. Furthermore, a focus on social disabilities may lead to mental health services prioritising resources to compensate for social inequalities: providing mental health services where what is necessary is employment, an adequate income, decent housing and proper education.

On the criterion of duration, *Building Bridges* (1996) cites 'periods which vary between six months and more than 2 years'. Although affording priority to those with long-term problems necessitates some criterion of longevity, this is problematic because long-term, effective support may in fact reduce needs. Waiting until a person has had difficulties for long enough to warrant prioritisation may incur further damage than would otherwise be necessary.

Defining serious mental health problems will always pose dilemmas, so it is perhaps unsurprising that for the purpose of this book we have not prescribed any particular definition of the population. In much the same way as local services develop their own criteria for prioritisation, the authors in this book have adopted their own definitions. These are not always explicit, but there is general acknowledgement of the need to consider a heterogeneous client group whose everyday lives are seriously curtailed by disabling cognitive and emotional difficulties. Although many will have a diagnosis of schizophrenia or affective psychosis, the population with serious mental health problems will include people with a range of diagnoses all of whom have high levels of need as a result of the disabling impact of their problems.

The contributors use a variety of terms to describe people who have serious mental health problems: users, patients, clients and consumers. This reveals aspects of each writer's philosophy of mental health care and is perhaps representative of the wide-ranging beliefs held by different professionals about the nature of mental health. It was our deliberate intention at the outset to ensure a contribution from all disciplines involved in the care and treatment of people with serious mental health problems – particularly given the increasing attention being paid to the principles of effective multidisciplinary teamwork. Thus, as a group, the authors represent psychology, psychiatry, nursing (including primary health care), social work, occupational therapy and pharmacy, although we should acknowledge the lack of a general practitioner perspective.

The book begins with a consideration of the principles of working with people who have serious mental health problems and firmly places the needs and – perhaps most importantly – the wishes of people who use services as the central consideration in all ensuing discussion. Indeed, the importance of these principles is confirmed throughout the text as authors repeatedly emphasise the need to heed clients' views and wishes, the need to work collaboratively with other service providers, and the importance of a comprehensive range of resources. In Chapter 2 with Julie Repper, Rachel Perkins writes as a service user, a psychologist and clinical director of Rehabilitation and Continuing Care Services to advocate a social disability and access model as a means of facilitating access to roles, relationships, activities and facilities within the social world. This provides a framework within which specific interventions can be offered and legislative requirements met – with due regard to issues of power, choice and civil rights.

In Chapter 3, Edward Peck describes the evolution of the organisational framework within which mental health services are provided and discusses the role and characteristics of different purchasers with an emphasis on the importance of collaboration. Assessment of need and contracting for services are considered in detail, with enumeration of the challenges that face purchasers, and, more unusually, suggestions of ways of overcoming these challenges.

Steve Onyett and Helen Smith draw on their extensive work on community mental health teams and mental health service development to examine the function and organisation of community mental health teams in Chapter 4. They provide a useful critique of the issues to be addressed in order to improve the effectiveness of community mental health teams, and they offer five possible approaches for collaboration between primary and secondary care services. The latter issue is developed further in Chapter 5 in which Liz Armstrong describes the role of the primary health care team in the care of people with serious mental health problems, and draws on practical examples and research to make recommendations for better integration between mental health services and primary care services.

The final two chapters in the first section of the book examine aspects of research in the domain of serious mental health problems. Richard Ford and Edana Minghella propose a pragmatic approach to the evaluation of mental health services; they deliberately avoid theoretical explanation and emphasise the contribution that service evaluation can make to service development. As well as offering advice regarding the process of successful external evaluation, they illustrate the flexibility and practical usefulness of their model through a case study of its use. Andrew Healey and Martin Knapp provide an important overview of the economic evaluation of mental health services. The service costs of mental illness were estimated as amounting to over £4.5 million in 1986 yet there exists surprisingly little information about the relative costs and benefits of interventions and services. Healey and Knapp examine the purpose, modes and application of economic evaluation in mental health services, concluding that more work needs to be done in this area and the findings should be used to inform decisions in policy and practice.

The second part of the book examines in more detail specific interventions and approaches for working with people who have serious mental health problems. Gráinne Faddon leads this section with conclusive evidence of the effectiveness of family intervention. However, as she points out, there are clearly problems to be overcome if families are to receive effective interventions in routine clinical settings: ongoing training and supervision of staff, organisational support, and fidelity to the specific interventions shown to be effective are important in this regard. There is also only limited evidence of efforts to implement this work with people who do not have a diagnosis of schizophrenia. These conclusions offer useful insights into the difficulties of research implementation – an issue which is discussed in more detail in the final chapter.

In Chapter 9, David Kingdon takes a broader look at the application of cognitive behaviour therapy with people who have serious mental health problems, including those with a diagnosis of personality disorder and affective disorder. He goes beyond research and theory to provide detailed practical descriptions of a cognitive approach illustrated with useful case examples. Again, the final message of this chapter is the need to use cognitive interventions as just one part of a multidisciplinary, collaborative approach within a comprehensive range of services.

Max Birchwood and his colleagues examine early intervention in psychotic relapse. Although they focus on cognitive approaches to the management of early warning signs, if the full potential of early signs monitoring is to be realised, services need to be based on a philosophy in which the client is the expert and the clinician's role lies in using and developing this expertise in the prediction of relapse and appropriate intervention. Widespread systems need to be introduced in local services to ensure that assessment, monitoring and education become a routine part of clinical practice. Indeed, this review clearly indicates the importance of a flexible and responsive service in which communication between all involved is crucial.

Although many of the authors emphasise the importance of medication, Peter Pratt (Chapter 11) cautions that the aim of drug treatment must be to achieve a balance between the consequences of the illness and the consequences of the treatment. Ultimately it is the patient who will decide where this balance lies, but they can only make real choices about their treatment if they are given accurate, adequate and accessible information. Once more, the significance of the patient's experiences and wishes are emphasised. This theme is continued in Steve Morgan's chapter on risk management: rather than reduce risk by limiting liberty, opportunities and choice, the management of risk is best achieved through an enabling and collaborative approach between workers and clients within a strong network of services with careful systems of communication. This chapter not only addresses the assessment and management of suicide and violence, it also examines the problem of self-neglect. Although this is not unusual in people who have the 'negative' symptoms frequently associated with long-term and serious mental health problems, it is rarely addressed in its own right. Steve Morgan illustrates the manifestations and management of self-neglect in a case study. He also draws attention to the need for healthcare workers to examine their own levels of tolerance against objective levels of risk before intervening.

If the research and practice evidence presented in this book is to find its way into routine practice there is clearly a need for further training of multidisciplinary staff, at all levels of the service, in service structures, general approaches and specific interventions for working with people who have serious mental health problems. Kevin Gournay reviews the current position in relation to training; as yet, there is little evidence of the success of educational initiatives in changing services, and there is no consensus regarding the content, level or target audience of such training. Although an important area to consider, it is clear that there is much work to be done in addressing these questions.

In the final chapter of the book, the complex relationship between policy, practice and research is examined with reference to the foregoing text. There is extensive research evidence and policy guidance to inform services and individuals working with people who have serious mental health problems, but it is not widely implemented in local settings. Many of the impediments to the development of effective services are clear: fundamental and ongoing changes in mental health services are making new demands on ill-prepared staff, purchasers of mental health services have different priorities and agendas, local populations have a complex range of needs and wishes, and despite the notion of the NHS as a service free to everyone who needs it, limited resources require a system of prioritisation. However, there are examples of good practice within local services for people who have serious mental health problems, and it is these that must be followed. Work needs to be undertaken to identify and evaluate ways of ensuring that available evidence is implemented. It is with this purpose that the book concludes, providing a final summary of the main issues to be addressed at the levels of policy, purchasing, providing and using community services for people who have serious mental health problems.

*REFERENCES*

Bachrach, L. L. (1988), Defining mental illness: a concept paper. *Hospital and Community Psychiatry*, 40, 234–235.

Department of Health (1991), *Report for Health: an R&D Strategy for the NHS*. London: HMSO.

Department of Health (1995), *Building Bridges, A Guide to arrangements for inter-agency working for the care and protection of severely mentally ill people*. London: HMSO.

Perkins, R. and Repper, J. (1998), *Choice and Control. Dilemmas in community mental health care practice*. Oxford: Radcliffe Medical Press.

Powell, R. and Slade, M. (1995), Defining severe mental illness. In: Thornicroft, G. and Strathdee, G. (Eds) *Purchasing Mental Health Services*. London: Cambridge University Press.

**CHAPTER 2**

# Principles of Working with People who Experience Serious Mental Health Problems

## Rachel E. Perkins and Julie Repper

*KEY ISSUES*

♦ The aims of work with people who experience serious mental health problems.

♦ Models of work with people who are seriously disabled by enduring mental health problems.

♦ Forming effective relationships.

♦ Issues of choice and power.

*INTRODUCTION*

People with the cognitive and emotional difficulties associated with serious mental health problems often experience life in a way that is profoundly different from most other people. Although appropriate support and interventions might help them to cope with their difficulties, they often continue to experience problems in some areas of their lives. Since most professional training focuses on time-limited interventions designed to remove a person's problems, workers may feel helpless and hopeless when confronted by people whose perceptions are often shared by no-one else and whose problems do not resolve with their ministrations.

The purpose of this chapter is to address the principles underlying work with people who are seriously disabled by ongoing mental health problems. It will begin by an examination of the aims of such work, followed by a critical appraisal of the models that might be adopted. An approach which focuses on social disabilities, and the commensurate need for access to social relationships, facilities and activities will be outlined as a useful integrative model for work. Issues relating to the formation of effective relationships that can promote access, as well as implications in relation to choice and power, will be considered.

*WHAT ARE WE TRYING TO ACHIEVE?*

In working with people who experience serious ongoing mental health problems the first question that must be asked is 'What is this work designed to achieve?' It is not possible to decide what should be done, or how it should be done, unless the intention of the endeavour is clear. Often these aims or purposes are not overtly considered. It is common for disagreements between different groups and agencies to arise as a result of conflicting ideas about the purpose of both services and work with the individuals they serve.

At a societal level, mental health services have long faced contradictory sets of demands. On the one hand – fuelled by media portrayals of people with serious mental health problems as universally dangerous, antisocial and unpredictable – there is considerable public concern about the presence of people with serious mental health problems in their communities (Dear and Gleeson, 1991; Dear, 1992). The consequent demands on mental health services to ensure public safety are reflected in mental health legislation. On the other hand, there has been pressure from an increasingly powerful mental health user/survivor lobby and a general societal trend towards 'consumerism', which has led to demands for mental health services to be responsive to the wishes and preferences of those who use them.

Ensuring public safety and responding to the wishes and preferences of service users represent different aims that often require different courses of action. Such conflicting demands need to be explicitly addressed by mental health workers as they profoundly affect day to day judgements that have to be made, especially those concerning risk. If a person has a history of disruptive behaviour, is it 'safe' to accede to their wishes to go out of the hospital? If a person is going through an acute crisis is it 'safe' to go along with their wish to remain at home?

At a team and service level there are yet more choices that have to be made about the purpose of work with people who experience serious mental health problems. Numerous suggestions can be discerned in both literature and clinical practice (Anthony and Margules, 1974; Anthony, 1977; Bennett, 1978; Wolfensberger and Tulman, 1982; Shepherd, 1984; Perkins and Dilks, 1992; Perkins and Repper, 1996). These are shown in Box 2.1. Although all of these may seem desirable, it is often not possible to address them all and choices have to be made about priorities. In some settings,

**Box 2.1** Purposes of work with people with serious mental problems

- ◆ Minimising symptoms
- ◆ Preventing relapse
- ◆ Increasing independence from services
- ◆ Optimising functioning in normal social roles
- ◆ Living outside hospital – closing hospital beds
- ◆ Preventing admission to hospital
- ◆ Improving quality of life
- ◆ Increasing skills
- ◆ Accessing facilities, activities and relationships in the community

priorities are determined by external factors, such as closing large remote hospitals, but in most situations clinical decisions have to be based on the needs and priorities of individual clients. For example, a 30-year-old man, who had a diagnosis of schizophrenia of 12 years standing and had spent long periods in hospital, wanted a job, a home of his own, and friends and a social life. He was assisted to find a job and was doing this well while living in hospital. He also developed a circle of friends and was going out several times per week. He then wanted to move into a flat of his own, which he did. However, even with thrice weekly help from an outreach worker, his social activities dropped off under the demands of independent living. He also started turning up late for work and getting into arguments with his colleagues. Although he was managing his flat, he seemed unable to cope with the multiple demands of independent living, work and social activities. If the primary aim had been to enhance independence from services, then priority might be accorded to helping him to keep his flat. If the primary aim had been to optimise his social role functioning then his job and social networks could have taken priority. In fact, he decided that he wanted his friends and job more than he wanted the flat. Therefore he moved, not into hospital, but into a staffed, community facility where he had people around and help with day to day domestic chores. His work and social life picked up again.

Different clinicians may have different opinions about the aims of their work, and there are no 'right' answers. Decisions involve value judgements: increasing independence from services is not in any absolute sense better than optimising and maintaining role functioning. Problems arise when differing aims remain implicit rather than explicitly acknowledged. Most importantly, clients have views about what matters to them. Where decisions have to be made between different goals and priorities the individual concerned can judge what is important to them. With help, even the most seriously disabled person is able to identify many things that they want to do and achieve. These may not always accord with the priorities of professionals, but if clients are to have real choices, professionals cannot always expect to 'know best'.

***MODELS FOR*** Decisions about the aims of support are important, but it is also
***INTERVENTION*** necessary to have a model to guide the way in which a person's problems are understood, the priorities and interventions adopted, and how the success of interventions is judged. A variety of different models have been employed in work with people who have serious ongoing mental health problems (see Ekdawi and Conning, 1994 and Perkins and Repper, 1996 for critical reviews of disability, cure-based, needs, roles and normalisation models). However, like aims, these often remain implicit. This is problematic because whilst implicit, a model cannot be examined, negotiated, challenged or modified: a situation which leads to a great deal of 'blind doing' which can be as destructive as it is helpful.

***Cure-based*** Ideas about cure pervade most mental health services, and indeed
***approaches*** most health care, but they are not restricted to the 'medical model'. In most professional training, prospective clinicians are taught to identify a person's problems or symptoms whether in terms of neurochemical imbalances, faulty cognition, dysfunctional family relationships or disturbed intrapsychic processes. They then learn interventions to put things right: medication, cognitive therapy, family therapy, psychotherapy, counselling, advice and education. Although there are a variety of cure-based models, all share a common approach: focus on the identification of underlying problems and interventions (often time limited) to improve or remove them.

Clearly, interventions which have the potential to reduce particular problems or improve a person's ability to cope with their difficulties may be useful. However, cure-based models can be problematic in work with people who have disabilities arising from serious mental health problems.

♦ People whose problems are ongoing have often experienced many cure-based efforts and their disabilities remain. Continuing attempts to effect a cure can be demoralising for both clients and staff and may result in hopelessness when a cure is not achieved.
♦ A focus on 'cure' as the only way in which life can be meaningful and valuable implies that life with a disability is not worthwhile.
♦ Cure-based models have led to a prioritisation of treatment and a devaluing of support and care. Medication and other specific therapies with a 'treatment' label have a much higher status than

ongoing help with everyday activities. Such help and support are equally important.

♦ The status afforded 'treatment' means that ordinary activities tend to be labelled as 'treatment' or described in spuriously technical language: work therapy, gardening therapy, 'counselling', 'home management' and 'self-care'. This translation of ordinary activities into therapy devalues what clients do: they are not doing real work, it is therapy – good for them, not for the benefit of others. Staff do not do 'self-care' and their work is rarely construed as therapy despite its known protective effects against mental health problems (Smith, 1985).

♦ Therapy is typically time-limited. An intervention is deemed to have failed if the problems have not gone away, or if they recur when it stops. If a person's problems are ongoing then support needs to be ongoing.

*Skills-based approaches*    The development of skills – skills training – is very popular in services for people who have serious mental health problems (Anthony, 1977, 1979; Drouet, 1986). Offering a clear direction for work, this approach starts with the identification of a person's skills and skills deficits. The things that a person needs to learn are then broken down into their component parts and intervention takes the form of building up skills step by step, usually within a behavioural framework.

In many areas 'rehabilitation' has become synonymous with skills development, usually with a view to resettlement: a person is taught the skills they need to live independently and then moves out of the hospital, hostel or day facility. In community services much help with day to day activities is seen not as ongoing support to enable the person to do things, but as training the person to do them without help. Despite its popularity, a skills approach is fraught with problems.

♦ If a person has to acquire the skills of independent living as a prerequisite for community living then many people will remain in institutions. The evidence of problems in generalising social skills (Shepherd, 1977, 1978) indicates that even those people who are judged to have acquired sufficient skills for independent living in a sheltered setting will not necessarily be able to utilise these skills in other settings.

♦ If a certain repertoire of skills is necessary for community living then this implies that the disabled person must be rendered suitable to 'fit in' to the community, with little consideration of ways in which 'the community' can be rendered suitable to accommodate them.

♦ A skills-based approach can only be used where there is an identifiable skill that can be taught: this may be reasonable with mechanical skills like using a bus or boiling an egg, but is problematic in social and emotional areas where the specific skills are more elusive.

♦ All skilled performances, no matter how basic, involve more than the simple mechanical elements that are the focus of skills training. Cognitive, judgemental and organisational skills are critical – what to do when, how much, adjusting behaviour in response to feedback – yet traditional skills training focuses only on the mechanical elements.

♦ Skills training has offered little in relation to helping people to cope with the experience of mental health problems and all that they imply (Perkins and Dilks, 1992; Perkins and Repper, 1996). The ways in which a person copes are important in determining the extent to which they are disabled by their problems (Wing and Morris, 1981; Shepherd, 1984; Taylor and Perkins, 1991; Perkins and Moodley, 1993).

♦ A skills approach can lead to the inappropriate prioritising of interventions: a focus on those areas where there is an identifiable skill to teach. Often this leads to a mismatch between client priorities (to feel better, get more money, have friends) and those of staff (budgeting skills, domestic skills, cooking skills, social skills).

It is sometimes argued that, as skills training is based on an educational model, it has the advantage of giving the client the valued role of student, with staff as instructors or facilitators. The role of medical, or psychology, or nursing student may be valued, but these hardly parallel skills training in mental health services. This usually involves teaching things that most adults can already do: it can be very demeaning, as an adult, to be taught to shave, wash up, go on a bus. The relative roles of staff (as teachers) and clients (as learners) devalue the client: staff have skills to teach, clients have not and must learn.

The situation would be quite different were a more commonplace, adult model of help adopted. Many people get help with day to day activities, e.g. from service washes, cleaners, cafés. This support does not demean the person receiving it: in every case, the person getting help is in charge, says how things should be done. Mental health workers could offer practical help with specific tasks in the same manner, or, at the very least 'being with' and 'doing with' rather than 'instructing' and 'supervising'.

***Needs approaches***   Concepts of need are very popular. There is a desire to develop 'needs led services': define the needs of service users and develop treatment and support that is responsive to these (Wing and Morris, 1981; Bennett, 1978; Shepherd, 1984; Brewin *et al.*, 1987, 1988; Thornicroft *et al.*, 1992).

Needs approaches try to move away from the problems and deficits on which cure and skills approaches are predicated, towards consideration of the complex requirements of individuals. They open the possibility of a range of ways in which a person's needs, once defined, can be met: not simply treating symptoms or teaching skills, but also providing supports, aids and adaptations in the environment. This avoids many of the problems inherent in problem/symptom based approaches. For example, if a person cannot cook, training is one option but there are many other ways to ensure nutritional needs are met: cafés, meals on wheels, take-aways and so forth.

Despite the advantages of needs-based approaches, their usefulness depends on the way in which need is defined. The term 'need' is used to refer to very different things. On the one hand, it encompasses everything from basic physiological necessities (food, water) to complex psychological needs (love, esteem, belonging) (Maslow, 1970). On the other hand, it is used to refer to ways of organising services to ensure that basic human needs are met, thus people are said to 'need' a day centre, hostel or medication. When needs assessment in mental health services involves evaluation of needs for specific services (Brewin *et al.*, 1987, 1988; Clifford, 1989) the devalued status of people with serious mental health problems is reinforced. A special breed of human being is created – 'the mental patient' – who, quite unlike other people, needs hostels, day centres and the like. Indeed, defining needs in terms of services available works against the development of new and innovative ways of helping people. A hostel is one way of meeting a person's needs for such things as food and company, but it is not without problems like ghettoisation and segregation. There are other ways of ensuring that such needs are met (which may have less deleterious side effects) that are obscured if the person is simply deemed to need a hostel.

A further question to consider in relation to a needs-based approach is: Who defines a person's needs? Often clients and mental health workers have different views of need. A client may say that they are tired and need to stay in bed until lunch time whereas staff, aware of the detrimental effects of doing nothing (Wing and Brown, 1970) say that the person needs to get up and do things. Petersen *et al.* (1996) have shown that staff tend to focus on the basics of everyday life (health, hygiene, domestic chores) whereas clients prioritise those things that 'make life worthwhile' (work, relationships and so forth). There are many 'interested parties', but it is not clear whose opinions of need should take precedence.

Any definition of need inevitably involves political and ethical judgements. A 'civil rights' position might claim that people with serious mental health problems have a right to be part of communities. A 'paternalist' perspective might argue that there is a duty to protect those who are vulnerable from themselves and from potentially harmful situations. The needs defined would be quite different, depending on the perspective adopted.

Despite the problems in defining needs, it is evident that many of the requirements of people with serious mental health problems remain unmet. However, a way of thinking about needs is required that does not generate a special category of 'mental patients' who have needs that the rest of the population do not share. One possibility is shown in Box 2.2 (adapted from Perkins and Repper, 1996).

**Box 2.2** Meeting needs

◆ Needs relate to more than safety and physiological necessities of life. They include love, affection, belonging, esteem and respect (Maslow, 1970).

◆ People with disabilities arising from serious mental health problems differ from others, not in terms of their needs, but in terms of their ability to meet these needs with the ordinary resources available.

◆ People with serious mental health problems are often deprived of the means on which most people rely to meet their needs: work, an adequate income, home and family, relationships and social activities. Many unmet needs arise not from serious mental health problems themselves, but from the stigma, poverty and exclusion that so often accompany them.

◆ The primary role of mental health workers is to assist people to access the ordinary activities, facilities and relationships through which most people's needs are met.

*Social disability and access*    Ideas about social disability in relation to serious ongoing mental health problems have been developed from the work of Wing and his colleagues (Wing and Morris, 1981). Within these models a person is seen as socially disabled if they are unable to perform socially to the standards they expect of themselves or that others expect of them. These disabilities arise from three sources: the cognitive and emotional difficulties themselves; the way in which the person copes with, or adapts to, their problems; and social disadvantages that predate, and/or are consequent upon, the difficulties.

Although cognitive and emotional difficulties – concentration problems, cognitive confusion, unshared perceptions, depression, mood swings – can be socially disabling in and of themselves, other factors are at least as important. The way in which the person copes with their problems substantially influences their level of disability (Shepherd, 1984). For example, a person may consider being 'mad' so awful that they reject the idea that they have any problems at all and are thus reluctant to accept support that could help them to make the most of their life. Given the way in which mad people are treated, this response is understandable. Others may see themselves as entirely hopeless and useless as a result of their mental health problems, lose confidence entirely and stop doing things for fear of making a bad situation worse.

The social disadvantages which are so often attendant on serious mental health problems can be more disabling than cognitive and emotional problems or the person's adaptation to these. Some disadvantages, like poor education, disrupted family relationships, sexual abuse, racism, poverty, poor housing, predate the mental health problems and mean that the person has fewer personal, social and material resources with which to cope with the difficult experience of serious mental health problems. In addition, or alternatively, having serious mental health problems is almost invariably accompanied by numerous social and economic disadvantages, such as unemployment, loss of home, disruption of family relationships and social networks, poverty, stigma, rejection, exclusion difficulties, each of which is disabling in and of itself but when combined with cognitive and emotional difficulties is doubly difficult.

A disabilities approach offers a broader perspective, encompassing social and psychological factors as well as the specific cognitive and emotional difficulties associated with mental health problems. However, it can tend to result in long lists of problems that give little guidance about the directions that intervention might take. Perkins and Repper (1996) have, therefore, described an extension which parallels perspectives within the physical disability arena. The main tenets of this social disability and access model are as follows.

♦ Disabilities cannot be defined in a vacuum. A person is only disabled in relation to a particular social or physical context and the demands and expectations it comprises.
♦ A person who experiences the cognitive and emotional difficulties associated with serious mental health problems is socially disabled in much the same way that someone with mobility or sensory difficulties is physically disabled. A person with physical limitations is unable to negotiate the 'normal' (able-bodied) physical world without help, support and adaptation of that world. The handicap that someone with, for example, mobility problems experiences is far greater in the absence of adaptations such as ramps, mobility aids, wide door ways, transport and the like. These accommodations ensure access to roles, activities, facilities and relationships in an able-bodied community.

♦ A person who experiences the cognitive and emotional difficulties that characterise serious mental health problems is unable to
negotiate the 'normal' (able-minded) social world without help,
support and adaptation of that world. Accommodations and
support which ensure access to work, housing and social/
leisure activities facilitate access to roles, activities, facilities
and relationships in an able-minded community.
♦ The support required by any individual to gain access to
activities, facilities, roles and relationships might include specific interventions to reduce the cognitive and emotional difficulties associated with their mental health problems and enable
them to maximise their role within the community. But it will
also involve working within that community to reduce the social
and economic disadvantages associated with social disability:
facilitating access to housing, work, full benefits and other
ordinary activities and supports to ensure that their needs are
met in the same way as they are for the rest of the population.

The basic premise of this social disability and access approach is
that support should be directed towards ensuring that people with
ongoing and serious mental health problems can lead the lives they
wish to lead. Such a model has several important implications.

First, the person, their interests, preferences and social circumstances are central. In ensuring access, the first question is 'access
to what?'. There are many different and intersecting communities
each comprising a myriad different roles, activities and possibilities: in reality 'the' community does not exist. Different people
have different identifications, and desire different roles. Some may
seek communities based on race, culture or religion, others on
politics, others may identify themselves as lesbian or gay, yet others
seek like-minded drinkers at the pub, pool players, body builders.
Some may value work roles, others may prefer home life and
domestic pursuits. The individual's preferences and characteristics
must determine the community to be accessed.

Second, a range of different interventions, supports and strategies can be utilised. A disability and access perspective does not
require a choice between medical, social and psychological
approaches. These may all be useful; decisions need to be based
on the extent to which access is facilitated. For example, a
particular medication may facilitate access to work by reducing
symptoms, but it may also inhibit such access with its side effects.
Practical help may enable a person to go to the pub, but it may also
inhibit access by attracting negative attention.

Third, the focus shifts from changing the disabled individual to
changing the community in which they function. To always have to
change to 'fit in' is devaluing, implying that there is something
wrong with the person that has to be put right before they are
acceptable. In the presence of ongoing disability it is not always

possible to change in the manner required. The essence of an access model is that at least as much attention must be paid to providing supports, help and adaptations in the community; changing the demands of different situations so that a person can be accommodated. This is commonplace in the area of physical disability but is relatively rare in the mental health field where people are largely excluded unless they are willing or able to change.

'But they are unrealistic' is something that is frequently said of people with serious mental health problems, despite the fact that the aspirations they espouse are typically things that many people take for granted: work, home, family, friends. To deem someone unrealistic is a destructive mistake: a way of ignoring what they want that can lead to their rejecting the help that is offered. If services will not help you to do what you want, why should you use them? Even if that which a person desires seems a long way off, it is almost always possible to help them to move towards it. For example, one seriously disabled young man with both mental health problems and drug misuse (and a string of convictions) wanted to be a film producer. He was helped to embark on this road by attending an adult education video class. Since he could not go on his own, a staff member went with him. This served the dual purpose of increasing his understanding of film making, and facilitated better relationships with staff: they were helping him to do something that he valued.

*RELATIONSHIP FORMATION*    Whatever the model of work adopted, success will in large measure be determined by the quality of relationship between mental health worker and client. An 'effective relationship' is not an easy thing to define. However, in the context of people who are severely socially disabled, it might best be judged in terms of the extent to which the person is facilitated in living the life they wish to lead and achieving their own goals. Towards this end, the relationship must provide a safe environment in which the person can think about what they want to do, mobilise their personal resources and work out ways of circumventing their limitations. This can be a difficult process and trust is critical.

Relationships cannot be divorced from the context in which they occur: the possibilities of an effective alliance are enhanced or constrained by the characteristics of the worker, the client and the situation. For example, the relationship between a young African Caribbean man and an older white female worker will differ from a relationship where both are of African Caribbean origin. Similarly, relationships with a person who is compulsorily detained are different from those with someone in voluntary contact with services. Honesty is important. The element of compulsion and the sense of anger, unfairness and injustice that the detained person may understandably feel require empathy and understanding rather than refutation and justification of detention. If worker and client differ in terms of such things as age, gender, culture and race, it is incumbent on the worker to appreciate and explore these differences and their implications so that they can offer support in an acceptable manner.

Although every relationship is an individual affair, there are several factors that may contribute to success (Perkins and Dilks, 1992; Repper *et al.*, 1994; Perkins and Repper, 1996).

*Understanding experiences from the client's perspective*

Esso Leete (1988) echoes the sentiments of many people who experience serious mental health problems when she says: 'I can talk, but I may not be heard. I can make suggestions, but they may not be taken seriously. I can voice my thoughts, but they may be seen as delusions. I can recite experiences, but they may be interpreted as fantasies. To be a patient or even an ex-client is to be discounted.'

Most interviewing and information gathering in the field of mental health is not designed to enable a person to describe and understand their experiences but to enable the worker to categorise the person's experiences within the framework they are using (organic/diagnostic, psychodynamic, cognitive, behavioural, systemic, etc.). Most of the language and theories used to explain mental health problems have been developed by people who have not experienced those things that they purport to describe. This leaves socially disabled people, whose lives and experiences may have been very different from those of people who are not so disabled, feeling isolated and misunderstood. They must speak in a foreign language, that of professionals, if they are to be heard.

Different people adopt different models for understanding what has happened to them: some may prefer organic constructions, others psychological, social, religious or spiritual formulations. People have a right to define their own experiences for themselves and it is rarely helpful – and more likely to be alienating – for the clinician to insist that their understanding is correct. Rather than insisting on a particular construction, it is more important for the worker to explore the client's understanding and seek room for manoeuvre that will enable the person to achieve what they want to achieve. It should also be emphasised that adoption of a particular model does not necessarily preclude interventions developed from different models. For example, it is entirely possible to adopt a social, or psychological model of distress and still take medication. The drugs may be seen as a way of decreasing immediate distress so that the person can address other difficulties.

Numerous diagnostic labels have been used to describe serious ongoing mental health problems, but these tell little about the individual or their personal reality. Concepts such as 'flight of ideas', 'delusions' and 'being in denial' fail to capture the rich complexity of serious mental health problems. The first task for a worker in forming an effective relationship is to understand the person's experiences from their own perspective. There are now numerous 'first person accounts' that can be useful (e.g. Schiller and Bennett, 1994; Jamison, 1995; Geller, 1995 (review article)) but these are not a substitute for detailed exploration of each individual's world, beliefs and perceptions, even when these are apparently shared by no-one else. The widely held axiom 'never collude with a delusion' is destructive of relationship formation: it prevents the worker from understanding the client and leaves the person feeling isolated and misunderstood. Some experiences may be terrifying, but it is important to remember that others may be profound and positive. As one man (cited by Perkins and Repper, 1996) said: 'It was that day when I could see the whole universe spread out in front of me. I just stood there in the ward and I could feel it all. It was the most wonderful day of my life.'

The meaning of being deemed 'mad' also requires attention. To have serious mental health problems is not a thing that anyone would wish for their nearest or dearest, or brag about in the pub. To be mad is to be very much a second class citizen who is both excluded and feared, and portrayed in the media as either a drooling long-stay patient with the compulsory 'half-mast' trousers or a dangerous murderer: images that are as inaccurate as they are cruel. The fear that such oppressive portrayals engender, and their impact on mad people's lives, should not be underestimated.

Although it is important for mental health workers to make efforts to appreciate the world from clients' perspectives, there are dangers. It is important to acknowledge the expertise of their clients that workers do not themselves share. No-one without personal experience of serious mental health problems can really understand what these are like, or what life is like with them. An empathic understanding involves humility; 'I know what you mean' is often an inaccurate and dismissive statement. The huge gulf between the experience of someone who has serious ongoing mental health problems and someone who has not must be accepted, respected and actively explored if an effective relationship is to be formed.

There are people who have a better understanding of the experiences of people who have serious mental health problems: others who have experienced similar difficulties. As Deegan (1993) has argued:

> No-one ever came to me and said 'Hey, I know what you're going through... But I've been where you are today... And I'm going to tell you there is a way out...' All I knew were the stereotypes and what terrified me was that professionals were saying I was one of them. It

would have been good to have role models – people I could look up to who had found a good job, or who were in love, or who had an apartment or a house of their own, or who were making a valuable contribution to society.

'Self-help', assistance from peers, the expertise of experience, all have a central role to play in making the most of life with a disability. People with serious mental health problems can often help each other at least as well as mental health workers and without the undesirable side effects. An example of this can be seen in the Hearing Voices Network.

It is possible to increase the skill base available in mental health teams by actively recruiting, as clinicians, people who have themselves experienced mental health problems.

> An important step in moving toward a client-centred mental health system is to employ people with psychiatric disabilities as staff members in mental health agencies. Including consumers among staff will provide an enriched program both for staff members and for people who receive mental health services. Hiring a person with psychiatric disability will provide a powerful role model for your agency's clients. It also will help staff to gain a deeper understanding of psychiatric disabilities. (Shepherd, 1992).

The employment of people who have serious mental health problems is commonplace in some areas of the USA (Sherman and Porter, 1991; Woodward *et al.*, 1991) and is beginning to happen in the UK (Perkins *et al.*, 1997).

*Realism*   Mental health workers need to be realistic about the very slow (and sometimes non-existent) pace of change that they can expect, and the fact that crises, relapse and deterioration can and do happen. Helping someone to maintain their work, social network, accommodation, relationships and activities, and to minimise the disruptive effect of crises and difficulties on these, is central. However, workers all too easily feel disheartened and demoralised when, despite all their hard work, a client fails to make progress or gets worse. It is impossible to see the prevention of deterioration, or the minimising of disruptive consequences, in the same way as improvement can be evaluated. Effective relationships with people who have serious ongoing mental health problems must support a person through the bad times as well as the good in order to help them to do the things they want and live the life they want to live. A clinician who gets fed up when things are going badly, or dispirited when progress is slow, is not a useful ally for the person who must live with ongoing disabilities.

*A long-term perspective*   If someone has serious ongoing mental health problems, then a long-term perspective is essential. It takes time to form a relationship with someone who has often experienced years of difficult relationships within mental health services and fractured social networks outside. Yet it is the understanding that this relationship will exist over a long period of time which allows various approaches and interventions to be tried, without limits on time, or impatience for evidence of success. Years rather than months are often necessary to see changes in the lives of these people (Harding *et al.*, 1988), consequently, rather than seeking evidence of improvement, staff need to find reward in other aspects of this work, for example: the privilege of knowing someone whose life has been so different from that of most people; the innovation required to ensure they have access to the facilities, activities and relationships they desire and helping them to work out ways of living with their problems; pleasure in the satisfaction that people experience when, after years of trying, they manage to achieve something they really want.

***Client-centred flexibility***    An individualised approach tailored to the clients' preferences, circumstances and resources is critical. Predetermined agendas and adherence to traditional, formal, therapeutic models can be destructive if not impossible. Many different therapeutic approaches, social supports and forms of practical help may be useful in helping the client to achieve what they want, but they need to be employed in a sensitive manner. Individuals differ in many ways, as indicated in Box 2.3.

These differences need to be explored with the client, and respected, if an effective alliance is to be formed. However, it is worth remembering that it is almost invariably easier to give help than to receive it. When we help someone else we feel good, valuable, worthwhile. When we cannot do something, especially something that everyone else seems to be able to do unaided, we feel deskilled, useless, stupid. Facilitating people with serious mental health problems, who have themselves been on the receiving end of help, to do something to assist others can be enormously valuable.

**Box 2.3** Individual differences

Individuals differ in terms of:

◆ The way in which they understand their problems and what has happened to them

◆ The things they want to achieve

◆ The sort of help and support they want

◆ The sort of person they wish to get different assistance from

◆ The way in which support is offered.

Not only are there differences between clients, the possibilities for each person differ over time. Serious mental health problems are not static, they fluctuate markedly over time, therefore interventions and supports must be continually varied. For example, when someone's 'voices' are particularly troublesome, they may find it difficult to manage more than a cursory conversation, but can use some practical help with shopping, cleaning, etc. When their voices are not so problematic they may be able to consider ways of coping with their voices, or they may want support in trying to understand what has happened to them and work out what the future holds, but they will probably be able to manage the practicalities of day to day life quite well.

Client choice and self-determination are at the heart of effective relationships: the extent to which a person receives the support they want in the way they want it to achieve the things they want to achieve. There is a shift from the professional as expert telling the patient what to do, to the professional placing their professional expertise at the disposal of the client who can use it to help them achieve what they want. Yet there are difficult issues of power involved here. If clients have the right to make choices about what happens to them, then workers' power to determine what happens is reduced. It is towards these issues that the last part of this chapter will be directed.

*POWER, CHOICE AND INFORMATION*

Despite increased attention to the views of clients and to choice, many service users continue to view services as coercive and offering few options (Lindow, 1993; Lucksted and Coursey, 1995). The concept of choice is only meaningful if people have the right to make what workers consider to be 'wrong' or 'bad' choices. It is always hard to watch – or even support – someone in doing something that you think will not be good for them; yet, if people are to be assisted to live the lives they want to lead and have access to the roles, relationships and activities that they desire, mental health workers must be prepared to do this. Obviously there are times when a 'duty of care' requires prohibition of a chosen course of action – a worker may not help someone kill themselves or harm others – but these are rare. More commonly the likely outcomes of the client's choices are both less dramatic and less certain, as for example when a person wants to try living without medication or wants to move into a flat of their own.

The vast majority of people with serious mental health problems are, most of the time, not subject to powers of coercion under mental health legislation. Nevertheless, these powers can act as an important (implicit or explicit) back-up threat to deprive clients of choice and force them to do what the professional thinks best ('If you don't do this then...'). Because of this, and other structural inequalities of power and information, clients often need explicit permission to disagree with a worker: active encouragement to develop their own goals and solutions.

Legislation is not the only way in which mental health workers exert power. Lucksted and Coursey (1995), in a survey of mental health service users, found that: 'Overall, the type of behaviour most commonly identified as pressure or force consisted of efforts to verbally persuade respondents that the unwanted treatment was in their best interest.' There are many ways in which mental health workers exercise their power and deprive service users of any real choice, for example:

◆ Simple disbelief: the view that what people with serious mental health problems say must be taken 'with a pinch of salt' because they are, after all, mad.
◆ 'You only think that because of your illness': dismissing people's opinions as a reflection of their psychopathology.
◆ 'Yes dear, how interesting': humouring the person, listening politely and then taking no notice.
◆ Repeated verbal persuasion: sometimes referred to as 'counselling', but often more akin to bullying.
◆ 'I am the expert and you are just the patient': using professional power to assert that the mental health worker knows best.
◆ Limiting information about the options available. This can occur in two ways: first, by simply not giving people the information they need about choices available to enable them to make a judgement; second, by presenting information in an indigestible, incomprehensible or spuriously technical manner so that the person is not able to understand and make use of what they are told.
◆ Limiting the person's ability to opt for the choices available. As well as simply depriving people of information about the range of choices, this most often occurs in two ways. First, when support is made contingent on the person doing what the worker considers best: 'You can go and find somewhere else to live if you want but I won't help you because I think you should stay in the hostel'. Second, when one form of help is made contingent upon another: 'There's no point in me coming to see you unless you take your medication', 'You can only come for lunch at the day centre if you attend one of the groups'.

By whatever means, power is often exercised from the best of motives: the worker believes they are acting in the person's best interests. However, the negative consequences of doing this are threefold. First, clients are deprived of choice and control over their lives: the views and preferences of an already devalued group of people – those with serious mental health problems – are further devalued by those who are supposed to help them. Second, a significant number of people reject support that they see as controlling and failing to meet their needs. Third, a significant number of people are rejected and excluded because mental health workers consider that they 'abuse' the help that is offered, that is, use services in an 'inappropriate' manner.

These two latter issues are particularly important in relation to those people whom mental health services most manifestly fail. There is increasing concern about people who 'fall through the net', although many might more accurately be said to have actively 'jumped out of the net' or been 'pushed out of the net'. Hirsch (1992) has described:

> A group of patients who are hard to sustain in a meaningful clinical alliance with psychiatric services... These patients do not engage in treatment, are often not at home when doctors, nurses or social workers visit, and may abuse alcohol [or drugs]... They sometimes end up with no home of their own.

Such clients have often been involved in a power struggle with mental health services: trapped in a cycle of compulsory inpatient admissions interspersed with rejecting, or being rejected by, community services. Often these problems are met with demands for greater powers to compel: supervision registers, supervised discharge and so forth. However, it seems unlikely that further control will generate the necessary meaningful alliance of which Hirsch (1992) speaks.

A more productive approach, at both an individual and a service level, is to really begin to provide such support and services on clients' own terms, in a manner that is acceptable to them and of a type that meets their needs (as they see them). In some instances, the legal and resource constraints on professionals will mean that clients' wishes will be over-ridden, but this can become the exception rather than the rule. Although choices are often constrained, they are rarely absent. In order to exercise choice and so take a part in deciding what sort of support they would like, clients need to know what the various options are: it is not enough to simply list them, clients will need help to understand what each choice means. Where it is necessary, the constraints can be honestly explained to clients rather than obscured in the persuasive rhetoric of professional expertise and clients' supposed 'best interests'.

*CONCLUSION*    In working with people who experience ongoing social disabilities as a consequence of their serious mental health problems, clinicians need first to consider what they hope to achieve with their endeavours. A 'social disability and access' model which parallels approaches in the physical disability arena offers a potentially useful integrative framework. Thus a range of interventions, approaches and forms of support can be implemented to facilitate access to those roles, relationships, activities and facilities in the social world through which their needs can be met.

Such an approach involves changing the social world to accommodate the disabled individual rather than always changing the individual to 'fit in' (and excluding them if they do not). This means that interventions not only focus on the individual, enabling them to take up roles and responsibilities within a variety of living, working and social settings, they also involve changing the expectations, demands and supports available within the community of their choice to ensure access.

If socially disabled people are to have access to ordinary roles, relationships and opportunities, they also need to have the same choices as non-disabled people and this has implications for the power of professionals. People with serious mental health problems can only have control over their lives if they can pursue options of their own choosing rather than those which professionals think best.

*DISCUSSION QUESTIONS*

♦ What are the core tenets of the social disability and access model?

♦ What are the advantages of this model compared with other popular approaches for working with people who have serious mental health problems?

♦ What principles can help the worker to engage in a trusting relationship with clients?

♦ In what ways are choice and self-determination frequently limited within services?

♦ How can clients gain more control over their own lives?

*FURTHER READING*

♦ Geller, J. L. (1995) First person accounts of psychiatric illness and treatment: Reviews of recent books, *Psychiatric Services*, 46, 1080–1087.
A review of recent publications by people who experience mental health problems. In itself this gives a useful insight into the breadth and variety of difficulties experienced and perceptions of the support received. However, a much clearer picture will be gained by reading a selection of the accounts reviewed here.

♦ Hirsch, S. (Chair) (1992) *Facilities and Services for the Mentally Ill with Persisting Severe Disabilities*. Working Party Report on behalf of the Royal College of Psychiatrists.

Although somewhat dated, this is a useful review of the problems faced by services attempting to meet the needs of the most seriously disabled clients, and the extent to which this limits the support available for the clients themselves.

♦ Perkins, R. E. and Repper, J. M. (1996) *Working Alongside People with Long Term Mental Health Problems*, London: Chapman & Hall.

This is a practical guide for those working with people who are socially disabled by serious mental health problems on a day to day basis. Based upon the social disability and access model introduced in this chapter, it outlines the ways in which acceptable and effective support can be provided to enable users to gain control of their own lives as far as possible.

*REFERENCES*   Anthony, L.A. (1977), Psychological rehabilitation: a concept in need of a method. *American Psychologist*, 1977, 658-662.

Anthony, L.A. (1979), The rehabilitation approach to diagnosis. *New Directions in Mental Health Services*, 2, 25-36.

Anthony, L.A. and Margules, A. (1974), Toward improving the efficacy of psychiatric rehabilitation: a skills training approach. *Rehabilitation Psychology*, 21, 101-105.

Bennett, D. (1978), Social forms of psychiatric treatment. In Wing, J. K. (Ed) *Schizophrenia: Toward a New Synthesis*. London: Academic Press.

Brewin, C.R., Wing, J.K., Mangen, S.P. *et al.* (1987), Principles and practice of measuring needs in the long-term mentally ill: the MRC needs for care assessment. *Psychological Medicine*, 17, 971-981.

Brewin, C.R., Wing, J.K., Mangen, S.P. *et al.* (1988), Needs for care among the long-term mentally ill: a report of the Camberwell High Contact Survey. *Psychological Medicine*, 18, 457-468.

Clifford, P. (1989), *Evaluating the Closure of Cane Hill Hospital: Plans for Residential Services and the Long-Stay Population*. London: National Unit for Psychiatric Research and Development.

Dear, M. (1992), Understanding and overcoming the NIMBY syndrome. *Journal of the American Planning Association*, 58, 288-300.

Dear, M. and Gleeson, B. (1991), Community attitudes towards the homeless. *Urban Geography*, 12, 155-176.

Deegan, P.E. (1993), Recovering our sense of value after being labelled. *Psychosocial Nursing*, 31, 7-11.

Drouet, V.M. (1986), Individual programme planning with long stay psychiatric patients. *British Journal of Occupational Therapy*, 52, 11-15.

Ekdawi, M. and Conning A. (1994), *Psychiatric Rehabilitation: A Practical Guide*. London: Chapman & Hall.

Geller, J.L. (1995), First person accounts of psychiatric illness and treatment: reviews of recent books. *Psychiatric Services*, **46**, 1080-1087.

Harding, C.M., Brooks, C.W., Ashikaga, T. *et al.* (1988), The Vermont longitudinal study of persons with severe mental illness II: Long-term outcome of subjects who once met DSM III criteria for schizophrenia. *American Journal of Psychiatry*, 144, 727-734.

Hirsch, S. (Chair) (1992), *Facilities and Services for the Mentally Ill with Persisting Severe Disabilities*. Working Party Report on behalf of the Royal College of Psychiatrists.

Jamison, K.R. (1995), *An Unquiet Mind: A Memoir of Moods and Madness*. New York: Alfred A. Knopf.

Leete, E. (1988), *The Consumer Movement and Persons with Mental Illness*, Presentation at the 12th Mary Switzer Memorial Seminar in Rehabilitation, Washington DC, June 15-16.

Lindow, V. (1993), A service user's view. In: Wright, H. and Giddey, M. (Eds) *Mental Health Nursing: From First Principles to Professional Practice*. London: Chapman & Hall.

Lucksted, A. and Coursey, R.D. (1995), Consumer perceptions of pressure and force in psychiatric services. *Psychiatric Services*, 46, 146-152.

Maslow, A. (1970), *Motivation and Personality* (2nd edition). New York: Harper & Row.

Perkins, R.E. and Dilks, S. (1992), Worlds apart: Working with severely socially disabled people. *Journal of Mental Health*, 1, 3-17.

Perkins, R.E. and Moodley, P. (1993), Perceptions of problems in psychiatric inpatients: denial, race and service usage. *Social Psychiatry and Psychiatric Epidemiology*, 28, 114-119.

Perkins, R.E. and Repper, J.M. (1996), *Working Alongside People with Long Term Mental Health Problems*. London: Chapman & Hall.

Perkins, R.E., Buckfield, R. and Choy, D. (1997), Access to employment: a supported employment project to enable mental health service users to obtain jobs within mental health teams. *Journal of Mental Health*, 6(3), 307-318.

Petersen, K., Shah, R. and Perkins, R.E. (1996), Whose care plan is it anyway? The extent to which staff, client and relatives' views are reflected in care plans. Submitted to *Health and Social Care in the Community*.

Repper, J., Cooke, A. and Ford, R. (1994), How can nurses build trusting relationships with people who have severe long term mental health problems? Experiences of case managers and their clients. *Journal of Advanced Nursing*, 19, 1096-1104.

Schiller, L. and Bennett, A. (1994), *The Quiet Room: A Journey Out of the Torment of Madness*. New York: Warner Books.

Shepherd, G. (1977), Social skills training: the generalisation problem. *Behaviour Therapy*, 8, 100-109.

Shepherd, G. (1978), Social skills training: the generalisation problem – some further data. *Behaviour Research and Therapy*, 116, 287-288.

Shepherd, G. (1984), *Institutional Care and Rehabilitation*. London: Longman.

Shepherd, L. (1992), *So You Want to Hire a Consumer? Employing People with Psychiatric Disabilities as Staff Members in Mental Health Agencies*. Burlington, Vermont: Center for Community Change Through Housing and Support.

Sherman, P.S. and Porter, R. (1991), Mental health consumers as case management aides, *Hospital and Community Psychiatry*, 42, 494-498.

Smith, R. (1985), Bitterness, shame, emptiness, waste: an introduction to unemployment and health. *British Medical Journal*, 291, 1024-1028.

Taylor, K.E. and Perkins, R.E. (1991), Identity and coping with mental illness in long-stay psychiatric rehabilitation. *British Journal of Clinical Psychology*, 30, 73–85.

Thornicroft, G., Brewin, C.R. and Wing, J.K. (Eds) (1992), *Measuring Mental Health Needs*. London: Gaskell/Royal College of Psychiatrists.

Wing, J.K. and Brown, G. (1970), *Institutionalism and Schizophrenia*. London: Cambridge University Press.

Wing, J.K. and Morris, B. (1981), *Handbook of Psychiatric Rehabilitation*. Oxford: Oxford University Press.

Wolfensberger, W. and Tulman, S. (1982), A brief outline of the principle of normalisation. *Rehabilitation Psychology*, 27, 131–145.

Woodward, M.K., Kane, G., Porter, R. *et al.* (1991), *Training Consumer Colleagues*. Colorado: Regional Assessment and Training Center.

# CHAPTER 3

# Purchasing Mental Health Services

## Edward Peck

**KEY ISSUES**

- ◆ The origins and motives of *Working for Patients* and *Caring for People*.

- ◆ The characteristics of Health Authorities, Social Service Departments and GP Fundholders as purchasers of care.

- ◆ Approaches to the assessment of need for mental health services.

- ◆ Types of contract for mental health services.

**INTRODUCTION**

The aim of this chapter is to introduce the role of purchasers of mental health services (Health Authorities, Social Services Departments and GP Fundholders) and map the development of purchasing of mental health services in the UK since 1989. This evolution has had cultural, structural and clinical implications which will be explored; but it is the cumulative effect of these implications that this chapter will seek to demonstrate. Given the breadth of the field and the limited space available, references will point to accessible sources of further reading.

The publication of *Working for Patients* (Department of Health, 1989a) and *Caring for People* (Department of Health, 1989b) ensures that 1989 will be remembered as a watershed in the development of the organisational arrangements within which mental health services are provided. One of the major purposes of the proposals contained in the White Paper was to challenge the cultural assumptions which guided managerial and professional behaviour in health and social services; although the exact nature of that cultural change was always difficult to predict. Roger Freeman, then Under Secretary of State at the Department of Health, admitted as much when he acknowledged that he had no idea what health services would look like in 1995 (Peck, 1996).

However, he was right to believe that the complexity and pace of change faced by health and social services during the 1990s would exceed that of the previous four decades. In the process many of the consequences of the reforms outlined in the two White Papers, in particular those arising out of *Working for Patients* (Department of Health, 1989a) have evolved over the course of the subsequent years in a manner and at a speed that has often been difficult to keep pace with, especially for clinicians working in the field and for users of services. This chapter will update the story to mid-1996.

*THE ORIGINS OF THE WHITE PAPERS*

The origins of *Working for Patients* (Department of Health, 1989a) and *Caring for People* (Department of Health, 1989b) are both similar and different. Similar in the sense that both had their roots in concerns about the effectiveness of public spending, different in the amount of time spent addressing the potential solutions, and the amount of detail provided about those solutions.

In January 1988, it was announced that a Cabinet review into the NHS, chaired by the Prime Minister, Margaret Thatcher was to be established. The review was prompted both by a series of reports from the presidents of three Royal Colleges on alleged under-funding in the NHS and by hostile media reporting of delays in treatment for children awaiting heart surgery. The review was therefore clearly propelled by a financial agenda (Ham, 1994, p. 3). This agenda initially comprised two items: the overall level of funding and the potential sources of that funding.

Subsequent debate about these two issues was constrained, however, by powerful forces; first, by the overall financial strategy of the government towards public sector spending, and second by the perceived political vulnerability of the government on the NHS. By August 1988 little progress had been made, and Kenneth Clarke was appointed Secretary of State for Health with the task of taking forward and publishing the review. In considering options, both Thatcher and Clarke were influenced by the ideas of Enthoven (1985) who had proposed an internal market in the NHS where the purchase of health care was separated from the provision of health care.

In the account of the review in her memoirs, Thatcher (1993) records that, 'Professor Alain Enthoven of Stanford University had been advancing ideas about creating an internal market in the NHS, whereby market disciplines would be applied even though a full-scale free market would not' (p. 607). For the Prime Minister, the attraction of Enthoven's concept lay in the opportunity to 'work towards a new way of allocating money within the NHS, so that hospitals treating more patients received more income' (p. 607). This concept of 'money following the patient' was a powerful one in the formulation of the internal market. Clarke later revealed that he was attracted to such an internal market because 'it tried to inject into a state-owned system some of the qualities of competition, choice, and measurement of quality that you get in well-run, private enterprise' (Roberts, 1990, p. 1384). Thatcher (1993) reveals the haste with which the White Paper was put together, with the first draft only being produced four week before publication, with the so-called 'wild card' of GP fundholding apparently entering the picture very late in the day. It is important to recognise that, in the end, as Klein (1989, p. 238) notes, 'a policy review launched in an attempt to devise a new funding system ended up by saying nothing about how to finance the NHS'. *Working for Patients* envisages the purchase of health care services being the responsibility of Health Authorities and GP fundholders, with the provision of health care being managed by self-governing (later NHS) Trusts. The relationship between the purchasers and providers would be handled through contracts for care.

The financial concern that prompted *Caring for People* lay in the ready, and open-ended, availability of social security benefit payments for residential care for the elderly, and other client groups. In a report entitled *Making a Reality of Community Care*, the Audit Commission (1986) pointed out the cost to the government of this availability, and the perverse incentive it gave, in particular, to elderly people, their carers and their social workers, to arrange entry into residential care rather than consider support in their own homes, support that would be paid for by Local Authority Social Services Departments. Furthermore, many psychiatric patients resident in hospital were discharged to such residential care; Murphy (1991, p. 74) maintains that 'the NHS effectively shuffled off high-cost in-patients to a low-cost system remote from the statutory services'. As a consequence, the payments from the social security budget to home owners soared during the 1980s without the government being able to impose any ceiling. Murphy (1991, p. 68) records the enthusiasm for such transfers, 'health and local authorities faced with strict budgetary constraints quickly came to realise that, if they discharged patients into the community, the funding responsibility would pass elsewhere'. This enthusiasm was not shared by the government; just as nature abhors a vacuum, so the Treasury abhors a government budget without a predetermined limit.

In order to address this problem, in 1988 the Department of Health asked Sir Roy Griffiths to investigate and recommend solutions. The ensuing report, *Community Care: Agenda for Action* (Department of Health, 1988), suggested that social services departments should be given the responsibility for assessing client needs and putting together care packages, within which residential care would be one potential component. Crucially, access to public financial support for residential care would be channelled through Local Authorities, cash-limited, and only made available after thorough assessment and exploration of alternatives. As Sir Roy noted:

> the role of social services authorities should be reoriented towards ensuring that the needs of individuals ... are identified, packages of care are devised and services coordinated; and where appropriate a specific care manager is assigned ... as to residential accommodation social services authorities would be responsible for assessing whether a move to such accommodation was in the best interests of the individual and what the local authority would be prepared to pay for (Department of Health, 1988, p. vii).

These ideas form the backbone of *Caring for People* (Department of Health, 1989b).

*Caring for People* envisaged Local Authority Social Services Departments becoming purchasers of care from independent providers, as well as continuing to be providers of services. Resources were to be transferred from the social security benefits budget to the Local Authority Social Services Department budget, but cash-limited.

In summary, therefore: the NHS White Paper was based on consideration of the issues that in some instances lasted less than six months, could generously be described as broad-brush, left much of the detail to be worked out during implementation and proposed a new method of passing money through the system rather than advocating radical options for paying for health care (e.g. vouchers); the Social Services White Paper was based on consideration of the issues over a five-year period, was quite specific in its recommendations and proposed a new method of passing money through the system rather than radical options for paying for social care (e.g. insurance).

**HEALTH AUTHORITIES AS PURCHASERS**

Three quotations illustrate the three major features of health purchasing. The first quotation was made by Alan Langlands, subsequently Chief Executive of the NHS, to the Health Select Committee when it was investigating mental health services during 1993:

> We are listening to carers and users, the people whom we think know best about services (Department of Health, 1993, p. 13).

This quotation merits careful consideration; 'we', presumably meaning the NHS Executive, 'are listening to carers and users, the people whom we think know *best* about services' (emphasis added). This represents a significant change of emphasis for managers within health authorities; Harrison *et al.* (1992) characterise health management prior to 1989 as giving predominance to staff (usually medical staff) concerns as well as favouring incremental change. Langlands signalled that health purchasers should look outside the network of local health professionals for views and ideas that will shape health provision.

The second quotation is taken from one of a number of speeches made by the then Minister of Health, Brian Mawhinney, during 1993 when the NHS Management Executive was trying to accelerate the impetus of health purchasing:

> Purchasers need to shift away from the old style focus on institutions and service inputs ... purchasers have responsibility to force the pace of change (NHS Management Executive, 1993, p. 11).

He was not referring explicitly to mental health services in his reference to the old style focus on institutions, although it gives a clear indication that mental health services might expect to be in the vanguard of services where purchasers challenge existing service patterns and propose changes.

The third quotation is drawn from the *Health of the Nation*, a policy that has come to represent a new approach to health policy making and objective setting whereby health purchasers are obliged to address health needs and health gain rather than the maintenance of existing patterns of health provision:

> The key policy objectives ... are the need to identify main health problems and focus on them (Department of Health, 1991, p. vii).

The inclusion of mental health within the five priorities specified by the *Health of the Nation* has served to ensure that mental health has remained near the top of the agenda for health purchasers as they have been developing their approaches to purchasing in the 1990s. The importance of the targets for mental health within the Health of the Nation document is that they sustain mental health as a key priority area (rather than, necessarily, the nature of the targets themselves, which have been the subject of criticism).

All of these three features of health purchasing have, therefore, particular resonance for mental health services; if purchasers were going to respond to this emphasis on listening to users and carers, challenge existing patterns of provision and address the priorities set down by *Health of the Nation*, then mental health services were going to be in the forefront of development of new approaches to strategy development initiated by health purchasers. Mental health services have become, therefore, almost a pilot for the potential for health purchasing to demonstrate the characteristics represented in the three quotations. The new approach therefore offered a real opportunity for users, carers, commissioners, clinicians and managers to influence strategy development and implementation in a way that has not been traditional within the National Health Service.

However, the ability of health purchasers to seize this agenda, within a new health care system, has been seriously impeded by their initial neglect following the publication of the White Papers.

Certainly Health Authorities have been the victims of subsequent loss of organisational experience/expertise and continual structural realignment. At the same time, clinicians, who have been accustomed to exercising a leadership role within mental health services, have experienced a loss of authority and control which is not being shared by their colleagues within other health specialties. Thus an inevitable tension has been created with the new approaches to purchasing which could be destructive, if not well thought through, or constructive, if handled with care and skill.

## *SOCIAL SERVICES DEPARTMENTS AS PURCHASERS*

The purchaser/provider split within the National Health Service was *not* designed with mental health services in mind. Neither was the separation of assessment from provision in social services. The following quotation is taken from detailed national guidance issued subsequent to the White Paper, and it is very explicit about the benefit of separating the assessment of need from the delivery of services to meet that need:

> If services are to be made more responsive, it is necessary to identify the disparity between assessed needs and the currently available services. This is most effectively achieved where the responsibility for assessing need is separated from that of delivering or managing services (Department of Health/Scottish Office, 1991, p. 11).

It is possible to discern two responses to this guidance by social services departments which relate specifically to mental health. The first is to apply the guidance consistently across all client groups, regardless of the impact on relationships with mental health services, and more particularly, mental health teams. This approach reflects the fact that, for social services departments, nearly all of their activity involves mental health work whereas specialist mental health provision consumes a very small proportion of their budget. The second response has been to construct a more or less creative fudge where the roles of assessment and provision are not so clearly distinguished. This response is perhaps more sensitive to the organisational arrangements already in place for the multidisciplinary delivery of mental health services; but it is also vulnerable to challenge and (subsequent) change by incoming Directors of Social Services. This process has been given impetus by the creation of smaller social services departments in so-called unitary local authorities in many parts of the UK during the mid 1990s.

Nonetheless the introduction of care management has given renewed emphasis to the importance of assessing people's needs rather than assessing people's suitability for services. This emphasis has been enhanced where care managers have been given specific budgets to purchase services to meet those needs on an individual basis from a range of statutory, independent and informal sources.

Furthermore, the strategic aggregation of assessed needs for the purposes of defining future purchasing activity holds considerable potential for mental health services users – particularly given the emerging emphasis on the importance of social care for the sustenance of meaningful life in the community for large numbers of service users. This is discussed in more detail below.

A note of caution has been sounded, however, by Hudson (1996a) who reports 'worrying evidence that mainstream care management is faltering in practice' (p. 77). In each of the key activities of care management, assessment, care planning and care plan implementation he points out problems in practice, such as: reconciling needs with resources during assessment; producing purposeful plans during care planning; and dealing with the constraints of the set menu of provision during care plan implementation.

In addition, the introduction of care management into mental health services was consecutive, but not coordinated, with the implementation of the Care Programme Approach, which may have served to blunt its potential. It is also true, of course, that being assessed as having a particular need does not impart any right to have that need met; many SSDs have created euphemisms for unmet need, of which the most elegant is perhaps 'preferred option shortfall'.

## GP FUNDHOLDERS AS PURCHASERS

It would be an understatement to say that GP fundholding was *not* designed with mental health services in mind. GP fundholding was intended to challenge the assumptions and stimulate the behaviours of both health care providers and health care purchasers around elective surgery, as the following quotation illustrates: 'This reform will deliver better care for patients, shorter waiting times and better value for money' (Department of Health, 1989a, p. 48). General practitioners were empowered to open a second front with providers thereby challenging the strategic intentions of health authority purchasers.

GP fundholders do not approach mental health services with universally positive views of recent trends in mental health care, especially the growth of community mental health teams (CMHTs) (Peck, 1994). CMHTs are often viewed with suspicion by GPs because: they are frequently based around social services boundaries rather than GP practice lists; they are often led by clinicians or managers who are not doctors; and they sometimes offer direct access to users which can bypass the GP. Furthermore, when teams are put together utilising existing staff resources and are focused strongly on the long-term seriously mentally ill, GPs resent the apparent threat to community psychiatric nurses (CPNs) already attached to practices. In a recent survey (Marum, 1995), GP fundholders prioritised three objectives in relation to community mental health services: to protect or increase CPN time in the surgery; to increase the availability of practice-based counsellors; and to challenge sectorisation.

**CONTRASTING PERSPECTIVES OF PURCHASERS**
The purchasing of mental health services in any locality is, therefore, the responsibility of three distinct and disparate interest groups. The policy approach from the Department of Health has emphasised partnership between these interest groups alongside collaboration with providers, users, and carers. As the characteristics of these groups (highlighted in Box 3.1) contrast so strongly, any successful partnership approach has to be based on stable personal relationships developed in the pursuit of a clear and agreed process. The creation of stable relationships assumes a stability of personnel; such stability has not been much in evidence in either health authorities or social services departments since 1991 (Johnson *et al.*, 1997). The search for the perfect structure has become for many an organisational obsession and it has proved as elusive as the quest for the Holy Grail. Meanwhile GPs usually remain in one locality for a lifetime and grow increasingly, and understandably, cynical about the comings and goings of health and social services staff sent to plan strategy with them.

There are additional obstacles to effective partnerships; for instance, the financial rules governing the creation of community mental health services predate both *Working for Patients* and *Caring for People* and generate considerable activity and sometimes conflict between health and social services. (Audit Commission/Centre for Mental Health Service Development, 1995). At the same time, most local authorities and many health authorities have experienced reductions in revenue available to purchase services during much of the 1990s. Furthermore, the process and outcome of local partnerships are monitored separately by the NHS Executive (HAs) and the Social Services Inspectorate (SSDs). Hudson (1996b) has identified a number of key characteristics of successful partnerships from his field research on interagency collaboration. The most important of his findings would appear to suggest that:

◆ reciprocity is the basis of collaboration;
◆ collaboration must take place on the most suitable agreed point on the continuum which ranges from complete separatism to complete merger;
◆ clarity is required as to the partners in the collaboration;
◆ collaboration necessitates a shared expression of the purpose of the collaboration;
◆ trust is essential to the initiation and successful maintenance of collaboration.

In summary, therefore, the process of purchasing mental health services in a locality has to recognise and reconcile the challenges

**Box 3.1**  Characteristics of Mental Health Purchasers

| | Strategic focus | Approach to needs assessment | Contract tools | Contract monitoring |
|---|---|---|---|---|
| GP fundholders | Individual patient/ practice population | Individualistic/ anecdotal | Variety of contract-types for specific secondary services/ employment of staff/direct service provision | Direct through experience of referred patients and personal contact with providers |
| Social services care manager | Individual client who meets local eligibility criteria/ caseload of clients | Individualistic/ extensive assessment | Call off or spot purchasing contracts with specified suppliers/ direct provision | Direct through monitoring of care plan |
| Social services assistant director: Purchasing | Overall client group that meets local eligibility criteria/ caseloads of clients | Client group/ informed by extensive assessment | Block and cost and volume contracts with selected providers | Indirect through feedback from care managers/local financial and activity data collected |
| Health authority purchasers | Total population/ overall patient group that meets national priority criteria | Population and client group informed by views of GPs, social services colleagues, providers, users, carers, research, demography, etc. | Block and cost and volume contracts with selected providers/extra contract referrals | Indirect through local and national mechanisms created/local financial and activity data collected |

inherent in multiagency collaboration; each of the essential tasks described below will only be effective as part of such a process. The failures of coordination and communication highlighted in numerous reports into homicides by, and suicides of, people with serious mental illness (e.g. Ritchie *et al.*, 1994) apply as much to purchasing as to provision. Such is the public, and therefore political, concern surrounding mental health services that there are regular calls for the merger of health and social care purchasing, the most recent of which led to a Department of Health review of joint purchasing, and the inclusion of the option of a united purchasing agency in the Green Paper issued in 1997 (Department of Health, 1997). However, the challenges can be met and a summary of one proven process, developed and refined in use by the Centre for Mental Health Services Development (CMHSD) has been described by Smith (1995). The following sections focus on two issues specific to purchasing not dealt with elsewhere in this book: assessment of need and contracting for services.

*ASSESSMENT OF NEED* *

The theory is simple enough. Purchasers have the responsibility to assess the overall needs of their local population and to use this information to define contract specifications and determine priorities for service development. There is also a requirement, under the NHS and Community Care Act, for community care plans to be based on an assessment of the care needs of the local population. The policy guidance states that assessment in community care plans should identify 'the care needs of the local population taking into account factors such as age distribution, problems associated with living in inner city areas or rural areas, special needs of ethnic minority communities, the number of homeless or transient people likely to require care' and, from April 1993, show: 'how the care needs of individuals approaching them for assistance will be assessed, and how service needs identified following the introduction of systematic assessment will be incorporated into the planning process' (Department of Health/Scottish Office, 1991, pp. 41–62).

Yet, despite a wealth of guidance on needs assessment, there is strong evidence that the 'Procrustean' approach to service planning and commissioning continues. Procrustes, a figure from Greek mythology, had a special bed which his guests had to fit exactly; too long and he chopped off their feet, too short and he stretched them until they fitted. Many people with mental health problems will strongly suspect that Procrustes is alive and well and commissioning their local services. The few studies undertaken in this area (for example Rogers *et al.*, 1993) suggest that people overwhelmingly find that they have to 'fit in' with what is offered to them. Stated

---

* This section draws on Hayward *et al.* (1993).

needs go unrecognised or, at worst, are ignored. Little wonder that users and their carers feel themselves luckless guests on an unchanging bed of professional skills. Indeed, the Department of Health has acknowledged that the service they receive 'is often more the reflection of historic circumstance, local service availability and provider priorities than a reflection of need' (Department of Health/Social Services Inspectorate, 1993, p. 34). If purchasers are to resolve this predicament they must get to grips with the complexity of assessing local need.

*GP fundholders* According to Department of Health data, every GP has around 450 people on his or her list with a 'minor' mental health problem and, on average, seven with a 'major' mental illness. Presentations have been estimated at around 240 people with non-psychotic mental health problems in one year. Even accepting the suggestion that GPs fail to detect 50% of the mental health problems that enter the surgery (Wright, 1993), the assessments made by GPs will inevitably emphasise the importance of dealing with anxiety, depression and general unhappiness. Nevertheless, the assessment of need in primary care is an idiosyncratic affair, with wide variations in both the competence of GPs to identify mental distress and then to respond appropriately to this distress.

The position is also very inconsistent for people with a long-term mental illness. In a recent survey, 25% of GPs reported that they did not know how many people with long term mental illness were on their practice list (Marum, 1995). Furthermore, the same survey showed that less than half of the fundholders who responded specified the Care Programme Approach (CPA) as a requirement of secondary care providers in their contracts despite NHS Executive guidance. The involvement of most GPs in the CPA for individual clients is negligible; one survey reports only 59 out of 369 GPs as being prepared to act as CPA keyworkers (Strathdee, 1992). However, there are a number of recent initiatives which aim to improve the assessment skills of GPs, including the Defeat Depression Campaign; the development of GP-friendly screening tools; and the development of GP facilitators for mental health, building on the proven role of facilitators in assisting GPs in the management of chronic conditions. For a more detailed examination of the interface between primary care and secondary care in mental health see the CMHSD Mental Health Review (1996).

*Care managers* In contrast, social services care managers use formal assessment procedures authorised by their employing authorities. However, as well as being an evaluation of the social care needs of a person with mental health problems, the assessment also establishes the eligibility of that individual to receive services against criteria laid down by the authority. Usually expressed as a series of bandings,

**Box 3.2** Summarised priority bandings of a social services department

BAND 1  Highest priority: Adults who are assessed as being highly vulnerable and dependent and where the absence of continuous support would result in an immediate and continued risk to life or rapid deterioration in condition. These adults would normally have an assessed need to be admitted to residential or nursing home care.

BAND 2  Adults who are assessed as having a high level of need and for whom, in the absence of frequent and regular support, there would be a severe and sustained effect on their ability to self-care which could result in significant risk to themselves or others.

BAND 3  Adults who experience episodes of poor functioning or ongoing disability which, without regular support, can place them at risk or significantly impair their independence. They may be unable to perform essential self-care tasks or may be substantially restricted in doing so.

BAND 4  Adults who do not need daily assistance with personal care but whose lives without some support would be restricted in consequence to continuing ill health or disability.

BAND 5  Adults who experience occasional or recurring problems or disability during which time their ability to live fully independently or care for themselves properly without some service is decreased.

BAND 6  Adults who may be experiencing some occasional problems or require assistance with mobility. Alternatively isolation may be identified as a significant factor.

BAND 7  Adults whose *only* requirement is for domestic cleaning or a service not provided by the Social Services Department.

these criteria prioritise the needs of the more severely mentally ill; the bandings of one typical authority are presented in Box 3.2.

The needs of users are recorded in a care plan, along with information detailing services identified to meet need and, in theory, the gap between need and services available. Following recent legal challenges, these gaps (or unmet need) are not always shared with users in their version of the care plan. In practice, users not falling within Bands 1–3 in Box 3.2 may be unlikely to receive services from social services departments.

*Health purchasers*  Health purchasers are responsible for the assessment of needs of the population; this is a major challenge to which they were initially ill-placed to rise.

The major reason for this early failure of needs assessment was an over-reliance on an underdeveloped quantitative methodology which meant that health authorities acquired, at best, only half the picture. There remain two distinct approaches to needs assessment: a qualitative approach which focuses on what people say they (or their relative) need; and a quantitative approach which assesses how many people may have those needs.

The first approach yields data about the range and content of people's needs but not about the numbers of people likely to use services and may fail to identify unmet need, particularly among those not in contact with the health services. The second, the quantitative approach, predicts how many people will use services but not what needs the services should be addressing. Both these approaches are necessary for a comprehensive assessment of need as they are two sides of the same coin.

The Department of Health recognises the need to fuse these two approaches. The NHS Executive, in tackling this task, describes three separate but linked elements in the process of needs assessment (Box 3.3).

However, these elements do not adequately develop a *shared* understanding of what constitutes the major needs of people using services within a locality. The approach can therefore fall prey to

**Box 3.3** Elements in the process of needs assessment

1. Epidemiological assessments based on the ability to benefit from health care which reflect what is known about incidence, prevalence and the effectiveness of treatment including cost effectiveness.

2. Comparative assessments by which district health authorities look at performance, price and utilisation to indicate the needs for change (such as the use of demographic data and health service indicators).

3. Corporate views which take account of the interests of:
   – Local people
   – GPs
   – Providers and their clinical staff
   – Other local agencies (family health screening authorities, local authorities etc)
   – Regional Offices and the NHS Executive.

the dangers of traditional planning whereby 'needs' are supplanted by other features that determine the shape of the service, such as the age groups concerned, location, time of day, professions involved or groupings of disabilities.

When working to develop a mental health strategy, there is a clear need to integrate both these qualitative and quantitative approaches to needs assessment into one coherent process. The following paragraphs explore qualitative approaches before moving on to quantitative approaches.

There are three major tools in the assessment of qualitative needs: first, the needs of individuals identified in the care management and care planning process; second, the use of the stakeholder conferences; and third, the construction of focus groups. As care management and care planning have already been extensively discussed above (and see also Chapter 4), this section will focus on the use of stakeholder conferences and focus groups.

The aim of a stakeholder conference is to determine the broad parameters of need which will form the basis of all future strategy development. It involves gathering together those with a major 'stake' in the service and jointly defining and agreeing upon the needs of people with mental health problems. Stakeholder conferences can have either a locality focus or a client group focus. The debate takes place within a framework where everyone's contribution is of equal value. Everyone listens and takes responsibility for their opinions and everyone is there as an individual not as a representative. The emphasis is on seeking and articulating different views but reaching a consensus is not important.

This principle only works if it is practised with the belief that people who have used mental health services have expertise to contribute to the process of planning and managing services which is derived from their sometimes considerable experience. It is important to guarantee adequate representation of both minority populations and women. This may be achieved by inviting relevant community groups and ensuring that, as far as possible, the participants as a whole reflect the multiracial and multicultural characteristics of the area.

All participants are encouraged to state what they perceive people's needs to be. An approach described within the Developing Integrated Services in the Community (DISC) framework can be employed (Peck and Smith, 1991; Johnson *et al.*, 1997). There can be a tendency to jump straight to a service response, such as 'they need a day centre'. However, participants are encouraged to think beyond a *solution* (i.e. the day centre) in order to identify the underlying need (i.e. meaningful day time activity) (Box 3.4). The approach is therefore based on 'ordinary' understandings of need (see Chapter 1) rather than on clinical notions of diagnosis or other specialist knowledge about mental illness.

This separation of needs and solutions is essential. Failure to

**Box 3.4** Example

100 people in a given area have a diagnosis of schizophrenia; planning usually proceeds on the basis of assumptions about service response – 20 acute beds, 70 day hospital/day centre places, 100 outpatient appointments and so on. However, this is not information about people's needs; how many of those 100 people need help in finding a job, in making friends, in using the adult education or leisure services, in shopping and caring for themselves adequately, in finding decent accommodation?

distinguish between the two will mean that solutions will nearly always be based on existing service models rather than thinking of truly new ways of meeting the particular needs of individuals.

Additionally, stakeholder conferences highlight the value of involving people with direct experience of the service as users or carers. Without such an input, it is not possible to identify needs effectively nor to move imaginatively towards a new pattern of services. Involving people in this way also circumvents many of the problems of working with users and carers.

Focus groups can also be used to assist in understanding the nature of need, to identify gaps in services, and to share ideas for future services. Separate focus groups can be held with each of the major players in the services (users, carers, GPs, voluntary organisations, ethnic minorities, service providers from health and social services). Focus groups have some similarities with other group methods but are distinctive in the following respects: explicit attention is paid to consumers rather than to professionals (the consumer is regarded as the expert); the groups can provide insights into attitudes, perceptions and opinions; and discussions in the groups are recorded using a tape recorder thus avoiding the distractions of note taking and flip charts.

Experience suggests that focus groups allow issues to be explored in more depth although the benefit of dialogue between the major players is lost. Thus the qualitative approach of stakeholder conferences and focus groups identifies what people feel their needs are but does not necessarily identify the number with that need and may not adequately identify current unmet need. These issues can be addressed by a more quantitative approach.

The starting point for the quantitative assessment of mental health needs is epidemiological data from studies conducted in both the UK and abroad. These provide incidence and prevalence rates for diagnostic groups such as schizophrenia and depression, usually derived from special studies of small and relatively discrete populations. These studies show that the prevalence estimates for mental illness diagnoses vary widely from place to place and hence cannot usually be applied directly to the population involved in qualitative needs assessment. The quality of the estimates that can be derived from such approaches has been markedly improved by the publication of the Office of National Surveys (ONS) study of psychiatric morbidity in Great Britain commissioned by the Department of Health (Meltzer *et al.*, 1994).

These broad epidemiological estimates must be refined so that they relate more closely to the population involved in the qualitative exercise. Two complementary approaches can be used: data on the size and characteristics of the population and mental illness specific data.

Data on population size and characteristics include demographic information and more specific census-derived variables which have been shown to be related to mental illness and also to mental health services use. Such indices comprise, for example, social isolation and deprivation and composite scores such as the UPA-8. The most recent census (1991) provides relatively up to date data on all these indicators. There are examples of software packages (e.g. MINI – Mental Index Needs Index) that attempt to link population size and characteristics directly to requirements for service. Useful as such packages may be, they should be used with caution as they tend to move straight from population figures to numbers of places in treatment settings (e.g. acute admission beds/residential care) and are reliant on a number of assumptions.

Mental illness specific data are often less directly related to diagnosis but can help to refine estimates by providing information as to the likely 'size of the problem' in a particular area. Data of particular use here may include the following:

*Service utilisation and provision data*  Although this will not address unmet need or patients who are not in contact with psychiatric services, a large proportion of the seriously mentally ill are likely to be currently in contact with services or to have had contact in the past. Where registers exist these can be particularly helpful and a knowledge of the location of the old long-stay hospitals will indicate where local prevalence in the community may be higher as a result of the relocation of former long-stay residents. Information about the current use of services will not, of course, address the issue of estimating unmet need.

*General practice data*  The increase in computerisation of general practice data will provide an ever more useful source of information, particularly if standard diagnostic criteria are used. Of particular help here may be practices who are involved in the General Practice National Morbidity Surveys. It is also likely that fundholding practices will increasingly hold high quality data, and perhaps have conducted a needs assessment exercise on the practice population. A high proportion of the seriously mentally ill may also be identified relatively easily through general practitioners especially given the increasing usage of diagnostic codes by GPs during patient consultations. For less sophisticated practices, repeat prescription data can be reviewed together with appointment or visit lists which may prompt the memories of GPs to help identify such patients. Assessing one or two 'typical' local practices can, therefore, provide a useful check on the estimates of the prevalence in the local population.

*Local surveys*    Useful data may be available from surveys carried out for other purposes, using standard instruments (e.g. the SF36) or undertaken specifically to determine the prevalence of mental illness in a particular subgroup of the population (e.g. using the GHQ). They may then be interpreted in conjunction with models of filters to care.

These two approaches, using population and mental illness specific data, lead to a 'patch specific' numerical estimate of the number of mentally ill at a given level of severity. They may also indicate areas of particular uncertainty in the epidemiological prediction which can be addressed by further specific local work. Standardised survey instruments, which do not necessarily need to be administered by professionals trained in psychiatry, may be particularly useful here. This quantitative approach based on diagnostic groups, will not of itself, however, identify the precise requirements for different types of local services. It is important to remember that needs assessment is an art not a science.

*CONTRACTING FOR SERVICES**    The specification for services, and the subsequent contract, is the link between purchaser and provider, the assessed need and the service to meet that need. At the same time, the contract attempts to delineate the balance for a particular service of the three corners of the iron triangle: quantity, quality and cost. It can be difficult to achieve a balance that satisfies all parties to the contract: purchaser, provider and user.

*Compile specifications*    The specification for service is the key document in the contracting process, because it enables the purchaser to detail the quantity of service, the quality of service and the money available for a service, i.e. it is the document that attempts to balance the three points of the iron triangle. In theory the specification is the product of the purchaser. In practice, however, providers play a central role in the development of most specifications. There are two main reasons for this role. First, the production of a comprehensive specification is a time-consuming process, as the above section on needs

---

*This section draws on Peck and Smith (1991). The author also acknowledges the contribution of Sheila Howells to this section.

assessment indicates. The capacity and capability of all purchasers, health authority, social services department or GP fundholder, are stretched by this process and there is an obvious temptation to seek assistance from the prospective provider(s), particularly where there is only one realistic source of provision. The provider(s) too will be keen to offer help as the more influence the provider(s) exercises over the specification the more certain their own future. The purchaser also needs to know that the provider is willing and able to deliver the quantity and quality at an agreed price and also that all clinical staff in the provider agency are willing and able to deliver the contract.

The extent to which purchasers decide to involve providers in the compilation of specifications (Box 3.5) may depend on a number of factors.

**Box 3.5** Compilation of specifications

- Many purchasers, in particular health purchasers, face a monopoly supplier whose managers and clinicians may be long-standing colleagues. In these circumstances, the purchasers may attempt to negotiate changes with the provider through the process of agreeing specifications (or contracts). If purchasers have undertaken a comprehensive needs assessment, and thought through the implications for services, they will have more confidence in introducing new requirements for providers in specifications or contract negotiation. It is pointless for purchasers to issue specifications to monopoly providers which those providers cannot or will not deliver.

- On occasions purchasers, in particular social services departments charged with stimulating the growth of independent provision of social care through spending 85% of the standard transitional grant (STG) in the private sector, may use specifications as the basis for competitive tenders from a number of providers. In these circumstances, consultation about the specifications may be more difficult to conduct in a manner which is seen to be even-handed.

- The potential number of competing providers should also help the purchaser decide on the degree of detail in the specifications, and therefore the amount of provider involvement in the compilation. Purchasers facing a monopoly supplier may be more inclined to detail the nature of the service required, whereas in a competitive situation purchasers might only outline the values and function of the service and expect suppliers to transform these into detailed proposals for service.

**Box 3.6** Nature of standards

There are four types of standards which could be included in a specification.

♦ Inputs, e.g. training requirements of staff employed in a sheltered work project.

♦ Processes, e.g. all referrals to a sheltered work project will be assessed within 'x' working days of receipt of referral letter.

♦ Outputs, e.g. provider will deal with at least 'x' number of users in each financial year.

♦ Outcome, e.g. 'x' % of users of the sheltered workshop will be placed in paid work in each calendar year.

In order to stimulate independent providers, social services departments must approach specifications in a manner which encourages new suppliers. One way of achieving this aim is to divide services into discrete components covered by separate specifications or to break purchasing decisions into individual specifications relating to a single aspect of a service for an individual user. Such microspecifications are often the outcome of individual assessments and care plans put together by care managers.

Health authorities, social services departments and GP fundholders may all decide to invite tenders from providers against macrospecifications. This is an increasing trend, and reflects the assertiveness of purchasers as well as their occasional frustration with the quality of service provided by current providers. However, purchasers need to be aware of the potential problems of such an assertive approach; for instance, where statutory providers have lost an element of mainstream service to independent providers, there may be a tendency for the previous providers to influence referral patterns to undermine the impact of the new provider.

Whichever of the above approaches is adopted, the cornerstone of the specification will be the quality standards which the purchaser lays down for the provider to meet. The purchaser needs to be clear about two basic issues: the nature and the number of standards to be specified (Box 3.6).

*Nature of standards* There is a growing belief that 'outcomes' represent the most valuable approach and 'inputs' the least valuable. However, reliable outcome measures in mental health services are proving difficult to develop. It is essential that any measure used fulfils the following criteria: it should be capable of unambiguous interpretation; changes in the measure score should be capable of unambiguous interpretation (e.g. increase = good, decrease = bad); systems developed to measure outcome are under the control of the provider.

There is an increasing emphasis from the Department of Health on evidence-based purchasing. In particular, the outcomes of purchased interventions should be understood by purchasers. However, little research evidence in mental health convinces all parties; in particular, there is a strong resistance among many clinicians to copying models from elsewhere – what could be called the 'it wouldn't work here' syndrome – even when purchasers demonstrate enthusiastic support for new 'evidence-based' models. On occasions where the clinical research evidence appears to demonstrate clear outcomes there are often other influences on decisions. This aspect of outcomes – 'whose outcome is it anyway?' – is illustrated by generic counselling in primary care: clinical research indicates that such counselling is typically no more effective than doing nothing. GP fundholders often understand this fact but they also know that one proven impact of the provision of counselling is that the number of consultations with GPs reduces and for GP fundholders this constitutes an excellent outcome. Furthermore, counselling is often requested by patients in the surgery and provision in primary care is an immediate method of responding to that request.

***Number of standards***  The more detailed the specification, the more standards of service are likely to be included. However, this may invoke the law of diminishing returns whereby the more measures that are included, the less chance there is that any will be monitored adequately. The important discipline here is to focus on those measures which really indicate the provision of a high quality service for users. The specification will also need to explain how the purchaser intends to monitor the standards.

***Select contract form and funding method***  There are a number of forms of contracts and payment systems. The contract form and method of paying providers will have a major impact on the nature and development of services. This section briefly describes the options.

### 1. Facility-based payment
This has been the common method of funding mental health services. A facility receives a fixed sum of money to provide what is usually an ill-determined service, often a number of places or beds, to a specific catchment area. Clearly, purchasers will continue to buy beds and associated services in such facilities for some time, but this should be within the context of a clear performance payment and quality standards.

### 2. Programme payment

This method provides revenue for a particular programme of care services, usually in the community, and states in general terms the client group which the programme should serve. Sometimes purchasers fail to stipulate requirements sufficiently explicitly or monitor them effectively.

### 3. Cost per case payment

This is the retrospective method of payment and, as the name implies, involves reimbursement of costs for treating individual clients. This is a method being increasingly deployed by care managers and GP fundholders and by health authorities purchasing extracontractual referrals (ECRs) from the independent sector.

### 4. Performance payment

This method rewards the achievement of explicitly stated and agreed objectives and/or outcomes. It can be introduced into most other forms of payment systems as a major incentive for suppliers to focus on quality.

### 5. Cost and volume

This method specifies the purpose of the service, number of patient episodes and overall expected cost.

### 6. Capitation payment

Capitation can be defined as a method of payment for services in which an individual is paid a fixed amount for specified users to be provided with a service over a given time period without regard to the number and nature of services provided to each user.

### 7. Block payment

A block approach identifies the type of service, a defined population and an overall funding level. It is still the most common form of health authority mental health contract.

The three forms of contract favoured by the Department of Health are cost per case, cost and volume and block. Box 3.7 presents the advantages and disadvantages of each method outlined above.

In a recent review of health authority contracting in mental health, Howells (1996) summarised the current process as being 'unsophisticated and highly unsatisfactory' in a number of respects:

♦ contracts are overwhelmingly block contracts;
♦ contracts are measured in meaningless currencies (e.g. finished consultant episodes);
♦ contract negotiations take place at the margins of activity whereas core activity continues unchallenged;
♦ contract monitoring focuses on activity (i.e. numbers) and not on quality of care or on clinical outcomes;

**Box 3.7** Advantages and disadvantages of three contractual approaches to services for long-term users in mental health services

| | Advantages | Disadvantages |
|---|---|---|
| **Block** | | |
| Purchaser | Easy to negotiate Unpredictable use of service therefore cheapest and lowest risk option for expensive services (e.g. inpatient admission) | Buy total service even though may not require certain components of the service Less opportunity to develop specific services No gain if service uptake lower than historical usage |
| Provider | Guaranteed income Potential financial gain if future use lower than recent use Easy to negotiate Easy to cross-subsidise | Potential that services unable to meet demands of all purchasers who have block contract |
| **Cost Volume** | | |
| Purchaser | Guaranteed access to traditional usage enables purchaser to start to develop alternative solutions for certain patients and therefore to offer wider range of choice of service options Ceiling on price | Historical prediction of need would have to prove accurate and alternatives would need to substitute for traditional services; if need outstrips specified volume then purchaser would pay a premium for any cases beyond that quantity |
| Provider | Guaranteed income level Opportunity to charge at premium rate for service delivery above specified volume (extracontractual referrals) | Less opportunity in system for cross-subsidy Volume purchased might not produce sufficient income to guarantee current levels of service provision Substitute services may be purchased from alternative providers |
| **Cost per case** | | |
| Purchaser | Pay for what is used (and no more) Increased opportunities for service innovation locally and therefore increased service choice; in particular if linked to microspecifications | If the purchaser remains high service user of traditional services this will prove more expensive solution as unit costs per user will be above those under a block or cost and volume system |
| Provider | Clear emphasis on the purchaser developing alternative services which may act as stimulus to change No penalties for non-achievement of block or cost and volume contracts | Potential competition and loss of guaranteed income; in particular purchasers may seek to reduce overheads attributed to each case Complicated to administer |

♦ contract monitoring does not establish whether individual or population needs are being met;
♦ contract monitoring does not compare cost or clinical effectiveness across providers.

Howell identified a number of potential alternative currencies based on, for instance, outcomes or care packages. The problematic nature of outcomes discussed above may be addressed by the Health of the Nation Outcome Scales (HoNOS). Developed in response to the need to measure the *Health of the Nation* targets for mental illness, HoNOS is a ten-point health and social functioning scale which measures user improvement, or deterioration, over time. The problematic nature of care plans discussed above may be addressed by the introduction of user-based approaches to monitoring of care packages which answer fundamental questions such as: did the user agree a care plan which he/she felt addressed the central problems; were the promised services delivered; and did the services help with the problems?

GP fundholders face a similar set of problems, although some are becoming more proactive in changing away from block contracts to cost and volume, and specifying very precise outputs (e.g. information to be contained in assessment reports from mental health teams). The Department of Health has been clear that social services department care managers should be moving towards cost per case spot purchasing (e.g. Department of Health, 1994) but Hudson (1996a) expresses doubts about whether sufficient social services departments have clear purchasing frameworks that facilitate spot purchasing. Clearly, such individualistic approaches to purchasing appeal to GPs as well as care managers, but for providers represent a major source of uncertainty.

Importantly, partnerships in purchasing must include partnerships in monitoring of providers. The integration of the care programme approach (CPA) with care management in mental health offers the opportunity for such joint monitoring, although there remain cultural (e.g. confidentiality) and practical (e.g. IT) obstacles to the sharing of assessments, care packages and reviews at a clinical level which therefore impede their use by purchasers.

*CONCLUSION*   This chapter has mapped the major issues in the evolution and current position of purchasing of mental health services. In so doing, it has focused on the specific areas which provide the policy and managerial context for the work of clinicians. Further evolution is inevitable, but the past and present provide important constraints on the shape of the future.

*DISCUSSION QUESTIONS*

◆ What were the factors that led to the publication of *Working for Patients* and *Caring for People*?

◆ What were the main proposals in the White Papers and what alternatives might the government have considered?

◆ What are the major differences between health authorities, social service departments and GP fundholders as purchasers and how do these differences inhibit or enhance collaborative approaches to purchasing mental health services?

◆ What are the problems with current methods used to assess needs and how might these problems be solved?

◆ What are the advantages and disadvantages of the various types of contract used to purchase mental health services?

◆ In what ways is the purchaser/provider split of benefit to service users either now or in the future?

*FURTHER READING*

There is a wealth of material available which concerns the recent developments in purchasing in the National Health Service which includes the following.

◆ Klein, R. (1995) *The Politics of the NHS*. London: Longman.
This book is updated regularly and provides both the historical context and a balanced account.

◆ Smith, R. (1994) *A Practical Guide to Fundholding*. London: Blackwell.
Describes GP fundholding well.

◆ Thornicroft, G. and Strathdee, G. (1996) *Purchasing Mental Health Services*. NHS Executive, Leeds: HMSO.
Thorough and provides a wealth of references.

◆ *Community Care Management and Planning Review* – published bi-monthly by Pavilion Publishing, Brighton.
There is less material which describes purchasing in local authorities, but this is a useful source.

*REFERENCES*

Audit Commission (1986), *Making a Reality of Community Care*. London: HMSO.

Audit Commission/CMHSD (1995), *Caring for Citizens*. London: CMHSD.

Centre for Mental Health Service Development (CMHSD) (1996), *Mental Health Review*, Vol. I, no. 3. Brighton: Pavilion Publishing.

Department of Health (1988), *Community Care: Agenda for Action*. London: HMSO.

Department of Health (1989a), *Working for Patients*, Cmnd 555. London: HMSO.

Department of Health (1989b), *Caring for People*, Cmnd 849. London: HMSO.

Department of Health (1991), *Health of the Nation*, Cmnd 1523. London: HMSO.

Department of Health/Scottish Office (1991), *Care Management and Assessment - Managers Guide*. London: HMSO.

Department of Health/Social Services Inspectorate (1993), *Health of the Nation Key Area Handbook: Mental Illness*. London: Department of Health.

Department of Health (1994), *Implementing Caring for People: Care Management*. London: HMSO.

Department of Health (1997), *Developing Partnerships in Mental Health*. London: HMSO.

Enthoven, A. (1985), *Reflections on the Management of the NHS*. London: Nuffield Provincial Hospitals Trust.

Ham, C. (1994), *Management and Competition in the New NHS*. Oxford: Radcliffe Medical Press.

Harrison, S., Hunter, D., Mornoch, G. and Pollit, C. (1992), *Just Managing: Power and Culture in the National Health Service*. London: Macmillan.

Hayward, P., Peck, E. and Smith, H. (1993), Qualitative and quantitative approaches to needs assessment in mental health: creating a common currency. *Journal of Mental Health*, 2, 287–294.

Health Select Committee (1993), *Report of the Inquiry into Mental Illness Services*. London: HMSO.

Howells, S. (1996), Contracts and Mental Health. Presentation to the CMHSD/NHS Executive North West Regional Office Conference, Manchester.

Hudson, B. (1996a), Care management: is it working? *Community Care Management and Planning*, 4, no. 3, 77–84.

Hudson, B. (1996b), Partnerships in purchasing: are there any lessons from the theory? Presentation to CMHSD Annual Conference, Sheffield (Summary available from CMHSD).

Johnson, S., Ramsey, R., Thornicroft, G. *et al.* (1997), *London's Mental Health*. London: Kings Fund.

Klein, R. (1995). *The Politics of the NHS*. London: Longman.

Marum, M. (1995), *The NAFP Straw Poll*. The Fundholding Summary. (February)

Meltzer, H., Gill, B. and Petticrew, M. (1994), *OPCS Surveys of Psychiatric Morbidity in Great Britain, Report 1: The Prevalence of Psychiatric Morbidity among adults aged 16–64, living in private households in Great Britain*. London: HMSO.

Murphy, E. (1991), *After the Asylums*. London: Faber and Faber.

NHS Management Executive (1993), *Purchasing for Health: A Framework for Action*. London: HMSO.

Peck, E. (1994), Community Mental Health Teams. *Journal of Mental Health*, 3, no. 2, 151–156.

Peck, E. (1996), Power and Decision-making in the NHS. Unpublished PhD Thesis, University of Newcastle.

Peck, E. and Smith, H. (1991), *Contracting In Mental Health Services: A*

*Framework for Action*. Bristol: National Health Services Training Directorate.

Ritchie, J., Dick, D. and Lingham, R. (1994), *The Report of the Inquiry into the Care and Treatment of Christopher Clunis*. London: HMSO.

Roberts, J. (1990), Kenneth Clarke: hatchet man or remoulder? *British Medical Journal*, 301, 1383–1386.

Rogers, A., Pilgrim, D. and Lacey, R. (1993), *Experiencing Psychiatry*. London: Macmillan.

Smith, H. (1995), Strategic planning of mental health services. *Community Care Management and Planning*, 3, no. 1, 3–14.

Strathdee, G. (1992), Liaison between primary and secondary mental health teams. In: Jenkins, R. *et al*. (Eds) *The Prevention of Depression and Anxiety*. London: HMSO.

Thatcher, M. (1993), *The Downing Street Years*. London: Harper Collins.

Wright, A. (1993), *Depression Recognition in General Practice*. London: Royal College of General Practitioners.

CHAPTER 4

# The Structure and Organisation of Community Mental Health Teams

## Steve Onyett and Helen Smith

*KEY ISSUES*

- ◆ The purpose of community mental health services
- ◆ The function and organisation of community mental health teams (CMHTs)
- ◆ Improving the effectiveness of CMHTs
- ◆ The relationship between primary care services and CMHTs
- ◆ The importance of effective relationships between staff and users.

*INTRODUCTION*

At a time when the rhetoric of preventing people 'falling through the net' is at the forefront of policy imperatives, that net often appears distinctly patchy for people with the most severe and long-term mental health problems (Mental Health Foundation, 1994). Some are asking whether the net is concerned with their safety, or their capture and containment (Crepaz-Keay, 1994). This chapter examines the ways in which continuous, coordinated and effective service provision can be achieved in this context. It does this by first considering the functions that services should be achieving for service users. It then examines how effectively these functions can be met by community mental health teams (CMHTs) and the implications for practitioners working within these teams. The development, structure and operation of these teams is explored and recommendations made for future development.

**WHAT SHOULD SERVICES BE ACHIEVING FOR PEOPLE?**

Although the move to community care has underpinned government policy-making for over three decades, it is only in the last decade that the development of community-based mental health services has become widespread. The Department of Health has sought to support this move through, for example, the inclusion of mental illness in the *Health of the Nation* key target areas, the creation of the National Mental Health Task Force, the allocation of specific resources (e.g. the Mental Illness Specific Grant and the Mental Health Challenge Fund), and the introduction of initiatives such as the Care Programme Approach and care management.

However, the diverse needs of people with mental health problems mean that mental health care is only partly about statutory services. Many of the factors which contribute to an individual's well-being – good housing, a job, adequate income – are not, or cannot be provided by mental health services alone. Services need to create the conditions which enable people to have access to – and use – these opportunities. Failure to do this will mean that people's level of disability (that is, the social effects of their mental distress, see Chapter 2) will remain unnecessarily high (Peck and Smith, 1991). Furthermore, the long-term nature of many people's mental health problems means that services have to be flexible enough to respond to an individual's changing needs over many years.

CMHTs are 'often viewed as the way to start community care – as cornerstones for new types of services in the community, and the focal point for a locally based range of services' (Ovretveit, 1993). There is no national consensus about how this might be achieved. Some CMHTs will attempt to provide services directly to too broad a range of people, often leading to the relative neglect of people with the most complex health and social care needs. Others may define their role and their client group very narrowly, but in a local context where the needs of the large numbers of people presenting with significant distress in primary care are inadequately served. In the context of a primary care-led NHS in which GPs increasingly shape service development, such a service is unlikely to remain viable over the long term. This chapter looks in detail at the development and operation of CMHTs as a way of evaluating their potential to achieve the ambitious aims that are often defined for them.

**THE SOCIAL POLICY CONTEXT FOR CMHTs**

The development of CMHTs in the UK has mirrored the development of community mental health centres (CMHCs), case management and assertive community treatment in the US. CMHCs aimed to provide services to a broad range of people, backed by an ideology concerned with promoting access for all, and offering an alternative to the 'medical model' (Dowell and Ciarlo, 1983). A review of British CMHCs in the mid-1980s highlighted a range of different approaches but a shared commitment to moving the 'centre of gravity' of psychiatric services from institutional settings to a more accessible local environment (McAusland, 1985). They often placed great emphasis on health promotion and community development work. These aims have been strongly criticised as overambitious and naive (Peck, 1994; Sayce *et al.*, 1991; Patmore and Weaver, 1992), but the subsequent changes in direction have led others to lament the shift away from a concern about the effects of social inequalities on mental health and appropriate community development (Samson, 1995). As with the American CMHCs (Dowell and Ciarlo, 1983), there is evidence that CMHTs developed in the UK did not place sufficient emphasis on people with severe and long-term mental health problems, tending to favour working with people who were perceived as having more tractable problems (Sayce *et al.*, 1991; Patmore and Weaver, 1992).

In the early 1970s, the US identified case management as the social policy response to the need to target people with the most complex mental health and social needs, while helping them navigate a fragmented and uncoordinated network of providers (Onyett, 1992). In the early 1990s, both the care programme approach (CPA) and social services-led care management were introduced as the British response to similar problems in service provision (Department of Health, 1990a). Despite concerns about overlap and confusion, little useful clarification of the relationship between these two initiatives was provided at the time. Indeed, the then Secretary of State for Health defined care management as 'Any strategy for managing and coordinating and reviewing services for the individual client in a way that provides for continuity of care and accountability to both the client and the managing agency' (Department of Health, 1990a, Appendix B, 1). This is a definition that clearly also encompasses the CPA. Care management guidance stressed the coordinating and purchasing role in social care, while at the same time, exhorting close partnerships with health services (Department of Health/Social Services Inspectorate, 1991). More recently the stated purposes of supervision registers (an elaboration of CPA; NHSE, 1994) include: providing a care plan that aims to reduce risk; regularly reviewing care needs; maintaining contact; providing a point of reference for relevant and authorised health and social services staff; planning for the facilities and resources necessary to meet need; and identifying those patients who should receive the highest priority for care and active follow-up. These functions have all been previously described as the remit of care management (Department of Health/Social Services Inspectorate, 1991).

In practice, the implementation of care programming and care management in mental health services has been slow and patchy. There were widespread concerns about confusing guidance, lack of resources for implementation, burdensome paperwork and the removal of social workers from direct client contact and multi-disciplinary teams to a middle-management resource-rationing role (Schneider, 1993; Marshall, 1996; North and Ritchie, 1993; Anonymous, 1995; Social Services Inspectorate, 1995). This culminated in a statement in the long-awaited *Building Bridges* guidance to the effect that: 'For people subject to the CPA, in essence the key worker and care management functions are the same. Both involve coordinating the delivery of an agreed care plan. One way of looking at the CPA is as a specialist variant of care management. ... In well integrated systems, it is quite possible for the care management function to extend in whole or part to health services as well, and for health professionals to be designated as care managers' (Department of Health, 1995, p. 56–57).

CMHTs are the obvious vehicle for such integrated practice. *Building Bridges* and the subsequent *Spectrum of Care* guidance makes explicit the role of CMHTs as the cornerstone of specialist mental health service provision (Department of Health, 1996). Indeed the latter is highly prescriptive on the subject: 'CMHTs cover defined population groups. This means each team is responsible for delivering and coordinating a specialised level of care. The teams include: social workers; mental health nurses; psychologists; occupational therapists; and psychiatrists' (Department of Health, 1996, p. 5).

## ORGANISATION AND OPERATION OF CMHTs

West (1994) provides a useful framework for considering team effectiveness. It has three main components:

1. Task effectiveness: the extent to which the team is successful in achieving its task-related objectives;
2. Mental health: the well-being, growth and development of team members;
3. Team viability: the probability that the team will continue to work together and function effectively.

There is a paucity of research evidence to support the extent to which CMHTs are currently effective against these criteria, apart from accounts of isolated demonstration projects, or highly prescribed models of service provision, often from abroad. In 1993, two large-scale national surveys by the Sainsbury Centre for Mental Health attempted to capture data on the current organisation and operation of CMHTs (Onyett *et al.*, 1994, 1995, 1996). A total of 517 teams in 144 District Health Authorities were identified.* Key findings from these surveys and their implications are discussed with reference to the limited literature available in the area.

*Findings presented here are based on data from 302 teams of which a further 60 were sampled again to examine burnout, job satisfaction, team role clarity, personal role clarity, team and professional identification, sources of pressure and reward and features of practice (e.g. caseload size and composition).

*The dominance of the community mental health centre*

Community mental health centres were still the main base for teams (44% of all CMHTs). They were second only to primary care-based teams in having a low proportion of people with severe and long-term mental health problems on their caseloads (53% and 38% of caseloads respectively).* In keeping with the CMHC tradition of offering a service to a broad sample of the population, 57% of CMHTs (and 63% of CMHCs) were the 'first contact point for all mental health referrals in their locality or sector'. These teams had a significantly smaller proportion of people with severe and long-term problems on their caseloads than those that were not the first point of contact. However, an open referral system was not associated with a smaller proportion of long-term users. This accords with other findings that accepting referrals from a wide variety of sources, including self referrals, does not affect targeting, as long as effective gate-keeping is in operation (Marriott *et al.*, 1993).

Teams with the highest proportion of long-term users (66%) tended to be office-based teams without facilities for seeing users on-site. They appeared to place greater emphasis on providing services where they were needed (in the manner of assertive community treatment teams described below).

*Improved targeting and the provision of more relevant services*

A third of CMHTs reported that long-term users made up over two-thirds of the team's caseload. Teams offering access to clients after hours and at weekends (23% of sample), services for people whose behaviour is 'challenging' (31%), services particularly for people with severe and long-term mental health problems (89%), work opportunities (24%), services offering practical help with everyday problems (70%) and assessment of activities of daily living (89%) had a significantly larger proportion of people with severe and long-term mental health problems on their caseloads than those that did not. It is encouraging that large proportions of teams were offering these services with the worrying exception of out-of-hours access and work opportunities.

By far the majority (73%) of teams had direct access to beds via the medical member of the team. However, responsibility for ongoing planning of an individual's care was retained by the team in only 30% of cases. Along with increased outreach from teams to people's homes, there appears to be a need for increased 'in-reach' into inpatient services.

---

* Severe mental health problems were defined as a level of distress or disturbance that could normally result in a diagnosis of psychosis, psychiatric admission, or community-based interventions to prevent admission. Long term was indicated by intense service use (e.g. hospital admissions or weekly home visits) over six months or more. People suffering from organic illness, brain injury or extreme personal trauma were included.

*Weak operational and strategic management and the fragmentation of teams*

The influential study by Patmore and Weaver (1991) advocated clearly defined management of gate-keeping, allocation of referrals and case load management. However, two years later, even tasks such as deciding the target group or assessing the mental health needs of the local community, were undertaken by the 'team as a whole'. Deciding who the service is for is a major strategic decision that should not be left to the team itself. Similarly, responsibility for the allocation of cases to team practitioners was undertaken by the 'team as a whole' in 51% of teams; and in only 20%, by team coordinators or managers. The 'team as a whole' also dominated when deciding which referrals the team accepted day-to-day.

The team's senior doctor rarely had ultimate responsibility for management tasks except in the area of 'over-ruling the decisions of team members if necessary'. However, even on this task, professional line managers were most frequently assigned responsibility. They were also most frequently ultimately responsible for clinical supervision.

Teams remain fragmented. Only community mental health nurses and other nurses, social workers, occupational therapists and community support workers worked on average more than four days per week with the team. High levels of part-time working were strongly associated with a small proportion of long-term users on the team's caseload. If CMHTs are to be appropriately focused on people with the most complex and enduring needs, then staffing should reflect the need for continuous and coordinated care over the long term.

*The mental health of teams*

West's (1994) definition of successful teams stresses the mental health of team members and the long-term viability of the team. Generally job satisfaction was high among team members, particularly where they had a positive sense of belonging to the team and were clear about its role (Onyett *et al.*, 1996). However, 44% of the sample fell into the 'high' burnout category for emotional exhaustion based on norms for mental health workers; 45% of CMHNs, 54% of social workers and 12 out of 19 consultant psychiatrists fell into this category. This finding has been corroborated by another study using the same instrument with CMHNs (Carson *et al.*, 1995). When examining the reported sources of pressure and reward it was striking that contact with service users and clinical work features more highly as a source of reward than as a source of pressure. The major concern of team members was threats to their efficacy arising from lack of resources, work overload and bureaucracy. Being effective clinically and clinical contact itself were major sources of reward for staff. However, contact with team colleagues and multidisciplinary working was the source of reward that was cited most often. This is of interest given the very critical commentaries on the experience of team working (e.g. Galvin and McCarthy, 1994; Anciano and Kirkpatrick, 1990).

**THE FUTURE FOR CMHTs**

Readers may have been surprised not to have encountered a definition of CMHTs in the discussion so far. In fact, Onyett *et al.* (1994), when piloting their original minimal definition of a CMHT,* found in practice they needed to add another criterion: 'recognised as a multidisciplinary team of two or more disciplines by service managers'. In other words, CMHTs often recognised themselves as a CMHT purely because someone had told them they were a CMHT. In view of this ambiguity it is not surprising that CMHTs have been strongly criticised for being poorly planned and operated (Galvin and McCarthy, 1994; Peck, 1994). However, this is insufficient reason to reject them wholesale. We need to think about what they are supposed to be achieving for service users and plan accordingly, drawing upon what is known from existing research. The following draws out some major themes.

**The need to prioritise**

CMHTs' lack of targeting might be construed as a major reason for their partial failure in meeting the needs of people with longer-term problems. Targeting based on diagnosis alone gives virtually no information about the needs of people using the service. As Peck points out in Chapter 3, information about the number of people who might be expected to have a particular diagnosis is often used as a basis for planning the required service response, i.e. the number of beds, day centre places and outpatient appointments. However, this does not reflect people's needs in terms of the help they require to find a job, find suitable accommodation, make friends, use education services, shop or care for themselves adequately (Peck and Smith, 1991).

Defining long-term users is always difficult. In general, most scales are a balance of diagnosis, duration and extent of disability (see Chapter 1). This form of categorisation runs the risk of ignoring the differences between individuals and may conflate the separate issues of severity and longevity. However, consideration of disability does include the important consideration of how mental distress is impeding people's ability to perform their various roles. Targeting based on descriptive criteria much more accurately assesses the range of needs which a team can address, although this presupposes that teams have defined their eligibility criteria in terms of which needs they intend to meet, rather than simply what types of services they will provide.

**A focus on relationships**

It is a paradox that perhaps the most important aspect of teams is the extent to which they are able to promote successful individual

---

*For a team to fulfil criteria for the study it served adults with mental health problems as its identified client group, did most of its work outside hospitals (although it may be hospital based), had four or more members, and offered a wider range of services than just structured day care. Teams that were wholly dedicated to people over 75, people with drink or drug problems, or people with learning difficulties were excluded.

relationships between users and staff. Effective assessment, planning, service delivery and the continuity of contact required for ongoing monitoring and review all require that staff and service users want to stay working together. The importance of the working alliance between worker and user is emerging in a number of ways. British research on case management has stressed the importance of effective relationships, particularly when case management has been evaluated from a user perspective (Beeforth *et al.*, 1994). Working alliances may be slow and hard to achieve, but reap the benefits of increased adherence to medication regimes, the need for less medication and better outcomes in terms of symptomatology, quality of life and satisfaction with mental health treatment (Frank and Gunderson, 1990; Solomon *et al.*, 1995; Gehrs and Goering, 1994). A recent study also showed how the tendency to over-prescribe antipsychotics to black service users was ameliorated when efforts to engage users were rated higher (Segal *et al.*, 1996). Effective working alliances appear to be promoted by providing contact as soon as possible after the need for intervention has been identified (Axelrod and Wetzler, 1989) and proactively offering practical support and assistance (Repper *et al.*, 1994).

Although practitioners cannot avoid the tension between care and control, being fully aware of it is necessary for effective practice (Handy, 1990). Practitioners need carefully to balance the need to develop effective working relationships, with an ethical imperative to communicate their social control functions to service users. Much of the literature on the relationships between service users and practitioners assumes a psychotherapeutic stance, characterised by warmth, empathy and genuineness, and aims for a reciprocal partnership based on collaborative problem-solving (e.g. Mosher and Burti, 1989). As discussed in Chapter 2, this is clearly desirable but is more likely to be achieved when practitioners can authentically discuss those aspects of their roles that may be less attractive to service users, including the implications of their status as a mental health professional employed by a statutory body. It also includes the limitations on their role as an advocate for the user. Service users can then exercise maximum control over how they handle the relationship. Many service users may be reassured by the knowledge that control will be taken away from them in certain defined circumstances. This will certainly be preferable to springing it on them if the need ever arises. Others will exercise their right to try to avoid statutory services because they find this aspect of the relationship unacceptable.

*The need for assertive community treatment*  Assertive community treatment (ACT) is the deployment of a multidisciplinary team to serve a defined group of long-term users by providing assertive outreach *in situ*. Users are typically visited at home and contact is maintained during their involvement with other providers (such as inpatient care). Services aim to help users manage the symptoms of their disorder, improve their material and social environment and train in activities of daily living, social relations and work. To achieve intensive individualised services caseloads are generally low, in the region of one staff member to 10–12 users.

ACT has been rigorously evaluated since its inception with the seminal work of Stein and Test in Madison, Wisconsin (Stein and Test, 1980; Stein, 1990). ACT-style teams reduce in-patient bed use (Merson *et al.*, 1992; Burns *et al.*, 1993b; Dean *et al.*, 1993; Marks *et al.*, 1994) and, subsequent to discharge, they ensure that difficult-to-serve people maintain an adequate level of service contact (Ford *et al.*, 1995). Users and carers prefer the care provided by such teams when compared to care provided by standard services (Merson *et al.*, 1992; Dean *et al.*, 1993; Marks *et al.*, 1994). They are cost-effective (Burns *et al.*, 1993b; Knapp *et al.*, 1994) and positively evaluated by referrers (Onyett *et al.*, 1990). Recent reviews of the international literature justify the early optimism concerning the impact of ACT on improvements in clinical status, independent living, social functioning, occupation, adherence to medication regimes, quality of life and cost-effective service use (particularly concerning use of inpatient beds) (Burns and Santos, 1995; Bond *et al.*, 1995).

Identifying the active ingredient in change requires further research. One study achieved improved engagement, reduced bed use and increased cost-effectiveness simply by introducing home-based assessment involving a psychiatrist and other trained professionals within two weeks of referral (Burns *et al.*, 1993a,b). Another study stressed the importance of the CMHT controlling access to a wide range of resources, particularly inpatient care (Marks *et al.*, 1994). Introducing a recent review of ACT, Drake and Burns (1995) say of the US that 'No psychosocial intervention has influenced current community mental health care more than assertive community treatment' (p. 667). The same is far from true of the UK where such services are still very much the exception. Contributory factors are likely to include:

♦ a general concern among devalued staff to avoid working with other devalued members of society;
♦ lack of competence to deliver service provision to people with severe and long-term mental health problems in chaotic community settings;
♦ a concern to maintain professional autonomy that is incompatible with team working and the operational management of a team;
♦ lack of resources;
♦ poor management and supervision;
♦ difficulties effecting change within developed services;

♦ operational managers with a lack of vision and inadequate management skills;
♦ poorly developed strategic frameworks for purchasing mental health care.

As the key vehicle for coordinated provision, CMHTs become the forum where these problems are most evident. Abandoning the forum will only serve to disguise these difficulties. It is difficult to see how this would be in the interests of service users.

*Links with primary care*   The drive towards a primary-care NHS that characterised government policy in the early 1990s (notably in the form of GP fundholding) has been a significant factor in influencing the work of CMHTs. Since this is discussed in detail in Chapter 5, attention here is limited to the relationship between GPs and CMHTs. The financial mechanisms which have allowed GPs to buy community services, using money top-sliced from funds that would formerly have been allocated to Trusts, have placed many CMHTs in a contradictory position. A major issue is the difference in priority target groups between health authorities, who focus on people with the most complex health and social care need, and GPs, who have small numbers of long-term users, but large numbers of patients with less severe mental health problems. Also, the desire of many GPs to have a CMHN based in the surgery can lead to problems for a Trust in ensuring adequate staffing for CMHTs in relation to duty systems, crisis cover and key worker responsibilities. The difficulties in attempting to meet both sets of demands can lead to a dilution of care to those most in need, a confusion about the nature of GP-based work and difficulties for the team in coordinating the delivery of mental health care to the local population. It is presently unclear whether the introduction of locality commissioning will serve to attenuate these conflicting imperatives.

The tensions between the different stakeholder groups involved in purchasing may be addressed by careful coordination of who has responsibility for purchasing for the broad range of needs presenting in any given locality. Collaboration will also be promoted by an appreciation of the variety of different approaches to the provision of mental health services by, in and to primary care. It is possible to construe five major ways in which GPs and specialist mental health service providers, such as CMHTs, could collaborate (developed from Hughes *et al.*, 1992). These approaches are not exclusive and various combinations of each may be operating in any given practice.

### The 'increased output' approach
GPs in this model are encouraged to refer more to specialist services through better detection and referral on. The limited

capacity of specialist care makes this problematic. The average GP list is estimated to contain seven people with a major mental illness (Kendrick *et al.*, 1991). There is only about one Community Health Nurse (CMHN) to every five GPs. There would therefore be approximately 35 people with severe mental illness allocated to each CMHN – a full caseload before people with less severe mental health problems are included (Jenkins, 1992).

### The 'replacement' approach

Here specialist providers separate themselves from the hospital-based services and replace GPs as the primary provider of mental health care, usually through CMHTs. GPs do not favour this approach on the grounds that specialist services would simply be swamped (Hughes *et al.*, 1992). Arguably this is exactly what has happened with CMHTs becoming overwhelmed with referrals of people with comparatively minor mental health problems (Patmore and Weaver, 1991; Sayce *et al.*, 1991; Jackson *et al.*, 1993).

### The 'shifted outpatient' approach

In this approach mental health specialists re-locate their services into primary care settings. A limitation of single disciplines working in primary care with people with severe and long-term mental health problems is the recognition that their complex health and social care needs require a multidisciplinary response. There is evidence that unidisciplinary teams (e.g. of CMHNs) are ineffective as they cannot provide the range of care required (Muijen *et al.*, 1994). Primary care-based CMHTs lighten the GP-burden and meet more of the needs of people with severe and long-term mental health problems. However, there are also significant disadvantages. They are costly and have difficulty remaining targeted on people with the most severe problems rather than 'anxious and unhappy people with overwhelming social and domestic difficulties' (Jackson *et al.*, 1993). The national survey of CMHTs confirmed that those based in the primary care setting had the smallest proportion of people with severe and long-term mental health problems on the team's caseload compared with other locations (Onyett *et al.*, 1994). One primary care-based CMHT reported that its availability resulted in GPs doing less counselling and had no effect on the ability of GPs to detect or manage mental illness (Warner *et al.*, 1993). A recent study found that 40% of service users in contact with psychiatrists objected to the idea of seeing them at their local GP practice. This was because of fears that other general practice attendees would know they were seeing a psychiatrist, a concern to remain in contact with the hospital service and a desire to maintain a separation between their care from primary care providers and that received from psychiatry (Nazareth *et al.*, 1995).

### The 'liaison-attachment' approach

Hughes *et al.* (1992) found considerable support among GPs for this approach, whereby specialised services are provided through primary care but with the specific aim of developing the capacity of the primary health care team to work effectively with people with mental health problems. Some CMHTs have named link workers (usually CMHNs) for each practice in their locality. These link workers may undertake initial screening in the surgery and/or train other primary care workers, including GPs, to be more effective in initial screening and in making appropriate referrals to particular services. In Nunhead, in London, a CMHT has developed joint case registers with GP practices for those with long-term problems (Strathdee, 1993). Outpatient clinics are held in surgeries and named liaison nurses are attached to practices. A number of good practice protocols have been developed which are used for a joint audit of services. Close collaboration between GPs and mental health services has been shown to improve early detection and treatment of psychotic episodes in rural environments and improved outcomes for service users (Falloon *et al.*, 1990).

The role of specialist providers in training GPs remains problematic. For example, a recent randomised controlled trial of teaching general practitioners to carry out structured assessment of their long-term mentally ill patients achieved disappointing results (Kendrick *et al.*, 1995). Although the introduction of regular, structured assessments did have some impact on changes in medication and referral to CMHNs, overall they were felt by GPs to be too time-consuming and of little relevance to subsequent management. This was among a highly selected group of practices that were willing to take on the intervention in the first place. It is also important that the training of GPs does not undermine those features that make them accessible to service users. The proximity of GPs' view of mental distress to the lay view makes them attractive to users in comparison with psychiatrists (Rogers and Pilgrim, 1993) and it may be that we need to be cautious about devaluing this aspect of their practice when advocating initiatives aimed at improving their detection and management of mental health problems using methods derived from specialist provision (Rogers, 1996).

### The 'training' approach

In this approach the emphasis is on training GPs to identify and manage people with mental health problems but not necessarily working alongside them to do so. This approach is highly dependent on the motivation of individual GPs to take on this work. The research suggests that the numbers of GPs who would want to take on a 'keyworker' role with people with severe and long-term mental health problems is likely to be very small (Kendrick *et al.*, 1991). Since the beginning of the 1990s GPs have experienced an increased workload which has affected their work stress, job satisfaction and mental health (Sutherland and Cooper, 1992). There are no extra resources allocated for the extra time that GPs spend with people with mental health problems. Although GPs' training needs may be substantial, there is evidence that detection and screening is only of value when GPs are also equipped with resources to intervene, either themselves or by referral to others (Ormel *et al.*, 1990).

Overall, there emerges a need to avoid a simplistic dichotomy between primary care-based provision consisting mainly of talking treatments for people with comparatively minor mental health problems and specialist provision conducted in secondary care settings consisting of more complex interventions. People with severe and long-term mental health problems have always been largely served in primary care and the positive aspects of this care need to be preserved and built upon. Often this will involve specialist providers working with users in primary care settings. At the same time, there is a need to avoid specialist services becoming overwhelmed with people with mental health problems that do not require specialist multidisciplinary, multiagency input. Nor should the CMHT become a 'clearing house' for all mental health problems resulting in their becoming merely an assessment and allocation service. Targeted CMHTs appear to thrive in environments where purchasers have paid sufficient attention to developing alternative services to which GPs can directly refer people who may not require a multidisciplinary, multiagency response. Such services may take the form of dedicated counselling and psychotherapy services. One popular option is to establish teams of counsellors under the supervision and management of clinical psychology services (Burton and Ramsden, 1994).

Whatever the future role of GPs in purchasing via locality commissioning processes, the commitment to a primary care-led NHS remains in place and it will continue to be of utmost importance that GPs understand the role of CMHTs in helping to achieve a comprehensive mental health service for the residents of their locality.

*The need to integrate purchasing and provision* Complex health and social care needs demand coordinated access to a wide range of resources. This includes coordination of inputs from within the team, for example when a care manager or key worker involves other team members in the assessment. It also includes coordination beyond the team, for example when a care manager secures provision from other agencies. Ideally, health and social services staff should use the same core assessment process and access funds, where necessary, through a single procedure controlled by a senior worker. Thus, CMHNs would access care management funds in the same way as social workers. This promotes easier monitoring, the possibility of pooling information on met and unmet need and ensures equitable and accountable allocation of resources to all members of a team. Placing approval for funding at a higher level also avoids the conflict of interest that arises when a practitioner is both accountable for an assessment of need and the management of a limited budget. Focusing on access to funds, rather than actually shifting resources from health to social services or vice versa also avoids legal complications. Such arrangements are in the spirit of the early care management guidance which stated that although care management is a social services-led activity, the role itself could be undertaken by practitioners employed by other agencies (Department of Health, 1990b).

The ACT model described above is itself based on a need to integrate coordinating and providing functions. Some models of case management in the US, like care management in the UK, have emphasised the importance of coordination of services as a means of achieving positive outcomes for service users. Stein (1992) has highlighted the radical limitations of such an approach, arguing that coordination is effective only insofar as there are resources to deploy and agencies with an interest in collaborating. Where this is lacking, as it usually is, Stein stresses that mental health workers need to be able to step into the breach as providers when no other option is available. This is echoed by the disappointing outcomes of case management (or 'keyworking' under the UK system) when operated merely as a means of service coordination and follow-up outside of a multidisciplinary team context (Franklin *et al.*, 1987; Marshall *et al.*, 1995; Tyrer *et al.*, 1995). It is likely, therefore, that CMHTs need to straddle the purchaser–provider split, as they are both purchasers and providers of care as circumstances dictate.

Integration of CPA and care management in CMHTs requires the definition of a core role that is shared by all practitioners. This is not an argument for generic mental health workers but rather the definition of a shared platform on which more specialised skills can be developed. If that specialisation does not occur, the core rationale for multidisciplinary team-working – access to a diversity of skills, knowledge and experience – is sacrificed. Figure 4.1 provides a description of the diversity of tasks undertaken by members of ACT-style CMHTs based on the experience of the Early Intervention Service, an inner-London CMHT (Onyett, 1992).

Within this range of tasks, a core role that comprises both coordination within the team and beyond can be described. In common with an increasing number of services, this role is referred to as 'care coordination' (Onyett, 1995). Although introducing yet more new terminology, it does provide a descriptive term that avoids some of the confusion that arises when using the term 'key worker'. Although traditionally 'key working' has been a within-provider coordinating role (e.g. day hospital key worker, hostel key worker), the CPA guidance uses the term to describe an

**Figure 4.1** The main tasks of the care coordinator

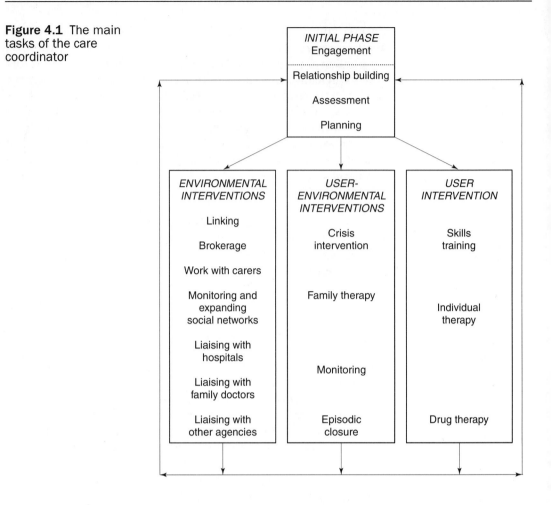

interagency role, thus creating the confusing situation where 'key workers' coordinate and monitor the outcome of input from other 'key workers'. The main tasks of the 'care coordinator' are described in Box 4.1.

*The need for relevant skills and services*
People with long-term difficulties only show improvements in clinical state or social functioning when they have access to relevant therapeutic input and practical assistance (e.g. Brooker *et al.*, 1994; Ford *et al.*, 1995). Teams must either deliver relevant interventions themselves or have access to them. The CMHT survey would suggest that social workers are important for ensuring continuity of care, psychiatrists are associated with easy access to hospital beds, and occupational therapists are associated with practical help with activities of daily living (Onyett *et al.*, 1994). Clinical psychologists may also be well qualified to work with people within complex systems such as their families, or in work contexts.

**Box 4.1** Care coordinating responsibilities

> *Coordinating care within the team*
>
> ◆ Carrying out core assessments.
>
> ◆ Ensuring that other team members contribute to a more comprehensive assessment as required.
>
> ◆ Collecting and maintaining information from other involved workers in the team for continued monitoring and review.
>
> *Coordinating care beyond the team*
>
> ◆ Achieving appropriate input from other statutory and independent providers. This may include the use of a devolved (preferably joint health and social services) budget.
>
> ◆ Monitoring the outcome of provision and feeding this back to team reviews. This will require regular and long-term contact with the service user.
>
> ◆ Ensuring that involved workers beyond the team are involved in team reviews and that the views of users, relatives and friends are represented.
>
> ◆ Collecting and maintaining information from others involved outside the team for continued monitoring and review.

However, it is not just diversity in disciplines that is critical. Attitudes and interpersonal abilities are also likely to be important. Community Companions in California is a successful, long-standing case management service (Williams *et al.*, 1994). They stress the need for diversity among team members in order to reflect the demographic characteristics of the locality and promote choice for service users. In selection they do not find educational level to be predictive of success and specifically avoid people who:

◆ lack optimism about the potential for service users to change;
◆ display patronising attitudes towards users;
◆ have difficulty working with a user-driven philosophy of care;
◆ are reluctant to help with necessary, but less glamorous activities;
◆ are reluctant to be available for occasional weekends or evenings.

Professional staff may find it more difficult to achieve these criteria than non-professional staff. Experience from the American CMHC movement would suggest the greater deployment of non-professional staff to promote access for disadvantaged groups and people from minority ethnic groups. Their advantages included an ability to identify with users through their cultural similarity, and skills in advocating on their behalf because of good local knowledge. They also achieve clinical outcomes that are equal to or better than those achieved by professional staff (for review see Huxley *et al.*, 1990). Similarly, UK studies of case management for older adults have stressed the benefits of being able to employ neighbours and others known to service users as providers (Challis and Davies, 1986). Services are increasingly employing current or ex-service users in case management roles (Sherman and Porter, 1991; Nikkel *et al.*, 1992). A recent randomised trial found them to be as effective as non-service users (Solomon and Draine, 1995).

The optimal mix of professional and non-professional staff in teams remains the subject of on-going research. It may be that non-professional staff will remain reliant on professional staff to provide the treament (e.g. psychotropic drugs) and therapy necessary for them to be able to provide effective support. Similarly, professional therapeutic interventions will be undermined if basic support and practical assistance is absent.

*The need for improved interagency coordination and collaboration*

Diversity and choice in provision allows increased opportunities for people with severe and long-term mental health problems to develop valued social roles. Befriending or citizen advocacy services may be particularly critical to helping people achieve such roles. Valued roles will also be easier to develop when maximum use is made of non-specialist facilities for accommodation, occupation and leisure. CMHTs need to ensure that they are fully aware of the ordinary facilities available. New services can usefully be developed jointly with non-mental health agencies using their ordinary facilities (McLean and Leibowitz, 1990). There is evidence that the greater use of ordinary facilities (e.g. for accommodation) may also increase cost-effectiveness (McCrone *et al.*, 1994).

*Opportunities for participation*

Differences in the exercise of power are inevitable and necessary both between team members (e.g. between a line manager and a junior subordinate) and, more contentiously, between users and providers (e.g. when a practitioner is convinced that a user is sufficiently at risk to instigate a formal mental health act assessment). CMHTs are certainly not egalitarian and rarely democratic. To argue otherwise is simply to mislead people. It is because of these real differences that checks and balances need to be in place to ensure that power is not abused, and that services are developed and delivered in a way that reflects the needs of service users. This requires that there are maximum opportunities for participation in decision-making on the part of users and team members. Effective participation requires that all participants are clear about where and how power is held within the team and the parameters within which they are operating. For users, participation includes maximum involvement in the planning and delivery of their own care and, increasingly, participation in planning, managing and providing care for others. Although improving, the national survey found such participation to be rare among CMHTs, with only 8% of teams involving users in a decision-making capacity in the running of the team (Onyett *et al.*, 1994). For team members, participation is simply the result of good management where staff do not feel that decisions are imposed without consideration or consultation.

***Stronger operational management at team level***

It will be clear from the foregoing that there is a challenging operational management and leadership role to be fulfilled at team level. Full elaboration of this role is beyond the scope of this chapter (Onyett 1995; Onyett *et al.*, 1997). Suffice to say, that in order to be tenable, the team manager or coordinator role needs to be supported by a strong mental health service strategy borne of a clarity of purpose among all the key agencies involved. Only then can this be translated into the robust operational arrangements of which the team coordinator/manager role will be the mainstay. For this to endure there must be a strong sense of ownership among key stakeholders of the CMHT and its aims. This will be fostered by continuous, high quality information on the operation of the team, the outcomes it is achieving and how this relates to changing patterns of needs in the locality.

## ALTERNATIVES TO CMHTs

Although difficult to define, it is possible to evaluate alternative approaches that aim to achieve continuous and coordinated care while avoiding certain features of team working. For example, Ovretveit (1993) coined the term 'network associations' to describe services where separate disciplines communicate without meeting, and do not share an operational policy. Their apparent popularity may be because they avoid operational management and promote maximum autonomy among practitioners. They have not been subject to outcome evaluation, although they resemble the control conditions of some of the studies cited above (e.g. Merson *et al.*, 1992; Dean *et al.*, 1993; Marks *et al.*, 1994). Brokerage schemes and single agency care management schemes are also non-CMHT alternatives that have not been systematically evaluated. Their application with other client groups highlights a number of difficulties such as neglect of issues of equity of resource allocation, and poor access to resources (Onyett, 1992).

## CONCLUSION

This chapter has explored, in detail, the development and operation of CMHTs, as one of the most common service responses to meeting the needs of people with mental health problems. From this discussion it can be concluded that for their effective operation such teams should:

1. Focus on people with severe and long-term mental health problems using unequivocal eligibility criteria based on a definition of people's needs and not simply diagnosis and/or intended service responses;
2. Ensure that joint commissioning (involving health, social services and GPs) delivers CMHTs with clear mandates in relation to organisational and financial responsibilities, realistic objectives – in terms of which needs are to be met and how – and adequate resources;
3. Achieve a team management role with enough authority to ensure that all the various disciplines within the team conform to an agreed operational policy;
4. Clarify shared core roles and responsibilities among team members and separate these from the specific, unique skills that individuals and disciplines contribute and clarify lines of accountability accordingly;
5. Provide the CMHT manager with enough time and resources to ensure that systems for monitoring allocation, case-loads and clinical review processes are in place;
6. Recognise the nature of the work and its demands and provide appropriate time, training and resources to ensure staff are able to retain a sense of competence, achievement and professional identity;
7. Involve service users in a variety of formats, and provide them with material and personal support to promote their maximum impact on the shape and relevance of the service;
8. Monitor, evaluate and develop team operations learning from the experience of all the major stakeholders.

Real innovation may require far-reaching changes, such as giving CMHTs a block budget (including local authority resources) to purchase all services for people with long-term problems, including inpatient care, thus greatly encouraging the development of alternatives to admission and reversing some of the perverse incentives that operate to keep people in hospital. Whatever their future, it seems that CMHTs are currently here to stay. They have the ability, through the combined skills and experience of team members, to greatly improve the lives of people with severe and long-term mental health problems. However, this will only be achieved through a clear sense of what users actually need and a creative and individualised response from committed and energetic staff.

*DISCUSSION QUESTIONS**

◆ Has the team successfully articulated its aims and the values that underpin them?

◆ Is this demonstrated in a service that achieves a powerful role for users in choosing the content and course of their involvement with the team?

◆ Is this demonstrated in good quality, enduring relationships between staff and users?

◆ Does the team manager have the authority to ensure that a person presenting with a pressing need is unambiguously allocated to a team member for immediate action?

◆ Do team members clearly understand their own roles and the roles of others?

◆ Does the management structure allow clear determination of who has authority over specific tasks?

◆ Does the management structure allow staff to maintain a sense of professional identification and development?

◆ Does the team recognise legitimate power relationships while actively confronting oppressive and illegitimate power relationships?

◆ Does the team attend to the needs of its own members by ensuring adequate support, supervision, resources and rewards? Is this reflected in staff recruitment and retention?

◆ Can the team manage poor staff performance without punishing?

◆ Can the team recognise and resolve conflicts? Can the team learn from its own experience and change accordingly?

*FURTHER READING*

◆ Ovretveit, J. (1993) *Co-ordinating Community Care: Multidisciplinary Teams and Care Management*. Buckingham: Open University Press.
Professor Ovretveit provides a detailed examination of the organisational and conceptual issues concerning multidisciplinary teams. Mainly, the work aims to capture the experience of a large body of developmental research in detailed models and descriptions. Extremely useful to someone developing operational policy but one that

* These questions were developed with Helen Wood of the Sainsbury Centre for Mental Health as part of a project on CMHT Management conducted by the Mental Health Foundation.

should be read alongside the more contextualised accounts provided by such commentators as Dave Pilgrim, Ann Rogers and Mick Carpenter.

◆ Pilgrim, D. and Rogers, A. (1993) *A Sociology of Mental Health and Illness*. Buckingham: Open University Press.

This very comprehensive and clearly written text provides an account of the social and political context of CMHT operation. It covers perspectives on mental health and illness, issues concerning the effects of social inequalities, the organisation and operation of the mental health professions and the development of the user movement.

◆ Carpenter, M. (1994) *Normality is Hard Work: Trade Unions and the Politics of Community Care*. London: Lawrence and Wishart.

A critical but constructive, even visionary, analysis of community care reforms from the political left. Some good cartoons too.

◆ West, M. A. (1994) *Effective Teamwork*. Leicester: British Psychological Society.

Although not specifically concerned with mental health issues, this small text provides an accessible account of the key psychological factors concerned with effective teamworking from perhaps the leading authority in the field of innovation and work groups in the UK.

◆ Onyett, S. R., Pillinger, T. and Muijen, M. (1995) *Making Community Mental Health Teams Work*. London: Sainsbury Centre for Mental Health.

This report details some of the research described here in more detail and in an easily digestible form. It provides further details of the research on burnout, job satisfaction, personal and team role clarity, team and professional identification among team members.

**REFERENCES**

Anciano, D. Kirkpatrick, A. (1990), CMHTS and clinical psychology: the death of a profession? *Clinical Psychology Forum*, 26, 9–12.

Anonymous (1995), Care-management: a disastrous mistake. *Lancet*, 345, 399–401.

Axelrod, S. and Wetzler, S. (1989), Factors associated with better compliance with psychiatric aftercare. *Hospital and Community Psychiatry*, 40, 397–401.

Beeforth, M., Conlon, E. and Graley, R. (1994), *Have We Got Views for You*. London: Sainsbury Centre for Mental Health.

Bond, G.R., McCrew, J.H. and Fekete, D.M. (1995), Assertive outreach for frequent users of psychiatric hospitals: a meta-analysis. *Journal of Mental Health Administration*, 22, 4–16.

Brooker, C., Falloon, I., Butterworth, A., Goldberg, D., Graham-Hole, V. and Hillier, V. (1994), The outcome of training community psychiatric nurses to deliver psychosocial intervention. *British Journal of Psychiatry*, 165, 222–230.

Burns, B.J. and Santos, A.B. (1995), Assertive community treatment: an update of randomised trials. *Psychiatric Services*, 46, 669-673.

Burns, T., Beadsmoore, A., Bhat, A.V., Oliver, A. and Mathers, C. (1993a), A controlled trial of home-based acute psychiatric services I: Clinical and social outcome. *British Journal of Psychiatry*, 163, 49-54.

Burns, T., Raftery, J., Beadsmoore, A., McGuigan, S. and Dickson, M. (1993b), A controlled trial of home-based acute psychiatric services II: Treatment pattern and costs. *British Journal of Psychiatry*, 163, 55-61.

Burton, M.V. and Ramsden, R. (1994), A survey of GP referral patterns to outpatient psychiatry, clinical psychology, community psychiatric nurses and counsellors. *Clinical Psychology Forum*, 13-17.

Carson, J., Fagin, L. and Ritter, S. (Eds) (1995), *Stress and Coping in Mental Health Nursing*. London: Chapman and Hall.

Challis, D. and Davies, B. (1986), *Case Management in Community Care*. Aldershot: Gower.

Crepaz-Keay, D. (1994), I wish to register a complaint ... *Openmind*, 71, 5.

Dean, C., Phillips, E.M., Gadd, E.M., Joseph, M. and England, S. (1993), Comparison of community based service with hospital based service for people with acute, severe psychiatric illness. *British Medical Journal*, 307, 473-476.

Department of Health (1990a), The care programme approach for people with a mental illness referred to the specialist psychiatric services. *DoH Health Circular*. HC(90)23/LASSL(90)11.

Department of Health (1990b), *Community Care in the Next Decade and Beyond*. London: HMSO.

Department of Health (1995), *Building Bridges: A guide to arrangements for inter-agency working for the care and protection of severely mentally ill people*. London: HMSO.

Department of Health (1996), *The Spectrum of Care: Local Services for People with Mental Health Problems*. London: Department of Health.

Department of Health/Social Services Inspectorate (1991), *Care Management and Assessment: Managers Guide*. London: HMSO.

Dowell, A. and Ciarlo, J.A. (1983), Overview of community mental health centres program from an evaluation perspective. *Community Mental Health Journal*, 19, 95-125.

Drake, R.E. and Burns, B.J. (1995), Special section on assertive community treatment: an introduction. *Psychiatric Services*, 46, 667-668.

Falloon, I.R.H., Shanahan, W., Laporta, M. and Krekorian, H.A.R. (1990), Integrated family, general practice and mental health care in the management of schizophrenia. *Journal of the Royal Society of Medicine*, 83, 225-228.

Ford, R., Beadsmoore, A., Ryan, P., Repper, J., Craig, T. and Muijen, M. (1995), Providing the safety net: case management for people with a serious mental illness. *Journal of Mental Health*, 1, 91-97.

Frank, A.F. and Gunderson, J.G. (1990), The role of the therapeutic alliance in the treatment of schizophrenia. *Archives of General Psychiatry*, 47, 228-236.

Franklin, J.L., Solovitz, B., Mason, M., Clemons, J.R. and Miller, G. (1987), An evaluation of case management. *American Journal of Public Health*, 77, 674-678.

Galvin, S.W. and McCarthy, S. (1994), Multi-disciplinary community teams: clinging to the wreckage. *Journal of Mental Health*, 3, 167-174.

Gehrs, M. and Goering, P. (1994), The relationship between the working alliance and rehabilitation outcomes of schizophrenia. *Psychosocial Rehabilitation Journal*, 18, 43-54.

Handy, J. (1990), *Occupational Health in a Caring Profession*. Aldershot: Avebury/Gower.

Hughes, I., Kidd, R., Cantor, R. and Killick, S. (1992), Do GPs want community mental health facilities? *Psychiatric Bulletin*, 16, 413-415.

Huxley, P., Hagan, T., Hennelly, R. and Hunt, J. (1990), *Effective Community Mental Health Services*. Aldershot: Avebury/Gower. Review in chapter six.

Jackson, G., Gater, R., Goldberg, D., Tantam, D., Loftus, L. and Taylor, H. (1993), A new community mental health team based in primary care. *British Journal of Psychiatry*, 162, 375-384.

Jenkins, R. (1992), Developments in the primary care of mental illness – a forward look. *International Review of Psychiatry*, 4, 237-242.

Kendrick, T., Burns, T. and Freeling, P. (1995), Randomised controlled trial of teaching general practitioners to carry out structured assessments of their long term mentally ill patients. *British Medical Journal*, 311, 93-98.

Kendrick, T., Sibbald, B., Burns, T. and Freeling, P. (1991), Role of general practitioners in care of long term mentally ill patients. *British Medical Journal*, 302, 508-510.

Knapp, M., Beecham, J., Koutsogeorgopoulou, V. *et al.* (1994), Service use and costs of home-based versus hospital-based care for people with serious mental illness. *British Journal of Psychiatry*, 165, 195-203.

Marks, I.M., Connolly, J., Muijen, M., Audini, B., McNamee, G. and Lawrence, R.E. (1994), Home-based versus hospital-based care for people with serious mental illnesses. *British Journal of Psychiatry*, 165, 179-194.

Marriott, S., Malone, S., Onyett, S. and Tyrer, P. (1993), The consequences of an open referral system to a community mental health service. *Acta Psychiatrica Scandinavica*, 88, 93-97.

Marshall, M. (1996), Case management: a dubious practice. *British Medical Journal*, 312, 523-524.

Marshall, M., Lockwood, A. and Gath, D. (1995), Social services case-management for long-term mental disorders: a randomised controlled trial. *Lancet*, 345, 409-412.

McAusland, T. (1985), *Planning and Monitoring Community Mental Health Centres*. London: Kings Fund Centre.

McCrone, P., Beecham, J. and Knapp, M. (1994), Community psychiatric nurse teams: cost-effectiveness of intensive support versus generic care. *British Journal of Psychiatry*, 165, 218-221.

McLean, E.K. and Leibowitz, J. (1990), A community mental health team to service revolving door patients: the Doddington Edward Wilson (DEW) Mental Health Team 1984-1988. *International Journal of Social Psychiatry*, 36, 172-182.

Mental Health Foundation (1994), *Creating Community Care*. Report of the Mental Health Foundation Inquiry into Community Care for People with Severe Mental Illness. London: Mental Health Foundation.

Merson, S., Tyrer, P., Onyett, S. *et al.* (1992), Early intervention in psychiatric emergencies: a controlled clinical trial. *Lancet*, 339, 1311-1314.

Mosher, L.R. and Burti, L. (1989), *Community Mental Health: Principles and Practice*. New York: Norton.

Muijen, M., Cooney, M., Strathdee, G., Bell, R. and Hudson, A. (1994), Community psychiatric nurse teams: intensive support versus generic care. *British Journal of Psychiatry*, 165, 211–217.

Nazareth, I., King, M. and Davies, S. (1995), Care of schizophrenia in general practice: the general practitioner and the patient. *British Journal of General Practice*, 45, 343–347.

NHSE (1994), *Discharge of Mentally Disordered People and their Continued Care in the Community*. HSG(94)5, Leeds: NHSME.

Nikkel, R.E., Smith, G. and Edwards, D. (1992), A consumer-operated case management project. *Hospital and Community Psychiatry*, 43, 577–579.

North, C. and Ritchie, J. (1993), *Factors Influencing the Implementation of the Care Programme Approach*. London: HMSO.

Onyett, S.R. (1992), *Case Management in Mental Health*. London: Chapman and Hall.

Onyett, S.R. (1995), Responsibility and accountability in community mental health teams. *Psychiatric Bulletin*, 19, 281–285.

Onyett, S.R., Pillinger, T. and Muijen, M. (1995), *Making Community Mental Health Teams Work*. London: Sainsbury Centre for Mental Health.

Onyett, S.R., Pillinger, T. and Muijen, M. (1996), Job satisfaction and burnout among members of community mental health teams. *Journal of Mental Health*, 6, 55–66.

Onyett, S.R., Standen, R. and Peck, E. (1997), The challenge of community mental health team management. *Health and Social Care in the Community*, 5, 340.

Onyett, S.R., Tyrer, P., Connelly, J. *et al.* (1990), The early intervention service: the first 18 months of an inner London demonstration project. *Psychiatric Bulletin*, 14, 267–269.

Onyett, S., Heppleston, T. and Bushnell, D. (1994), A national survey of community mental health teams. *Journal of Mental Health*, 3, 175–194.

Ormel, J., Van der Brink, W. and Koeter, M.V. (1990), Recognition, management and outcome of psychological disorders in primary care: a naturalistic follow-up study. *Psychological Medicine*, 20, 909–923.

Ovretveit, J. (1993), *Co-ordinating Community Care: Multidisciplinary Teams and Care Management*. Buckingham: Open University Press.

Patmore, C. and Weaver, T. (1991), *Community Mental Health Teams: Lessons for Planners and Managers*. London: Good Practices in Mental Health.

Patmore, C. and Weaver, T. (1992), Improving community services for serious mental disorders. *Journal of Mental Health*, 1, 107–115.

Peck, E. (1994), Community mental health centres: challenges to the new orthodoxy. *Journal of Mental Health*, 3, 151–156.

Peck, E. and Smith, H. (1991), *Contracting in Mental Health Services*. Bristol: NHS Training Directorate.

Repper, J., Ford, R. and Cooke, A. (1994), How can nurses build relationships with people who have severe and long-term mental health problems. Experience of case managers and their clients. *Journal of Advanced Nursing*, 19, 1096–1104.

Rogers, A. (1996), Loosening the bond: mental health, psychiatrists and primary care. *Mental Health Review*, 1, 5–7.

Rogers, A. and Pilgrim, D. (1993), Medical health service users' views of medical practitioners. *Journal of Interprofessional Care*, 7, 167–176.

Samson, C. (1995), The fracturing of medical dominance. *Sociology of Health and Illness*, 16, 245–268.

Sayce, L., Craig, T.K.J. and Boardman, A.P. (1991), The development of community mental health centres in the UK. *Social Psychiatry and Psychiatric Epidemiology*, 26, 14–20.

Schneider, J. (1993), Care programming: assimilation and adaptation. *British Journal of Social Work*, 23, 4.

Segal, S.P., Bola, J.R. and Watson, M.A. (1996), Race, quality of care, and antipsychotic prescribing practices in psychiatric emergency services. *Psychiatric Services*, 47, 282–285.

Sherman, P.S. and Porter, R. (1991), Mental health consumers as case management aides. *Hospital and Community Psychiatry*, 42, 494–498.

Social Services Inspectorate (1995), *Social Services Departments and the Care Programme Approach: an Inspection*. London: Department of Health.

Solomon, P. and Draine, J. (1995), The efficacy of a consumer case management team: 2-year outcomes of a randomised trial. *Journal of Mental Health Administration*, 22, 135–145.

Solomon, P., Draine, J. and Delaney, M.A. (1995), The working alliance and consumer case management. *Journal of Mental Health Administration*, 22, 126–134.

Stein, L.I. (1990), A historical review of the Madison model of community care. *Hospital and Community Psychiatry*, 41, 649–651.

Stein, L.I. (1992), On the abolishment of the case manager. *Health Affairs*, Fall, 172–177.

Stein, L.I. and Test, M.A. (1980), Alternative to mental hospital treatment I. *Archives of General Psychiatry*, 37, 392–397.

Strathdee, G. (1993), The Nunhead Service: A community mental health service with a focus in primary care. London: PRiSM Occasional Paper 13.

Sutherland, V.J. and Cooper, C.L. (1992), Job stress, satisfaction and mental health among general practitioners before and after the introduction of the new contract. *British Medical Journal*, 304, 1545–1548.

Tyrer, P., Morgan, J., Van Horn, E. *et al.* (1995), A randomised controlled study of close monitoring of vulnerable psychiatric patients. *Lancet*, 345, 756–759.

Warner, R.W., Gater, R., Jackson, M.G. and Goldberg, D. (1993), Effects of a community mental health service on the practice and attitudes of general practitioners. *British Journal of General Practice*, 43, 507–511.

West, M.A. (1994), *Effective Teamwork*. Leicester: British Psychological Society.

Williams, M.L., Forster, P., McCarthy, G.D. and Hargreaves, W.A. (1994), Managing case management: what makes it work? *Psychosocial Rehabilitation Journal*, 18, 49–60.

**CHAPTER 5**

# The Primary/Secondary Care Interface

## Elizabeth Armstrong

*KEY ISSUES*

◆ Communication

◆ Teamworking

◆ Education and Training

◆ Information

*INTRODUCTION*

In the last few years, as successive reforms have taken place within the National Health Service and Social Services, the role of primary care professionals, GPs, practice nurses and others, in the care of people with serious enduring mental illness has become much more obvious.* Frequent exhortations in government documents for all agencies concerned to work together in providing care has made secondary care services and local authority services more aware of the role of GPs, but it has also brought more tensions. GPs have been reluctant to take on what is widely perceived as more work for no additional reward, and professionals from the secondary care sector have found that working with GPs and primary care teams is not necessarily straightforward.

This chapter is concerned with primary care and the part which primary care teams play in the provision of care for mentally ill people. Although concentrating on those with serious mental illness, as that is currently defined, it also acknowledges the fact that the majority of people with any degree of mental health problem are cared for within the primary care system. The first half of the chapter looks at mental health and illness in primary

---

*People registered with a GP are normally described by primary care doctors and nurses as 'patients'. Health visitors, who work with well people and families, usually refer to their 'clients'. In this chapter these conventions have been followed. 'Service user' is a term rarely employed in primary care settings.

care, including the nature of the setting and the roles of primary care team members. This section includes a discussion about mental health in primary care; the lack of appropriate education and training available to primary care professionals is highlighted.

The second half of this chapter then examines national policy for those with mental illness, and the changes which have occurred over the last 30 years. The most important of these are seen to be the closure of the large, Victorian mental hospitals, the recent National Health Service reforms such as the purchaser/provider split and the introduction of GP fundholding, and the introduction of the care programme approach.

The conclusion, whilst acknowledging the problems which exist in improving the relationship between primary care and the secondary care services, also proposes some solutions. A number of models are emerging, and the picture is certainly not one of unremitting gloom. However, it is clear that further change and development are required, as services have not yet fully recovered from the revolutionary changes of the early 1990s. Further developments would clearly require sensitive management, and this has not always been a feature of recent upheavals.

## MENTAL HEALTH AND ILLNESS IN PRIMARY CARE

### What is primary care?

Primary health care, as its name implies, is the first contact service. It is primary care professionals, most often the general practitioner (GP), to whom people go when they first consider themselves to be in need of help for their health. GPs are, in the main, accessible to members of the public without referral. Everyone is entitled to be registered with a GP, and any person on a GP list may consult that doctor at any time. It is this accessibility and universality which distinguishes primary care from other parts of the National Health Service.

The average GP has about 1900 patients on his/her list. Unlike secondary care professionals, GPs do not 'discharge' patients at the end of an episode of illness. Any patient may consult again at any time. This also applies to other primary care workers, such as practice nurses, whose potential clientele includes anyone on the practice list, and health visitors whose caseloads traditionally include all families with children under 5 years, on the list of the practice to which they are attached. In inner city areas, where health visitors may work geographically, the caseload will be all families within the area and anyone else requiring health visiting help. Contact with a GP or practice nurse is generally initiated by the patient though patients may attend special clinics (for example, well woman) by invitation from the practice. Health visitors usually work more proactively, frequently making the first contact with their clients.

Not all primary care services are GP practice-based. Inner city geographically based health visitors will see some clients who do not have a GP, and occupational health services and the school health service might also be seen as part of primary care. This chapter will focus mainly on those parts of primary care that are centred on general medical practice, since this has been the main setting considered in national policy, but it is important that other settings are not ignored.

As well as providing the first contact service, primary care professionals, especially nurses, are also engaged in health surveillance (for example: cervical cytology), health protection (for example: immunisation) and health promotion as in advising on smoking cessation and nutrition. In addition they also provide a large amount of on-going care to people with existing illness and disability through chronic disease management clinics (especially for diabetes and asthma), in people's homes and in residential care of various types (Ross and MacKenzie, 1996). It is the last two of these activities which may be described as 'community care'.

The idea of community care has been around for at least 35 years. The large-scale closure of mental hospitals began in the 1960s following the then Minister of Health, Enoch Powell's Hospital Plan of 1962. This set in train a programme for the replacement of large mental hospitals and mental handicap hospitals by a network of community services to be provided by local health and welfare authorities. In describing this, Means and Smith (1994) contend that there have been problems with the definition of community care since as far back as 1961.

According to the 1989 White Paper *Caring for people*, community care means providing the right level of intervention and support to enable people to achieve maximum independence and control over their own lives. The White Paper envisaged a wide range of provision but also recognised that much 'community care' was, in effect, informal care by family members. The National Health Service and Community Care Act (1990) which followed the White Paper sets out the responsibilities of health and social services to provide care appropriate to the client's need.

It should be clear from the foregoing that community care responsibilities form only part of the work of primary care teams. Misunderstandings about this on the part of secondary care professionals and managers, many of whom come from secondary care backgrounds, are at the root of some of the tensions which arise between primary health care teams (PHCTs), community mental health teams (CMHTs), health authorities and trusts.

Freeling and Kendrick (1996) have placed the tasks of primary care within a preventive framework, here applied to mental health but equally applicable to all aspects of health care (Box 5.1).

General medical practice is a business with GPs as independent contractors to the NHS. This applies whether or not the practice is fundholding. Unlike most other health service workers, GPs are not salaried employees. Practice nurses are usually employed by GPs

**Box 5.1** Tasks of
primary care

♦ *Primary prevention* includes offering support to people at increased risk of mental illness, for example the unemployed, bereaved, new mothers, single parent families, isolated elderly and disabled.

♦ *Secondary prevention* includes early identification and effective treatment for mental illness. The general practice setting offers a non-stigmatising environment in which this can happen, but it is also essential that there is rapid and easy access to specialist support when it is required.

♦ *Tertiary prevention* is about the provision of on-going care and support for those with chronic illness and persistent disability. In many cases this will necessitate effective joint working between specialist services, local authority services and the PHCT. There also needs to be rapid access to help for those whose conditions are likely to relapse or recur.

not trusts. They are therefore outside the normal NHS management structure, and may have limited professional support though this varies. The difference in employment conditions for practice nurses and other community nurses may cause tensions and can mean that teamwork suffers.

*The primary care of mental health*

Secondary care professionals may believe that the role of the GP in the care of mentally ill people is new, and is mainly due to increasing numbers of mentally ill people being cared for in the community. This is not so. Goldberg and Huxley (1980) have used a series of levels and filters, which are illustrated in Box 5.2, to describe the ways in which people with mental illness obtain the care they require. Their model demonstrated clearly that the vast majority of people with mental illness are treated by their GP and are never referred to specialists. It has been estimated that GP consultations for mental illness outnumber psychiatric outpatient consultations by at least 10:1 (Jenkins, 1992a).

In addition, many inner city GPs complain of an increase in workload due to mental hospital closure and have been particularly concerned by an apparent increase in the numbers of mentally ill homeless people. It may not, in fact, be accurate to ascribe this increase to mental hospital closure. Craig and Timms (1992) reviewed a number of studies and concluded that the majority of homeless mentally ill people were not those who had been discharged as part of planned closure programmes. Most had never experienced long periods in hospital. These authors believed that what they have termed the 'crisis of visibility' is more the result

**Box 5.2** Mental illness: levels and filters

Level 1 The Community
        260–315/1000/year                                    First Filter

                                                             (Illness behaviour)

Level 2 Total mental morbidity – attendees in primary care
        230/1000/year                                        Second Filter

                                                             (Ability to detect disorder)

Level 3 Mental disorders identified by doctors
        101.5/1000/year                                      Third Filter

                                                             (Referral to mental illness services)

Level 4 Total morbidity – mental illness services
        23.5/1000/year                                       Fourth Filter
                                                             (Admission to psychiatric beds)

Level 5 Psychiatric inpatients
        5.71/1000/year

Source: From Freeling and Kendrick (1996) after Goldberg and Huxley (1980), with permission.

of long-term failures to provide adequate community services, and the closure of hostels which had previously acted as unofficial asylums for many mentally ill people.

Most of the mental illness dealt with by GPs is non-psychotic illness such as depression and anxiety. It is inaccurate to characterise this population as the 'worried well'. People attending their GP surgery with depression have been shown to have as many symptoms as those attending psychiatrists, and depression is a serious illness from which people do die (Mann, 1992). It has been estimated that around 5% of GP attenders will have major depression with a further 5% having symptoms just a little below the threshold for major depression. Another 10% will have milder illnesses. This represents 300–400 patients per GP (Paykel and Priest, 1992).

Numbers of patients with psychotic illness on the average GP list are likely to be relatively small, varying from about 4 to 12 (Strathdee and Jenkins, 1996). The variability depends on a number of factors including GP interest in mental illness, but the most marked differences are between rural areas and the inner cities. In a survey conducted in the South West Thames region (Kendrick *et al.*, 1991) those GPs with higher than average numbers tended: to be working in inner London and near large psychiatric hospitals; to have worked in hospital psychiatry posts; and to have psychiatrists visiting their practices.

There has been less research into the contacts that generalist community nurses have with mentally ill people, though a consideration of the part these nurses play in patient care suggests that it is probably substantial, and has been largely unrecognised. In the case of practice nurses, the 1993 census (Atkin *et al.*, 1993) estimated that about 40% were involved in the early detection of depression and anxiety. Significantly, this survey also showed that less than 2% of this group had obtained a qualification as a mental health nurse. There is also a great deal of anecdotal evidence, and some research, showing that practice nurses may be quite heavily involved in giving depot neuroleptic medication to patients with schizophrenia. A South London study has suggested that about two thirds of all practice nurses in one district may be undertaking this task for at least one patient, on a regular basis (Miller and Garland, personal communication). In an audit of patients receiving depot neuroleptic medication conducted in North Yorkshire (Hamilton, 1996), 59% of patients were receiving their injection from a practice nurse. The problem is therefore not confined to London. The nurses in Miller and Garland's study frequently lacked knowledge of the side-effects of medication and felt ill-equipped to assess mental state or social care needs.

Practice nurse awareness of the care programme approach may not be high. Although many patients prefer to receive their medication in the relatively non-stigmatising setting of their GP surgery, Repper and Brooker (1993) have pointed out that many patients in this situation will have no contact with other health service professionals, and their carers may also be isolated. Kendrick (1996) confirms this, pointing to research which shows that up to a third of patients with psychosis lose contact with specialist services within a year of discharge from hospital, and rely totally on their GP for care. Many practice nurses may also be taking blood tests to monitor lithium levels in patients with bipolar depression. Anecdotal evidence suggests that many nurses regard this as just another task, and again may be unaware of the needs of these patients.

District nurse caseloads traditionally include large numbers of elderly people. Not only is depression more common in older than younger people and the suicide rate higher, but these nurses will also be caring for considerable numbers of patients with dementia. The district nurse may be the only professional with whom the carer has contact. Contacts between district nurses, who are usually general-trained nurses and may have little psychiatric experience or training, and community psychiatric nurse (CPN) colleagues may be limited. Coordination of care for people with dementia was a particular concern in the report of the Mental Health Nursing Review Team (Department of Health, 1994a), but the role of district nurses was not specifically acknowledged.

Health visitors have an important role in the recognition and care of mothers with postnatal depression, other mental illness in the postpartum period and mental health problems in families in general. Although postnatal depression is, in the main, a primary care illness, in order for it to be adequately treated each district needs to have provision for those few mothers whose illness becomes more serious, and there needs to be an appropriate level of support and supervision for health visitors engaged in counselling for this condition (Cox and Holden, 1994).

*Mental health training in primary care*

Most primary care workers, including both doctors and nurses, are generalists who may have little or no formal training in psychiatry beyond that which they will have received in their basic professional education. Though many recognise the importance of mental health care for their patients, and may pay some lip service to concepts of the interdependence of physical and mental health, there may be little attempt in practice to bring them together. Many GPs and primary care nurses consider that they do practice in an holistic way but physical health care often takes precedence over mental health care. It is traditional to eliminate the physical before thinking about the psychological.

Jenkins (1992b) considers that it is the specialisation in medicine which occurred towards the end of the 19th century which led to the separation of mind and body in medical theory. This has encouraged the 'one-patient – one diagnosis' model which may cause serious disadvantage for those with multiple problems. She points to research showing that people with emotional disorders are high consumers of general practice time and that patients with identified psychiatric illness had illnesses in more categories per head than other patients consulting their doctors. She also believes that doctors miss disease because of a fixation with the 'one diagnosis' model. Psychiatrists miss physical illness and people with serious mental illness have higher death rates than the general population from common killers such as heart disease and cancers (Department of Health, 1992). Moreover, general physicians, including GPs, often miss mental illness especially emotional disorders.

Major concerns have been raised over many years about the ability of GPs to recognise depression. Research consistently shows that about 50% of those presenting to the GP with depression are not detected, though this is an average figure which varies widely and depends on many factors, including the interest of the GP (Tylee, 1996). Even people with recognised depression may receive suboptimal treatment. These concerns have led to the development of training programmes for GPs in the recognition and management of depression, but there have been some major difficulties with the take-up and implementation of such programmes. Turton *et al.* (1995) have described an assessment of the mental health training needs of general practitioners and point to a dichotomy between what they call perceived competence and actual competence. The GPs in their survey were confident of their ability to recognise depression, but felt least confidence in their skills of psychodynamic counselling and stress management.

Unsurprisingly, they were most interested in further training in those areas in which they felt least confident. This survey also confirmed that most GPs had no formal experience or training in psychiatry beyond their basic education. There was also no apparent link between formal psychiatric experience (usually hospital-based) and the range of skills needed for mental health care in general practice. As these authors point out, there are challenges here to GP educators in motivating GPs to receive training in an area where research suggests there is a need, but where there is lack of awareness of need. There is research demonstrating that appropriate training can lead to improvement in GP performance in both recognition and management of depression and also to better patient outcome (Gask, 1992).

Community nurse training needs in mental health have not been examined to the same extent but there are studies looking at practice nurse assisted care of patients with depression (Wilkinson, 1992) and there is research currently in progress looking at the use of problem-solving techniques with depressed patients. Health visitors, trained in fairly basic Rogerian person-centred counselling techniques, have been shown to improve the outcome for mothers with postnatal depression (Holden *et al.*, 1989). Much of the research into improving the skills of general nurses in mental health care has been generated by psychiatrists and other non-nurses. It usually involves grafting new skills on to nursing practice, but the skills often derive from disciplines other than nursing and may therefore not fit easily into existing work patterns. There is a widespread perception among researchers that practice nurses have more time than GPs. This may not be borne out in practice. Experience in facilitating change suggests that changes which do not threaten the status quo too much are more likely to be taken up than those that are more radical.

Community nurses have not necessarily been slow to recognise their needs for mental health training, but many barriers exist. There is still a lack of appropriate courses in mental health for nurses working in primary care, though this is changing. Equally serious is the lack of commitment to training for primary care staff by health authorities. Training budgets may be unrealistically small (ranging from £25–£400 per staff member per year in one health authority with clinical staff somewhere in the middle of the range) and budgets are often vulnerable when finances are tight.

Many nurses, especially practice nurses, complain that the attitude of GPs makes it hard for them to gain access to training. This is sometimes regarded by educators as a convenient excuse, but there is some support from at least two sources. Ross (1992) investigated the reason for poor take-up of a course in communication skills for practice nurses. Of the 18 nurses questioned, 10 said that their GP employers did not regard the course as a priority. Reported comments included 'You're paid to work, not go on courses'. A survey of GP attitudes to practice nurses (Robinson *et al.*, 1993) showed that less than half the respondents recognised lack of training opportunities as a barrier to role development for practice nurses.

**THE POLICY**
**CONTEXT** Nationally, it has been recognised that there is a huge need for improvements in the care of mentally ill people. A number of policy changes over recent years have affected the way care is provided, some directly, some less so. The main influences are shown in Box 5.3.

**Box 5.3** Influences on policy

- ◆ The closure of large mental hospitals and the increase in numbers of people with serious mental illness now cared for in the community.

- ◆ The purchaser/provider split in the NHS including GP fundholding and all the variants now arising.

- ◆ The care programme approach (CPA) and supervision registers.

**Mental hospital**
**closure** The large old Victorian institutions have been gradually closing over the past 30 years, though, in the 1990s the pace of closure has increased. In a recent review, Barak *et al.* (1996) although agreeing that there are considerable advantages to closing these hospitals in terms of improving the rights of individuals, reducing stigma and improving quality of life, nevertheless contend that the advantages must be weighed against some problems. They raise four questions: are suicide rates increased among patients cared for in the community; are criminal offences more prevalent among this group; what are the rates of re-admission to hospital; and is there a connection between closure of hospitals and homelessness?

In the case of suicide, these authors believe that the evidence is inconclusive, and they suggest that any link between hospital closure and increased criminality is, at best, indirect. They do point out, though, that inadequate outreach services and shortage of acute care beds may exacerbate the problem. Re-admission rates vary between several studies cited in this review and one American study has found that, after 5 years, many patients cared for in the community were functioning much better than was expected at the time of their discharge from hospital even though the services available to them were patchy. A British study has found that the risk factors for rehospitalisation (younger age, previous hospital admission, behavioural disturbances and a diagnosis of bipolar disorder) were not dependent on the environment in which care was delivered.

The link, if any, between hospital closure and homelessness has already been discussed. The above review suggests that where carefully planned programmes of re-provision exist, those with chronic mental illness are unlikely to become homeless. The authors emphasise that whatever the causes, rates of mental illness among the homeless are high. They believe that this group presents a major challenge to health and social services, particularly in ensuring adequate availability of acute care, and in community support systems.

*Purchasing mental health services* (See also the discussion by Peck in Chapter 3)

Two of the main priorities for the NHS in the 1990s are the development of primary care led commissioning and purchasing, under the GP fundholding scheme and more recent variants such as locality commissioning groups and fundholding consortia, and the implementation of community care policies in mental health (Strathdee and Jenkins, 1996). Primary care commissioning is not yet universal and health authority commissioning agencies are responsible for purchasing services for patients not covered by fundholding GPs. The variety of organisations responsible for commissioning of services makes planning by provider units quite complex, since they may have to satisfy the needs of several purchasers.

Requests for help to the mental health development officer of the National Primary Care Facilitation Programme (NPCFP) (Armstrong, 1994 unpublished) show that some fundholding GPs are dissatisfied with services they are asked to purchase; though a recently published survey (Corney, 1996) underlines the fact that many fundholders have been able to use their contracts to make changes in local services, often ensuring that they become more practice- rather than sector-based.

There is at least anecdotal evidence that many purchasing decisions are still based on inadequate assessment of need. Ford and Warner (1996) suggest that, with the current state of development of mental health information systems, it is rarely possible to find out anything other than the number of inpatient episodes in a given district. Many GPs, even those actively involved in commissioning services, may still lack basic information such as the numbers of people with serious mental illness on their lists. The survey by Kendrick *et al.* (1991) showed that although more than 40% of respondents indicated willingness to organise the care of these patients, with specialist back-up when necessary, almost none had specific practice policies by which this might be done.

Most agreed that these patients usually only came to their attention when a crisis arose.

Problems are not all one-sided. GPs (and health authorities) may lack information on which to base rational purchasing decisions, but there is also evidence from requests to the NPCFP that some trusts have adopted a 'take it or leave it' attitude to providing services, and expect to provide the same service to every practice in their district. This may be justified on the grounds of equity, but in reality, it can be far from equitable. All practices are not the same. Not only may different practices in the same locality have a completely different practice population in terms of factors such as deprivation and ethnic mix, but the levels of skill within the practice, and the interest of PHCT members in mental health will also vary considerably. A practice where at least one partner has experience as a psychiatric registrar, where there are regular sessions from a clinical psychologist, and perhaps a practice counsellor, will require a very different amount of input from the CMHT when compared with the practice where no psychiatric training has been undertaken and where awareness of psychological problems is low. Additionally, some services may still be provided 'because this is what we've always provided' rather than being based on good information about local need.

*Care programme approach*
Secondary care services, including psychiatrists, community psychiatric/mental health nurses and social workers attached to community mental health teams have been urged to prioritise the care of the most seriously ill. There is continuing debate about the definition of 'serious mental illness' (see Chapter 1), but it is widely considered that diagnosis is only one of several criteria which should be taken into account. Others would include duration and level of disability and also safety and the need for formal or informal care (Department of Health, 1995).

The care programme approach (CPA) was introduced in 1991 to provide a framework within which high quality care could be achieved. Though designed for people with severe mental illness, it was intended that its provisions should apply to all people accepted by specialist psychiatric services and all psychiatric patients being discharged from hospital. This was to ensure that no vulnerable person was able to slip through 'the safety net of care' (Department of Health, 1994b). It was never the intention that the CPA should apply only to people suffering from psychotic illness, though in some districts it has been interpreted in such a way that only those with a diagnosis of schizophrenia will qualify. Many psychiatrists and GPs are concerned that over-concentration on diagnosis as the sole criterion for deciding eligibility for services means that many seriously disabled people with neurotic illness will not receive the care they need. There are four elements to the CPA: systematic assessment of the patient's health and social care needs; a package of care agreed between patient, providers and the patient's GP; nomination of a key worker for regular contact; and regular review and monitoring.

One of the responsibilities of the key worker is to ensure that the patient is registered with a GP, and to work closely with the primary care team. Where the patient was initially referred to the specialist services by their GP, this should not present too many difficulties, unless the patient is being discharged to a different area. But it is undoubtedly working with GPs which causes the most difficulties to community mental health teams (CMHTs). There may be a number of reasons for this. Community psychiatric nurses may in fact have little community training and have moved into community work directly from hospital. It is therefore possible that many CMHT members give GPs little thought. One published description of the implementation of the care programme approach in one district says only that care plan summaries and reviews were sent to GPs 'bearing in mind restrictions on the confidentiality of some information' (Shepherd *et al.*, 1995). There is no other mention that GPs were involved in any decision making at all. Yet it is likely that, at least in some cases, GPs were expected to prescribe for these patients, perhaps depot neuroleptics subsequently administered by practice nurses. There is no mention in this article of this aspect of care other than a very brief reference to treatment compliance.

Many complain that it is impossible to get GPs to attend CPA meetings. Sometimes this is as simple a problem as arranging meetings at inappropriate times. 9 am on a Monday morning may seem perfectly reasonable to most CMHT members; to most GPs it is right in the middle of the busiest surgery of the week.

*Supervision registers*   The main legislation affecting mentally ill people remains the 1983 Mental Health Act which governs the circumstances under which they may be compulsorily admitted to hospital. Under section 7 of this act, a person discharged from hospital could be placed under a 'guardianship' order which means that the guardian (who could be a social worker or sometimes a relative) has the power to say where the person should live, and to require him/her to attend for treatment, work or education at a specific place. It does not mean that treatment can be given without consent (Drew and King, 1995). A more formal system of supervision registers came into force in April 1994. These registers provide a means by which health authorities can identify psychiatric patients who are considered to be at serious risk to themselves or to others. There is also a duty on provider units to ensure that services are available for this highly vulnerable group. Supervision register patients will also be entitled to a key worker through the CPA (Department of Health, 1995). GPs should always be aware when one of their patients is on a local supervision register. In any one district the number of people likely to qualify for the supervision register – provided the criteria are followed – is likely to be relatively small, but it will vary according to the nature of the district, particularly whether rural, urban or inner city.

**THE PRIMARY/
SECONDARY CARE
INTERFACE: SOME
SOLUTIONS**

Strathdee and Jenkins (1996) contend that mental health research has consistently found that failure to communicate leads to poor patient care, and to misunderstandings about roles and responsibilities. They suggest a minimum amount of information which primary care teams require about their own area. This is summarised below, with some additional practical points.

♦ How local mental health services are organised. Sector names and boundaries are important, together with the names of key clinical and managerial staff.
♦ A summary of the needs assessment for the area, including numbers of patients on the CPA and the supervision register, deprivation indices and any services which are planned.
♦ Their own sector team names, roles and contact numbers, including out of hours contact and crisis services. This is especially important in inner city areas where practices may often need to liaise with more than one provider. This is cumbersome and leads to inappropriate referrals, but whereas fundholding GPs may use their purchasing power to change such an arrangement, non-fundholders may be less able to influence services. Providers may wish to consider simplifying arrangements wherever possible.
♦ Directory of the services provided, both at CMHT level, and by local hospital units.
♦ Information booklets about the various therapies available.
♦ Named contacts to advise on appropriate referrals. This function may be performed by a link worker, by regular meetings between PHCT members and the CMHT which serves their area, or by other means. Different models are evolving.
♦ Process by which the PHCT will be updated when changes occur; for example a regular trust newsletter, meetings or training events.

**Written
communication**

Strathdee and Jenkins (1996) also point to many studies showing that referral letters often do not contain information which is vital to decision making, nor do replies from specialists necessarily contain information that the GP wants to know. They suggest the following is important to the CMHT in referrals: background information about family and social history and presenting problem; interventions that have already been tried, and the outcome; the reason for referral – this may be for advice on management which the GP intends to continue (and for the secondary care service to take over the care or even for the specialist to relieve the GP of care for a short time, for respite).

In a recent facilitation study (Armstrong, 1994), some GPs expressed dissatisfaction with letters they received from specialists in response to referrals. In particular, detailed assessments of family circumstances were said to be unnecessary repetition of things the GP, as the family doctor, already knew. What was actually required, it was suggested, was clear guidance on management. Strathdee and Jenkins (1996) consider that some other pieces of information are essential: indication of suicide risk; what the patient has been told about their condition; prognosis and likely effect on lifestyle; GP and PHCT role in management; what the specialist team will do and when and who is responsible for prescribing and monitoring.

*Facilitation*  Wide experience over many years by facilitators in primary care has emphasised that merely sending information through the post to GPs is largely ineffective (Armstrong, 1992). Facilitators work by personal contact to help practices develop quality care. Important methods include building links between organisations and individuals and providing education and practical help to enable changes to happen as quickly and painlessly as possible. Practical help might include providing templates and support in designing practice-based clinical guidelines, and in audit of care (see, for example, Wilson, 1994). Information about services can be disseminated via a facilitator and feedback can be encouraged. Increasingly, provider units and GP practices are seeing the facilitator role as a crucial element in helping to bring people together and improve the dialogue.

Facilitators may be trust or health authority employees working on full-time projects. They usually have no clinical role, but most are experienced clinicians. Those currently working in primary care mental health come from a variety of professional backgrounds, with the majority being nurses though not necessarily RMNs (Armstrong, unpublished). Others may combine a part-time facilitator role with clinical responsibilities. This can work very well provided there are clear barriers between the two roles, and protected time for facilitation activities. Facilitators are agents for change and it is vital, if change is to be accepted by all stakeholders and implemented, that the facilitator is able to maintain a neutral role serving the interests of no single person or organisation. The purpose is to bring people together so that they can do things for themselves 'making it easier to understand others and effectively work with others' (Thomas, 1994). If the facilitator is perceived as supporting the agenda of any single group, this purpose will not be achieved. For the facilitator this can be uncomfortable, and the need for neutrality may be neither well understood nor supported by managers.

*Specialist attachments to primary care*

Before the introduction of the care programme approach, many CPNs were working with PHCTs on attachment, in much the same way as health visitors and district nurses work. One effect of this was that many CPNs became drawn into providing care for people with less serious illness. This was often believed to be highly cost-effective, but Gournay and Brooking (1995) contend that this belief was based on no good evidence. Their own study showed no difference in outcome for patients with depression cared for by a CPN or a GP. Further, there was no relationship between clinical improvement and the amount of contact the patient had with a CPN, and patients seeing a CPN did not reduce their use of the GP. Though numbers in this study were very small, the authors state that there is very little other evidence that CPNs are cost-effective in generic rather than specialist roles.

Awareness that the CPN as a specialist is a scarce and valuable resource and may be best used in the care of the seriously mentally ill (Jenkins, 1992a), led to many CPNs being withdrawn from their general practice attachments, often to the dismay of GPs. Ironically, this withdrawal, although encouraging these nurses to prioritise people with serious illness, may also have adversely affected communication between specialists and PHCTs. It appears that some CPNs are now returning to GP practices, albeit with a much more clearly defined role, which may include acting as key worker for patients of the practice who are subject to the CPA, and being a named link person with the rest of the CMHT. Other, experienced, CPNs may be working as facilitators for part of their time.

The CPN with good links to GP practice will often be able to set up meetings which the GPs will attend, simply because he or she will better understand the realities of the GP's workload and practice organisation. Most GPs hold weekday surgeries from 8.30 or 9 to 11 am and about 4.30 to 6 pm. During the late morning they will be doing house calls, and in the afternoon there may be special clinics in the practice. It follows that the best time to ask a GP to attend a meeting is lunchtime, provided the venue is reasonably accessible from the practice. It is often more successful to arrange to hold the meeting on the practice premises especially for single-handed practitioners who may be unable, or unwilling, to attend meetings elsewhere without the payment of locum fees. The link person does not have to be a CPN. Occupational therapists or social workers could also fulfil this role.

There are many more psychiatrists working at least part of the time with primary care teams than in the past, but nationally the situation is highly variable. Many GPs welcome input from a psychiatrist, particularly in assessment and perhaps short-term treatment (Strathdee and Kendrick, 1996), but it may be more important to most GPs, that when they refer a patient to a specialist service, the patient is seen by an experienced practitioner, not a junior clinician who may have less experience than the referring GP (Strathdee and Jenkins, 1996).

***Shared care*** Diabetes and asthma specialists, and maternity services, have long been involved in developing shared care systems with primary care teams. Shared care is said to occur when 'the care of the patient is shared between individuals or teams which are part of separate organisations' (Pritchard and Pritchard, 1994). Clearly this could be the case for those people with serious mental illness in the community. However, some of the reported attempts to introduce shared care systems for mentally ill people have been less than successful. Essex *et al*. (1990) considered that shared care records were acceptable to patients and improved autonomy and communication. Professional and managerial attitudes were the main barrier to further development, but these authors believed that the difficulties could be overcome.

Pritchard and Pritchard (1994) have suggested seven steps to successful shared care (Box 5.4). It is clear that they believe it to be fundamental that all teams involved should indeed be teams with common goals, not simply groups of people working from the same building. The need for teamworking in mental health care was also a fundamental conclusion of the facilitator in the Kensington & Chelsea and Westminster Family Health Services Authority (KCW FHSA) Mental Health Facilitator Project (Armstrong, 1994). Subsequent experience by the present author in leading practice-based courses in primary mental health care has tended to confirm the view that when teamwork is effective patient care improves, but research is needed to properly evaluate such programmes.

Agreed guidelines, across all teams, also seem important as is the evaluation of the systems set up. Clinical audit is an essential part of

**Box 5.4** Seven steps to effective shared care

1. Effective teamwork in all teams.
2. Common understanding of the domain – a common language.
3. Locally developed and 'owned' guidelines.
4. Effective communication and learning – planning should be seen as a learning process.
5. Development of alternative pathways for shared care – involve patients.
6. Evaluate process and outcome.
7. Use audit to refine knowledge base and guidelines.

Adapted from Pritchard and Pritchard (1994).

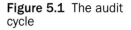

**Figure 5.1** The audit cycle

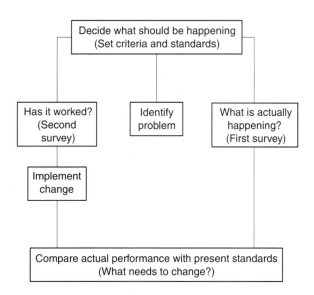

this process. Audit is not simply data collection, but should be seen as a cycle involving change and learning (Figure 5.1).

The comprehensive community-based approach to mental health care developed in Buckinghamshire and described by Falloon and Fadden (1993) involved working closely with primary care physicians, and seems to be the most highly developed form of shared care for mental health so far devised. The authors called their system 'integrated care'. They aimed to provide optimal clinical management for all the people who experienced mental disorders within a defined community. Key elements of the service were early detection and intensive interventions designed to minimise impairment, disability and handicap, minimise stress suffered by carers, and prevent future episodes as far as possible.

Their strategy involved a full range of community services including primary health care. The focus was on the provision of therapeutic interventions, largely family intervention, in a natural environment across biomedical, psychological and social management. They found that with this intensive system they required minimal mental hospital provision and that specialist day hospitals and outpatient clinics were rarely needed.

However, for this approach to work, extensive, on-going training of the specialist workforce in the latest cost-effective clinical management was required alongside specific training for PHCT members including GPs and community nurses.

***Education and training***
(see also Chapter 13)
Reference has already been made to deficiencies in training of both PHCT members and specialists. Over recent years there have been a number of efforts supported by the Department of Health to try to improve this situation, including the most recent which is a scheme devised by the Royal College of General Practitioners Unit for

Mental Health Education in Primary Care to train and support local doctor/nurse teams to act as education facilitators in their own districts. A few health authorities, notably Northampton, have set up innovative, practice-based training initiatives but nationally development is seriously hampered by lack of local commitment to training, short-term approaches and shortage of money to pay for it. When health authorities are in financial difficulties, it is often training programmes which are the most vulnerable to cuts and it is a scandal that much mental health training for primary care teams is currently solely provided and funded by the pharmaceutical industry.

*CONCLUSION*

This chapter has acknowledged that the relationship between PHCTs and other services for mentally ill people, both health and social services, may be an uneasy one, fraught with difficulty and misunderstandings. Cultural differences between different parts of the health service may lie at the root of at least some of the problems, but these are unlikely to change in the short term. They would matter less if they were openly discussed, accepted and understood. Key issues in improving the relationship are shown in Box 5.5.

**Box 5.5** Key issues in improving relationships

♦ *Communication* This means not only improving the formal referral procedures between PHCTs and CMHTs, but also more face to face contact between members of both services.

♦ *Teamworking* This seems crucial. Modern health care is too complex for any one professional to think that they have all the answers, but the reality is that many teams are teams only in name, and do not work cooperatively.

♦ *Education and training* Deficiencies in the knowledge and skills of all professionals concerned in the care of mentally ill people are widely acknowledged. Comprehensive, relevant and funded training programmes are essential. This is not just a one-off commitment which can be met by short-term projects.

♦ *Information* Lack of good information seriously hampers rational purchasing and meaningful planning. The means exist whereby information quality can be improved. Wider use of clinical audit could stimulate change relatively quickly.

**DISCUSSION QUESTIONS**

♦ How can managers in primary care and mental health services come together to facilitate better integration of services for seriously mentally ill people?

♦ How could practitioners themselves improve their access to appropriate training courses?

♦ What new strategies could be developed to improve understanding between specialist providers and primary care teams, and how could patients be involved in the process?

**FURTHER READING**

♦ Armstrong, E. (1995) *Mental Health Issues in Primary Care*. London: Macmillan.
A practical guide to coping with mental health problems for all members of the primary care team, especially practice nurses, this book will also help secondary care professionals to understand the primary care approach.

♦ Kendrick, T., Tylee, A. and Freeling, P. (1996) *The Prevention of Mental Illness in Primary Care*. Cambridge: Cambridge University Press.
The most comprehensive guide yet to dealing with mental health problems in primary care settings. Takes a preventive approach and contains much useful, practical, evidence-based help for GPs and primary care teams.

♦ Ford, R. and Warner, L. (1996) Reasoning the needs. *Health Service Journal*, 30 May, 24–25.
This article describes a straightforward method of assessing levels of need among mentally ill people which the authors believe could be widely applicable. May provide one way of ensuring that purchasing/commissioning decisions are based on needs assessment rather than guesswork.

**REFERENCES**

Armstrong, E. (1992), Facilitators in primary care. *International Review of Psychiatry*, 4, 339–342.

Armstrong, E. (1994), *The Kensington & Chelsea and Westminster Family Health Services Authority Mental Health Facilitator Project: report of the project facilitator*. Unpublished.

Atkin, K., Lunt, N., Parker, G. and Hurst, M. (1993), *Nurses Count. A National Census of Practice Nurses*. Social Policy Research Unit, University of York.

Barak, Y., Shamir, E., Trieman, N. and Elizur, A. (1996), From hospital to community: deinstitutionalisation in psychiatric services - a critical review. *Primary Care Psychiatry*, 2, 179–187.

Corney, R.H. (1996), GPs' views and use of adult mental health services in England and Wales: A survey investigating the effect of fundholding. *Journal of Mental Health*, 5, 489–499.

Cox, J. and Holden, J. (1994), *Perinatal Psychiatry: Use and Misuse of the Edinburgh Postnatal Depression Scale*. London: Gaskell.

Craig, T. and Timms, P.W. (1992), Out of the wards and onto the streets? Deinstitutionalisation and homelessness in Britain. *Journal of Mental Health*, 1, 265–275.

Department of Health (1992), *The Health of the Nation. A strategy for health in England*. London: Department of Health.

Department of Health (1994a), *Working in Partnership: a Collaborative Approach to Care*. Report of the Mental Health Nursing Review Team. London: Department of Health.

Department of Health (1994b), *The Health of the Nation, Mental Illness Key Area Handbook*. 2nd edition. London: Department of Health.

Department of Health (1995), *The Health of the Nation, Building Bridges*. London: Department of Health.

Drew, T. and King, M. (1995), *The Mental Health Handbook*. London: Piatkus Publishers.

Essex, B., Doig, R. and Renshaw, J. (1990), Pilot study of records of shared care for people with mental illnesses. *British Medical Journal*, 300, 1442–1446.

Falloon, I. and Fadden, G. (1993), *Integrated Mental Health Care. A Comprehensive Community Based Approach*. Cambridge: Cambridge University Press.

Ford, R. and Warner, L. (1996), Reasoning the needs. *Health Service Journal*, 30 May, 24–25.

Freeling, P. and Kendrick, T. (1996), Introduction. In: Kendrick, T., Tylee, A. and Freeling, P. (Eds) *The Prevention of Mental Illness in Primary Care*. Cambridge: Cambridge University Press.

Gask, L. (1992), Training general practitioners to detect and manage emotional disorders. *International Review of Psychiatry*, 4, 293–300.

Goldberg, D. and Huxley, P. (1980), *Mental Illness in the Community. The Pathway to Psychiatric Care*. London: Tavistock Publications.

Gournay, K. and Brooking, J. (1995), The community psychiatric nurse in primary care: an economic analysis. In: Brooker, C. and White, E. (Eds) *Community Psychiatric Nursing. A Research Perspective*, Vol. 3, London: Chapman and Hall.

Hamilton, L. (1996), *Audit of patients with schizophrenia on depot neuroleptics*. North Yorkshire Medical Audit Advisory Group.

Holden, J.M., Sagovsky, R. and Cox, J.L. (1989), Counselling in a general practice setting: controlled study of health visitor intervention in treatment of postnatal depression. *British Medical Journal*, 298, 223–226.

Jenkins, R. (1992a), Developments in the primary care of mental illness – a forward look. *International Review of Psychiatry*, 4, 237–242.

Jenkins, R. (1992b), A multiaxial approach to the primary care of schizophrenia. In: Jenkins, R., Field, V. and Young, R. (Eds) *The Primary Care of Schizophrenia*. London: HMSO.

Kendrick, T. (1996), Organising the care of the long-term mentally ill in general practice. In: Kendrick, T., Tylee, A. and Freeling, P. (Eds) *The Prevention of Mental Illness in Primary Care*. Cambridge: Cambridge University Press.

Kendrick, T., Sibbald, B., Burns, T. and Freeling, P. (1991), Role of general practitioners in the care of long-term mentally ill patients. *British Medical Journal*, 302, 508-510.

Mann, A. (1992), Depression and anxiety in primary care: the epidemiological evidence. In: Jenkins, R., Newton, J. and Young, R. (Eds) *The Prevention of Depression and Anxiety. The Role of the Primary Care Team*. London: HMSO.

Means, R. and Smith, R. (1994), *Community Care. Policy and Practice*. London: Macmillan.

Paykel, E.S. and Priest, R.G. (1992), Recognition and management of depression in general practice: consensus statement. *British Medical Journal*, 305, 1198-1202.

Pritchard, P. and Pritchard, J. (1994), *Teamwork for Primary and Shared Care. A Practical Workbook*. Oxford: Oxford University Press.

Repper, J. and Brooker, C. (1993), Valuable Insights. *Nursing Times*, 89, 28-31.

Robinson, G., Beaton, S. and White, P. (1993), Attitudes towards practice nurses - survey of a sample of general practitioners in England and Wales. *British Journal of General Practice*, 43, 25-29.

Ross, F. (1992), Barriers to Learning. *Nursing Times*, 88(38), 44-45.

Ross, F. and Mackenzie, A. (1996), *Nursing in Primary Health Care*. London: Routledge.

Shepherd, G., King, C., Tilbury, J. and Fowler, D. (1995), Implementing the care programme approach. *Journal of Mental Health*, 4, 261-274.

Strathdee, G. and Jenkins, R. (1996), Purchasing mental health care for primary care. In: Thornicroft, G. and Strathdee, G. (Eds) *Commissioning Mental Health Services*. London: HMSO.

Strathdee, G. and Kendrick, T. (1996), The regular review of patients with schizophrenia in primary care. In: Kendrick, T., Tylee. A. and Freeling, P. (Eds) *The Prevention of Mental Illness in Primary Care*. Cambridge: Cambridge University Press.

Thomas, P. (1994), *The Liverpool Primary Health Care Facilitation Project*. Liverpool: Liverpool Family Health Services Authority.

Turton, P., Tylee, A. and Kerry, S. (1995), Mental health training needs in general practice. *Primary Care Psychiatry*, 1, 197-199.

Tylee, A. (1996), The secondary prevention of depression. In: Kendrick, T., Tylee, A. and Freeling, P. (Eds) *The Prevention of Mental Illness in Primary Care*. Cambridge: Cambridge University Press.

Wilkinson, G. (1992), The role of the practice nurse in the management of depression. *International Review of Psychiatry*, 4, 311-316.

Wilson, A. (1994), *Changing Practices in Primary Care. A Facilitator's Handbook*. London: Health Education Authority.

CHAPTER 6

# Evaluating Community Mental Health Care

## Richard Ford and Edana Minghella

*KEY ISSUES*

◆ Evaluations must be driven by questions that need answers, not just data collection

◆ Evaluation is a political process where different vested interests come to light. The views of disempowered groups such as service users should be included

◆ The methods, and any measures used, must follow the questions being asked and be seen as tools for the evaluator, not as prescriptions

◆ The whole process of evaluation, and especially the presentation of findings, should be aimed at achieving maximum utility for further service development

*INTRODUCTION*

The move away from a hospital-based system of mental health care towards a service system that places users and the community at its heart has been on-going since the mid 1950s. The most obvious symbol of this development has been the reduction in hospital beds in England from 150 000 at their peak to below 43 000 in 1994 (House of Commons Library, 1995). The run-down in hospital services has been all too apparent, but the question of whether community care has fulfilled its intended purpose is less clear. Community care provides a more complex set of functions than the hospital. Many agencies are now involved, as care takes place in any and all community settings, and professional staff have diversified into a multitude of roles. Finally, the clientele for mental health services has become more varied and numerous (Goldberg and Gater, 1993).

This chapter aims to assist users, professionals and provider and purchasing managers in evaluating community mental health services. It therefore takes a deliberately pragmatic, as opposed to theoretical, approach and is based on the principle of maximising the contribution of service evaluation work to on-going service development (Patton, 1978). The nature and process of evaluation is first described and a quality improvement matrix is proposed. Although complex, the matrix is not offered as a 'high tech' prescription, but intended as an aide-memoire tool to assist those designing evaluations. This is followed by consideration of the evaluation questions that might arise, based on a case study example of a community crisis team. The methods and tools that could be used to answer these questions are briefly reviewed with an emphasis on standardised measures as useful tools that may or may not assist the evaluation process. Readers are cautioned against using measures unless as part of an evaluation driven by questions that people want answered: there is nothing more likely to 'queer the pitch' for evaluators than asking staff and users to help provide yet more data that seem to disappear into a black hole. The case study is then developed to give an insight into the utility of focusing on a small set of questions. The results of this case study example are presented to demonstrate the extent to which the original questions were addressed in a manner that generated useful information for future service development from various viewpoints. Finally, the recommended evaluation process is critically examined.

## THE NATURE AND PROCESS OF EVALUATION

There is considerable overlap between research, audit, monitoring, quality assurance and service evaluation. Their common foundation lies in the use of research methods of one kind or another for their tools. Service evaluation differs in that it seeks to determine the value of the service provided. It follows that service evaluation is not a neutral or 'value free' process: the different parties shown in Figure 6.1 have strong vested interests.

The evaluator needs to consider these potentially conflicting interests when establishing a study. For example, in the case study

**Figure 6.1** Values

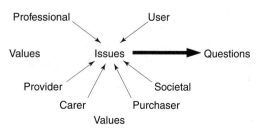

used in this chapter, the following values and vested interests might apply to the crisis service evaluated:

◆ Users – crisis service when and where I want it;
◆ Carers – support for me to survive the burden of supporting the user during crisis;
◆ General practitioner – quick response;
◆ Professional – job satisfaction;
◆ Purchaser – focus on SMI in keeping with *Health of the Nation* (Department of Health, 1993) objectives.

Different vested interests, and the values they carry with them, will influence the questions that the evaluation tackles. In practice, the evaluator will need to work with all parties in refining the questions that will drive the evaluation. Although agreement of evaluation questions is arguably the most important part of the evaluation process, it is the most problematic, not least because all groups do not have equal power or opportunity to influence the questions to be addressed. It may appear easier to avoid the questions stage and become task oriented by collecting data. However, without questions there will be no evaluation, just data. All too often health and social services have provided acres of computer print-out that provides no information that can be used for understanding or developing services. Data are not necessarily information. They only become useful when someone asks a question.

**WHAT QUESTION TO ANSWER**

Having stated that the identification and agreement of questions is the crux of a successful evaluation, and the most difficult part, a quality improvement matrix is offered as a tool. This matrix is designed to enable interested parties to examine the potential aspects of the service that might be evaluated and identify the questions they want answered. As such, it can function as a diagnostic instrument, but must not control the technician or limit ideas. Depending on the general remit of the evaluation, only selected parts of the matrix might be used. Typically, this would take place during an initial problem identification process facilitated by the evaluator through a series of one-to-one interviews, group meetings, focus groups, workshops or stakeholder conferences.

The evaluator needs to be aware of the politics of the process of evaluation. Those commissioning the evaluation are in a powerful position: in the case of internal research they may be the evaluator's line manager – allowing time-out and access to data sources; in the case of external evaluation, they generally control funding. What are the motives behind the evaluation? What do the commissioners hope to gain? What are the vested interests in the process of evaluation? What is the agenda of the evaluator? Independence for the evaluation should rightly be sought. The way to achieve the highest possible level of independence is for the evaluator to be aware of the potential bias from different interest groups, and from his or her own values.

To achieve a more balanced study there is merit in the evaluator giving additional weight and time to the views of less powerful or disenfranchised groups. Historically, service users and their carers have not been asked for their opinions and evaluations have omitted to take account of the experiences and views of those most closely involved in the service. Although users and carers should be involved in the process of establishing evaluations as well as in the subsequent process of investigation, it is unlikely that this will be immediately possible. It might more realistically be seen as a medium-term objective with ongoing efforts being invested in developing effective means of eliciting their views and, where necessary, equipping them with the skills and support needed to maximise the impact of their contribution. Similarly, the more powerful stakeholders (such as managers) need to develop ways of sharing power more equitably with less powerful groups (such as clinicians).

**USING THE QUALITY IMPROVEMENT MATRIX**

The quality improvement matrix (Box 6.1) has been developed with 'state of the art' community services in mind. Such services have now been described in the *Spectrum of Care* (Department of Health, 1996) following recommendations from the major reports of the 1990s (Mental Health Foundation, 1994; House of Commons, 1993; Audit Commission, 1994; Clinical Standards Advisory Group, 1995). The matrix was originally developed for the evaluation of the Sainsbury Mental Health Initiative. This initiative involved making grants worth £3m to eight areas over three years to develop community-oriented mental health services that could become demonstration sites.

The constituent parts and functions of a high quality service (Box 6.2) are represented on the horizontal axis of the matrix. The actual quality provided can be judged by examining the concepts listed on the vertical axis of the matrix (developed in Box 6.3).

**THE CORNWALL COMMUNITY TREATMENT TEAM**

In order to demonstrate and apply the principles and process of evaluation, a case study example of an evaluation of a community-based crisis team in Cornwall will be used throughout the rest of this chapter. The CTT was established in response to research evidence and consumer demands. Users and their carers would like mental health services to be available at all hours of every day of the year, and are increasingly making their views heard. For example a major goal of Mind's Break Through Campaign has been '24-hour access to crisis services in every area' (Open Mind, 1995). Often people must wait until their problems have created an emergency and they require input from their GP, approved social worker and

**Box 6.1** Matrix for measuring quality across the initiative sites: functions of care × quality

| Measures of quality | Initial assessment function (CT) | Preliminary outreach and engagement (CT) | Crisis related responses (CT) | Range of interventions (CT) | Liaison/ linking/ brokerage (CT) | Acute inpatient services (Service) | Range of housing (Service) | Day care/ training/ work (Service) | User involvement (All levels) | Advocacy (All levels) | Carer support (All levels) |
|---|---|---|---|---|---|---|---|---|---|---|---|
| Availability | | | | | | | | | | | |
| Accessibility | | | | | | | | | | | |
| Continuity of care | | | | | | | | | | | |
| Coordination | | | | | | | | | | | |
| Responsiveness | | | | | | | | | | | |
| Effectiveness | | | | | | | | | | | |
| Efficiency | | | | | | | | | | | |
| User satisfaction | | | | | | | | | | | |
| Carer satisfaction | | | | | | | | | | | |
| Staff satisfaction | | | | | | | | | | | |

Community team functions and service elements

Edana Minghella, January 1996

**Box 6.2** Community functions and service elements

Initial assessment function
    Entry into the specialist mental health services

Preliminary outreach and engagement function
    Overlaps with initial assessment but a specific function in assertive outreach

Crisis-related responses
    Includes crisis teams and community alternatives to in-patient care such as home treatment teams

Range of interventions
    Includes support, psychological, medication, social skills, physical health

Liaison/linking/brokerage
    Includes support with social and economic needs, linking across agencies and natural support systems, care management

Acute inpatient services
    Provision of hospital beds

Range of housing
    Residential, supported and other housing provision

Range of day services
    Includes the range of employment, training and day care provision, offering therapeutic, occupational and social opportunities

User involvement
    At service, group and individual levels

Advocacy
    Provision at all levels

Carer support
    Provision at all levels

duty consultant psychiatrist. This can then result in admission to an acute ward, sometimes compulsorily under the Mental Health Act. Users argue that this is expensive, often traumatic and does not meet their needs. Alternatives to acute inpatient care have been successfully developed in research studies such as the Daily Living Programme (Marks *et al.*, 1994). Users and their carers liked the service, use of inpatient beds was reduced and costs were cut (Knapp *et al.*, 1994).

**Box 6.3** Definitions of measures of quality

Availability
  Refers to service coverage generally.

Accessibility
  Refers to services being readily accessed by those who have mental health problems. Services need to be geographically accessible (or delivered at home), bureaucratically available (minimum bureaucracy), widely known about (cognitively accessible) and acceptable (psychologically accessible).

Continuity of care
  Defined at client level, refers to the cohesion between past and present care, congruent with and flexible to the therapeutic needs of the client.

Coordination
  Defined at a service level, involves collaboration between purchasers/commissioners, the broad spectrum of providers and service users, easy referral between services and effective communication between agencies. Duplication and gaps in service provision should be avoided.

Responsiveness
  Refers to the mandate to the mental health system to meet service needs of defined populations and subpopulations. It suggests the ability of services to be flexible, adapt, change and evolve in response to identified aggregated service user needs, i.e. service provision tailored towards a population needs assessment.

Effectiveness
  Refers to the extent to which desirable outcomes for service users are achieved through use of available resources. An effective service provides the most appropriate form of care or combination of care for each type of need.

Efficiency
  Refers to the volume of output achieved given the resources provided. It usually concerns resource allocation and costs.

In Cornwall, the Community Treatment Team (CTT) was established in 1992. They aimed to provide a 24 hour rapid response service to people with mental health crises, while giving top priority to those with serious mental illness. The team was staffed by six community psychiatric nurses, a clinical psychologist, a social worker and an occupational therapist. The team explicitly stated its aims as:

> ... to provide a rapid assessment and treatment service ... The team will operate 24 hours a day/seven days a week. ... to enable people suffering from mental illness to receive treatment in the least institutional environment possible, usually their own home. The CTT will therefore be targeting those people whose mental illness is such that it would otherwise have led to admission to hospital.

From the above information it can be seen that the CTT's work primarily fell into the third column of the matrix, 'crisis related responses', although the other three community team functions ('initial assessment', 'preliminary outreach and engagement', and 'range of interventions') also applied. For this evaluation the areas to be addressed related to the CTT's impact at the individual and service level. Questions might be selected from a list addressing the effect of the service on users and carers (in terms of effectiveness, efficiency, user and carer satisfaction, availability and accessibility, continuity and coordination), and its impact at service level (in terms of effectiveness, efficiency, coordination, responsiveness, accessibility and staff satisfaction). Issues to be taken into account in the evaluation of these questions are considered below, but it is first helpful to consider general methodological issues.

*A note on methods*   Having identified the questions, the most appropriate methods to maximise the amount of information available to address the questions can become apparent. Evaluation uses research methods to collect data that can then be analysed to provide information. A detailed discussion of research methods is beyond the scope of this chapter, but a few important points are worth making. In the same way as questions must be specific to each evaluation, so must the methods. Taking a broad perspective, questions will tend to fall into two main categories: those that require discovery and those that require testing methods. Qualitative discovery methods are most appropriate where less is known, for example investigating the perceived impact of a crisis team on other parts of the service. Such methods are also most appropriate for discovering the *type* of impact as opposed to the more quantitative *strength* of impact.

Where more is already known about the likely, or intended, impact of a crisis team, more quantitative methods are required. This usually involves some kind of comparison, often referred to as 'quasi-experimental designs' (Cook and Campbell, 1979). A descriptive survey could reveal the impact on bed usage over time; however, a more comprehensive evaluation of the impact of the crisis team requires comparison with an alternative, or with some kind of standard (Huxley, 1996). This may be a comparison with national averages or recognised best practice, often referred to as 'benchmarking', or a comparison with another local area that is as similar as possible except in having no crisis team, or an alternative model of crisis intervention.

*Impact of the crisis team for service users and their carers*

### What was the clinical outcome of receiving the crisis service? (Effectiveness)

In assessing clinical outcome, the focus should be on areas that are sensitive to short-term service impact. Active clinical symptoms could be measured, such as mood disturbance, hallucinations and delusions. Negative symptoms, such as apathy and withdrawal, social functioning and quality of life are less likely to be sensitive to change over the short-term and should not be included. Practitioners could complete the Health of the Nation Outcome Scale (HoNOS) or Manchester Scale, independent researchers could contact users and rate the Brief Psychiatric Rating Scale (BPRS) or users could be asked to complete the Symptoms Checklist (SCL30, SCL90) or the General Health Questionnaire (GHQ). Box 6.4 presents a brief review of the most commonly used standardised measures.

### Do users like the service and are they involved? (User satisfaction)

There are standardised measures available (CSQ or Verona) that may be useful if comparison can be made with some kind of control condition. To help further develop the service, qualitative questions are more informative. For the CTT evaluation, users were first asked a general question about their satisfaction with the care they had received. Following this, prompts were used to elicit satisfaction with frequency, length and number of visits. Finally, users were asked how they would like to improve the service.

### Can users and carers get the service at any time of day or night? (Availability and accessibility)

Team out of hours availability and team out of hours activity can easily be measured and many routine data systems now keep this kind of data. Wherever possible evaluators should try and support existing routine systems and not try and introduce yet another system, where the likelihood is that both systems will have poor completion rates. A fuller picture can be achieved by asking service users, their carers and their referrers how easy it was for them to access the service initially, and on an on-going basis. For the CTT evaluation GPs were asked if they preferred the CTT option to previous services, and if so why. GPs responded, without prompting, that it was the accessibility of the team that they appreciated; clearly accessibility was particularly important for them. An overt question on accessibility would not necessarily allow for such a conclusion on the importance of this aspect of the service.

**Box 6.4** Selected standardised measures

**User satisfaction**
*Client Satisfaction Questionnaire (CSQ)* (Larsen *et al.*, 1979)
Most frequently used brief tool. Data for comparison with previous studies can usually be found. On its own of limited value, unless accompanied by open-ended questions.
*Verona Service Satisfaction Scale (VSSS)* (Ruggeri and Dall'Agnola, 1993)
More detailed and becoming popular.

**Carer satisfaction and burden**
*Social Behaviour Adjustment Schedule (SBAS)* (Platt, 1985)
A broad instrument that includes the best available standardised measure for carer perceptions.

**Quality of life**
*Quality of Life Interview* (Lehman, 1983)
The most used measure; three UK versions available: Lancashire Quality of Life Interview (Oliver, 1991); Barry and Crosby, 1996; Adapted Quality of Life Interview (Ford, 1995).

**Symptoms**
*Brief Psychiatric Rating Scale (BPRS)* (Overall and Gorham, 1962)
Used in a large number of evaluations where a large proportion of the sample have a psychosis. Has to be rated by the evaluator who needs training. Clinical staff are relatively easy to train.
*Manchester Scale* (Krawiecka *et al.*, 1977)
A simplified version of the BPRS.
*Symptoms Checklist 30 or 90 item (SCL30; SCL90)* (Derogatis *et al.*, 1973; Derogatis and Melisaratos, 1983)
More frequently used in the US but sometimes used in the UK. Very simple self-completion questionnaires that have the advantage of including psychotic as well as neurotic symptoms.
*General Health Questionnaire (GHQ)* (Goldberg and Williams, 1988)
Very wide usage for mostly neurotic symptoms and has cut-off scores for 'caseness'. Must be purchased from NFER who also regulate use to ensure that the measure is only used by appropriate persons.

**Social Functioning**
*Life Skills Profile (LSP)* (Rosen *et al.*, 1989)
Developed in Australia for evaluating community care and therefore has advantages over many other measures which were developed for use in more institutional settings. Has 39 items and can be easily completed by a rater who knows the person well. Now used in many UK studies.

*(continued overleaf)*

**Box 6.4** (*continued*)

**Global Measures**
*Health of the Nation Outcome Scale (HoNOS)* (Wing *et al.*, 1995)
A well validated, and brief, 12-item measure. Includes risk behaviour, physical problems, symptoms and social factors. Staff making ratings do need training which can be obtained via the Royal College of Psychiatrists Research Unit.
*Camberwell Assessment of Need (CAN)* (Phelan *et al.*, 1995)
Similar coverage to the HoNOS. After rating the degree of problem in each area goes on to rate degree of unmet need for services.

**Staff Satisfaction and Burnout**
*Minnesota Satisfaction Questionnaire* (University of Minnesota, 1967)
Good conceptualisation of 'intrinsic' and 'extrinsic' factors involved in job satisfaction. Now broadly used in UK studies (e.g. Carson and Bartlett, 1993).
*Maslach Burnout Inventory* (Maslach and Jackson, 1986)
Good measure of emotional exhaustion, depersonalisation, and personal accomplishment.

***Does the service prevent unwanted events? (Effectiveness)***
The occurrence of unwanted events, such as admission to hospital, can be collated. Most hospital PAS (Patient Administration Systems) can provide these data. Senior manager support should be obtained as most IT (Information Technology) staff have many competing demands on their time.

Other unwanted outcomes, such as suicide, self-harm, physical health problems, relationship breakdown, job loss or homelessness could be measured. Such details may be difficult to collect reliably from service users alone, and multiple sources, such as information from carers and professionals, are preferable. Care should be taken in collecting appropriate information, bearing in mind the likely problems to be faced by the intended client group. If a problem, such as homelessness, is unlikely to occur whether someone receives the service or not, it may not be worth expending evaluation resources to collect the information. If two people in a control group and none in the experimental treatment group become homeless, the difference between groups is unlikely to reach significance. However, some very rare, but highly 'toxic' (Wykes and Carson, 1995) events, such as homicide and suicide, should still be recorded.

### *Can the user continue to receive appropriate services, where required, over the longer term? (Continuity)*

Where are people discharged to after receiving a crisis service and how long is the gap before they are seen? There is value in doing longer-term follow-up; for example, have people been re-referred to an acute response service within 6 or 12 months of original contact?

### *Is there coordination between all the services that an individual receives? (Coordination)*

Qualitative perceptions from users, carers, GPs and mental health professionals are of value. In the CTT study GPs were asked about their satisfaction with communication between the CTT and themselves on a five point scale. This quantitative rating was followed by an 'Any comments?' question. This proved very useful as GPs were satisfied with communication between the team and themselves, but confused by communication between different parts of the mental health service.

Alternative quantitative approaches can also be used. In a different study Warner *et al.* (1996) documented key worker contacts with other agencies in terms of written correspondence, 'phone conversations and meetings over a three-month period.

### *What is the impact on burden and satisfaction for carers? (Carer satisfaction)*

Again a mix of open-ended and standardised questions is most helpful. The most frequently used measure is the SBAS, but this is likely to need shortening and modification for each study.

### *What is the cost for each individual who uses the service in comparison to other services (or to no services)? (Effectiveness and efficiency)*

Cost evaluations can be limited to the service provided or extended to include all direct treatment costs and indirect costs, such as lost earnings from employment (Knapp, 1995). The minimal model for a crisis team should be to look at the cost of all acute response services. This could be extended to include the cost of all specialist mental health services. In turn, the cost of social care, primary care and general medical services could also be added. The principle should be to concentrate on collecting good quality service use data for services that are either frequently used and/or those with a high unit cost.

Once service use has been measured, a cost estimate for each unit of service used can be made. Ideally a 'long-run marginal opportunity cost' should be estimated (Knapp, 1995). In practice this is seldom practical. Local prices agreed between purchasers and providers are a good substitute if local conclusions are to be drawn. If broader generalisation is desired then national cost estimates are readily available (Netten, 1995).

*Impact of crisis teams at the service level*   Evaluations can also address questions at the service level. This is particularly important in terms of service sustainability. For example, the Daily Living Programme (Marks *et al.*, 1994) demonstrated benefits for the individuals who received the service. However, the service did not sustain. Audini *et al.* (1994) suggest that this may have been due to a less positive impact on the whole service. The service level questions and methods could be as follows.

### What is the impact on overall use of inpatient beds? (Effectiveness and efficiency)

At the individual level there may be less use of inpatient care for users of the crisis service. However, beds may be used by other people instead, leading to no change. This area is particularly important in relation to crisis services as it tends to be the 'purchaser's dream' to reduce expenditure on inpatient care, which in turn, even with an effective crisis service, becomes the 'provider's nightmare'. As described above, bed-use data can usually be obtained from PAS systems. The most helpful variables to request for each service user per admission are: individual identification number, to check for repeat admissions; date of admission and date of discharge, to look at rate of admissions and lengths of stay, as well as trends over time; and age, sex and diagnosis to examine case mix trends. Ideally data should cover the whole period during which the crisis team has operated and the two years before hand. This enables before and after comparison. Data should also be sought for neighbouring areas to further enhance comparison.

### Is there an integrated acute response service? (Coordination)

It follows from the discussion above on inpatient bed use, that a coordinated service, across a crisis team, acute wards, accident and emergency liaison, duty psychiatrist and duty approved social worker is essential. The methods are similar to those in section 6 of the Individual Level Impact. Again, much can be gleaned from qualitative interviews with different agencies or groups of staff trying to work with each other. For more quantitative data, referral patterns can indicate whether there are relationships between agencies. For particular relationships, say between the crisis team and inpatient ward, the amount of time spent in each others' environment is important.

### *What are the knock-on effects for other services? (Coordination)*

Crisis work tends to be short term and any team will have to work with other parts of the mental health service. In addition to the points described above, discharge patterns from the crisis team can be examined.

### *What is the impact on total service costs? (Effectiveness and efficiency)*

Cost at the individual service user level has already been discussed. At the service level the cost implications of a new service can be evaluated in many different ways. At the micro level, do costs shift to or from other parts of the acute response services? At the intermediate level, is there a shift in costs, and hence resources, between acute response service and continuing care? Finally, at the macro level, is there cost shifting between agencies, say between health and social services or between primary and secondary care?

With the separation of purchasing and provision under the 1990 NHS and Community Care Act, managers have greatly improved data on cost. On the downside, the Act also brought competition, and hence an unwillingness to share 'sensitive' cost information. Locally obtained expenditure information that includes estimates for management, maintenance, hotel, capital and other non-staff costs are always preferable. If such data are not available, the multiplication of units of service delivered by national cost estimates (Netten, 1995) may be sufficient.

### *Does the crisis service target and reach the intended client group? (Responsiveness and accessibility)*

As mental health services respond to focusing their care they are employing definitions of serious mental illness that include the concepts of diagnosis, disability and duration (Department of Health, 1995). Service use, in particular use of inpatient care, can be included in the definition as with the Audit Commission's (1994) 'ABC'. However, although use of inpatient services may be readily operationalised as a more concrete and available measure, such a definition is less helpful when the evaluation is examining a service that seeks to provide an alternative to inpatient care.

In practice, the concepts of diagnosis and duration can be measured by taking details from medical notes to enable a broad ICD 10 diagnosis and length of time in contact with services. Disability can be measured by asking keyworkers to complete a HoNOS or LSP. Further details on gender, age and ethnicity can also help in assessment of the responsiveness and accessibility of the service; for example, it may be that certain groups are not accessing the service. For the CTT study a crude definition of case mix for the CTT and the inpatient ward was provided by broad diagnostic grouping alone. In this way, it could be seen whether the inpatient ward and the CTT were working with the same client group.

### Is the intended service delivered? (Effectiveness and efficiency)

Ideally, a crisis team such as the CTT should be using an IT system that revolves around each individual service user and is capable of recording all staff activity undertaken on that person's behalf. Sometimes this can be as simple as recording the number of contacts. The evaluation can be extended if more details are available on the length of visit, where it took place and the content of the visit. The interventions being delivered can then be monitored to see if they match up to the team's aims.

### Are crisis staff happy, motivated and not under undue stress? (Staff satisfaction)

Many standardised measures are available (e.g. MSQ, Maslach, GHQ) and most are relatively easy to complete and analyse. However, standardised questions do not allow the evaluator to discover why people are dissatisfied or burnt-out. Qualitative interviews or the addition of one or more open-ended questions can be most valuable. Staff should be guaranteed anonymity when completing questionnaires and if the evaluator is a staff member an independent third party should be sought, who can receive returned questionnaires.

In summary, this is a broad range of possible individual level and service level questions. Any single evaluation may seek to answer a few of these questions. The precise questions to be answered will be influenced by different interest parties when establishing the evaluation, as outlined in the nature and process of evaluation section above. Also, the questions will need more specific framing on each occasion, in order to meet local requirements.

*Focusing on the most useful questions*   A steering group which included purchasers and providers was established for the CTT evaluation. The evaluation was commissioned from an external agency (The Sainsbury Centre for Mental Health) by the NHS Trust as the CTT provider, although this was in turn specifically funded by the local health authority. There was no direct user or carer involvement in the evaluation design. Managers were well represented as were senior clinical staff involved with the CTT. A full-time local researcher was employed on the project with back-up from more senior staff.

*Results*   For a full report on the CTT evaluation see Ford and Kwakwa (1996).

During 1993/94 the team received 543 referrals, GPs being the most common referral agents (Figure 6.2). This high number of referrals forced the team to provide a limited service with most clients being seen less than six times (Figure 6.3).

**Box 6.5** Key questions

The agreed evaluation focused on the following limited set of key questions.

◆ Is the intended service delivered?

◆ What is the impact on overall use of inpatient beds?

◆ Does the crisis service target and reach the intended client group?

◆ Do users like the service and are they involved? This included issues of accessibility and coordination, both from the user's perspective and the GP's perspective, as the main referral agent.

**Figure 6.2** Referrals

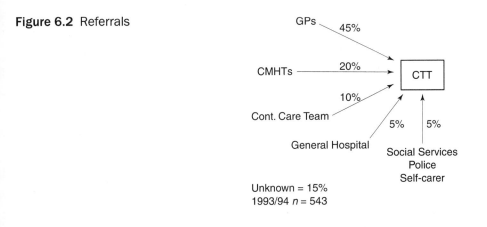

GPs
45%

CMHTs ——— 20% ——▶ CTT

10%

Cont. Care Team

5%    5%

General Hospital

Social Services
Police
Self-carer

Unknown = 15%
1993/94 n = 543

**Figure 6.3** Intensity of input

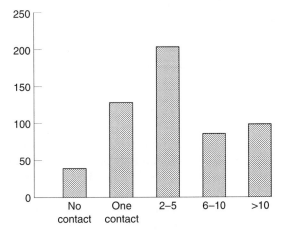

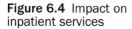

**Figure 6.4** Impact on inpatient services

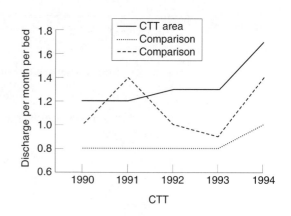

Rapid response and assessment were certainly provided, but few people went on to receive care of such an intensity that it could be seen as an alternative to inpatient treatment. The trend for this period was for the ward to receive an increased number of shorter admissions. However, as shown in Figure 6.4 this was part of a more general trend in the area. An examination of case mix for the ward and the CTT (Box 6.6) shows that the focus of the CTT's work was towards a group with less severe mental illness, as defined by diagnosis. In effect this crisis service opened up mental health services and made them available to a new population, mainly people with less severe illness referred by their GPs.

**Box 6.6** Inpatient/CTT comparison

| Contracts | Beds (n) | Days (%) | CTT (n) | (%) |
| --- | --- | --- | --- | --- |
| Psychosis | 5695 | 61 | 959 | 28 |
| Neurosis | 2866 | 31 | 1938 | 56 |

Service users and the main referral agents, GPs, were asked for their views of the service. All but 3 of the 30 randomly selected service users expressed high satisfaction with the care they had received from the team, particularly for its accessibility and 24 hour support to both clients and carers: 'I could ring anytime and someone always came if it was very urgent. They let you talk to them. Never pushed anything on to you.' However, some clients did not like the number of different staff providing care, as there was a loss of continuity and they may have had to recount events surrounding the crisis, causing them additional distress. Similarly there was criticism of the coordination of continuing support after the team had stopped working with them.

Out of 52 questionnaires sent to GPs, 31 were returned. Satisfaction levels were again high, with only 5 GPs expressing dissatisfaction with client care. In common with users of the service, GPs appreciated the improved accessibility. When asked specifically about communication one third of the GPs (10) were dissatisfied. For example, one GP was worried about the way people could receive a very short-term service from the CTT and then have a long wait for continuing care: 'I feel this is a good service, but I have concern over the interlude between the CTT and the local community mental health team.'

In summary, the 24-hour crisis team studied here provided an additional, and popular, service to people with less severe mental illness. An alternative to inpatient care was not provided and the use of inpatient care was not reduced.

## Evaluating the crisis team: implications for the evaluation commissioners

For commissioners of mental health services there is a difficult dilemma. Crisis services are demanded and may serve large numbers of less severely ill people who appreciate the care they receive. However, the resources needed to provide this additional service may be diverted from people with the most severe mental illness. Certainly decisions on where resources are spent should be explicit, rather than coming about as the unintended consequence of a novel development.

New resources for a crisis team are likely to have to be found from existing allocations. In reality the only potential source of funding is to reduce reliance on inpatient care. It is then essential that the service provides a community alternative. To do this the crisis function must focus on people with psychotic illness, who, as seen here, occupy the majority of bed days. Also, the service must focus on early planned discharge and intensive community follow-up. This promotes a focus on providing an alternative to acute inpatient care. Attempting to prevent admission cannot have such clear focus, as considerable triage and short-term working may be required with people who, in the absence of a crisis team, would not have required hospital care.

The existence of specialist teams, such as a crisis team, causes difficulties in providing continuity and coordination of care. To meet rising expectations for a 24-hour responsive service it may be more efficient to incorporate the crisis function into existing CMHTs. In this way service users and GPs only have one agency to contact. CMHTs could then filter referrals according to their needs for urgent care, treatment and continuing care. Filtering would need to be assisted by consistent priority setting through joint purchasing initiatives from GP fundholders, health authorities and local authorities. Referral protocols could then be established.

For the crisis function to be carried out by CMHTs, staff need to accept that they will have to work outside of Monday to Friday 9 to 5. Psychiatrists must also be full members of the team as they have essential assessment and treatment skills, as well as controlling admission and discharge from acute hospital beds. Training will also be required for all members of the team as they progress from providing a service that runs in tandem with hospital care, to one that seeks to replace much of it.

The evidence to date is clear. User demands for mental health crisis services cannot be met in full. Current resources will not allow for mental health services to be available to all people at all times. Commissioners need to ensure that focused alternatives to acute inpatient care are delivered. Providers must integrate the crisis function within the rest of their work so that continuity and coordination are achieved.

## CONCLUSION

This chapter has attempted to provide a pragmatic route to the evaluation of community mental health care. The process of establishing an evaluation has been discussed with the emphasis being placed on different values that may be involved in focusing on a limited set of questions to be addressed. It has also been emphasised that evaluations must have high utility in terms of future service development. To this end the service evaluation cycle must be completed (Figure 6.5). Completing this cycle is perhaps the biggest challenge of all, as the evaluation of services always carries with it either the explicit or implicit threat of change. As evaluations start with values so they also end with values and different interest groups will see the products of evaluations as more or less threatening, or desirable, to their own vested interests. In particular commissioners of evaluations need to be made aware of the political nature of evaluation from the outset. It is, however, this high utility, and its political nature, that can make service evaluation a powerful force for change in the pursuit of high quality community care for people with mental illness.

**Figure 6.5** Service evaluation cycle

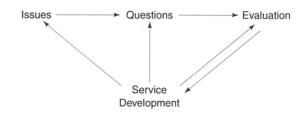

– therefore output focused

*DISCUSSION*
*QUESTIONS*

♦ In what way could your service benefit from evaluation? What issues need addressing?

♦ What are the key questions that could be posited for an evaluation?

♦ How can different vested interests, and the different values they bring, be included? In particular, how can service users be involved in the process?

♦ How might the process of evaluation, and the findings, fit into a broader framework of on-going service development and training?

*FURTHER READING*

♦ Cook, T. and Campbell, D. (1979) *Quasi-experimentation.* Chicago: Rand McNally.
A very detailed look at possible evaluation designs that takes one beyond consideration of randomised controlled trails. Considers questions of validity for all designs. Mostly readable but highly technical in places. Probably of most use to dip in and out of when designing new studies or looking at the threats to a completed study.

♦ Drummond, M. (1980) *Principles of Economic Appraisal in Health Care.* Oxford: Oxford University Press.
A brilliant overview of the concepts involved in health economics. In particular it is readable. A good introductory text that can be read from cover to cover. However, evaluators will have to read further before conducting their own economic appraisals.

♦ Gilbert, N. (1993) *Researching Social Life.* London: Sage.
This social research course textbook covers every topic from gaining access, through field work to statistical analysis and writing up. The use of examples helps make the book readable. Not to be read from cover to cover but very useful to look up the area of evaluation that one is currently concerned with.

♦ Lofland, J. and Lofland, L. (1984) *Analysing Social Settings.* Belmont, CA: Wadsworth.
If you want to know how it feels to do qualitative evaluations, this is the book. Its style engages the reader and there is a wealth of detail contained in a concise book. There are also very useful checklists for each stage of the process of evaluation.

*REFERENCES*   Audini, B., Marks, I.M., Lawrence, R.E., Connolly, J. and Watts, V. (1994), Home-based versus out-patient/in-patient care for people with serious mental illness. *British Journal of Psychiatry*, 165, 204–210.
Audit Commission (1994), *Finding a Place: A Review of Mental Health Services for Adults.* London: HMSO.

Barry, M. and Crosby, C. (1996), Quality of life as an evaluative measure in assessing the impact of community care on people with long-term psychiatric disorders. *British Journal of Psychiatry*, 168, 210–216.

Carson, J. and Bartlett, H. (1993), Stress and the CPN. *Nursing Times*, 89, 38–40.

Clinical Standards Advisory Group (1995), *Schizophrenia*: Vols 1 and 2: Protocol for Assessing Services for People with Severe Mental Illness. London: HMSO.

Cook, T. and Campbell, D. (1979), *Quasi-experimentation*. Chicago: Rand McNally.

Department of Health (1993), *Health of the Nation* Mental Illness Key Area Handbook. London, HMSO.

Department of Health (1996), *The Spectrum of Care*: Local services for people with mental health problems. Wetherby: Department of Health.

Derogatis, L.R., Lipman, R.S. and Covi, L. (1973), SCL-90: an outpatient psychiatric rating scale – preliminary report. *Psychopharmacology Bulletin*, 9, 13–28.

Derogatis, L.R. and Melisaratos, N. (1983), The brief symptom inventory: an introductory report. *Psychological Medicine*, 13, 595–605.

Ford, R. (1995), *Adapted Quality of Life Interview*. London: Sainsbury Centre for Mental Health.

Ford, R. and Kwakwa, J. (1996), Rapid Reaction, Speedy Recovery. *Health Service Journal*, 18 April, 30–31.

Goldberg, D. and Gater, R. (1991), Estimates of need. *Psychiatric Bulletin*, 15, 593–595.

Goldberg, D. and Williams, P. (1988), *A Users Guide to the General Health Questionnaire*. Windsor: NFER-Nelson.

House of Commons Health Committee (1993), *Better off in the community? The care of people with serious mental illness*. London: HMSO.

House of Commons Library (1995), Answer to parliamentary question on hospital closures.

Huxley, P. (1996), Social indicators of outcome at the system level. In: Knudsen, H. and Thornicroft, G. (Eds) *Mental Health Service Evaluation*. Cambridge: Cambridge University Press.

Knapp, M. (1995), *The Economic Evaluation of Mental Health Care*. Aldershot: Arena.

Knapp, M., Beecham, J., Koutsogeorgopoulou, V. *et al.* (1994), Service use and costs of home-based versus hospital-based care for people with serious mental illness. *British Journal of Psychiatry*, 165, 195–203.

Krawiecka, M., Goldberg, D. and Vaughan, M. (1977), A standardised psychiatric assessment scale for rating chronic psychotic patients. *Acta Psychiatrica Scandinavia*, 55, 299–308.

Larsen, D.L., Attkisson, C.C., Hargreaves, W.A. and Nguyen, T.D. (1979), Assessment of client/patient satisfaction: development of a general scale. *Evaluation and Program Planning*, 2, 197–207.

Lehman, A. (1983), The well-being of chronic mental patients. *Archives of General Psychiatry*, 40, 369–373.

Marks, I.M., Connolly, J., Muijen, M., Audini, B., McNamee, G. and Lawrence, R.E. (1994), Home-based versus hospital-based care for people with serious mental illness. *British Journal of Psychiatry*, 165, 179–194.

Maslach, C. and Jackson, S. (1986), *Maslach Burnout Inventory.* California: Consulting Psychologists Press.

Mental Health Foundation (1994), *Creating Community Care.* London: Mental Health Foundation.

Netten, A. (1995), *Unit Costs of Community Care* 1994/5. University of Kent: Personal Social Services Research Unit.

Oliver, J. (1991), The Social Care Directive: Development of a quality of life profile for use in community services for the mentally ill. *Social Work and Social Sciences Review*, 3.

Open Mind (1995), News item, 73, 8.

Overall, J.O.E. and Gorham, D.R. (1962), The Brief Psychiatric Rating Scale. *Psychological Reports*, 10, 799–812.

Patton, M.Q. (1978), *Utilisation Focused Evaluation.* Beverly Hills: Sage.

Phelan, M., Slade, M., Thornicroft, G. *et al.* (1995), The Camberwell Assessment of Need: the validity and reliability of an instrument to assess the needs of people with severe mental illness. *British Journal of Psychiatry*, 167, 589–595.

Platt, S. (1985), Measuring the burden of psychiatric illness on the family: an evaluation of some rating scales. *Psychological Medicine*, 15, 383–393.

Rosen, A., Hadzi-Pavlovic, D. and Parker, G. (1989), The Life Skills Profile: a measure assessing function and disability in schizophrenia. *Schizophrenia Bulletin*, 15, 325–337.

Ruggeri, M. and Dall'Agnola, R. (1993), The development and use of the Verona Expectations for Care Scale (VECS) and the Verona Service Satisfaction Scale (VSSS) for measuring expectations and satisfaction with community-based psychiatric services in patients, relatives and professionals. *Psychological Medicine*, 23, 511–523.

University of Minnesota (1967), *Manual for the Minnesota Satisfaction Questionnaire.* Minnesota: Work Adjustment Project, pp. 1–120.

Warner, L., Sathyamoorthy, G. and Ford, R. (1996), Mind the Gap. *Health Service Journal*, 5 September, 26–27.

Wing, J.K., Curtis, R. and Beevor, A. (1995), Measurement for Mental Health: Health of the Nation Outcome Scales (HoNOS). College Research Unit, pp. 33–46.

Wykes, T. and Carson, J. (1996), Psychosocial factors in schizophrenia: implications for rehabilitation and community care. *Current Opinion in Psychiatry*, 9, 68–72.

# CHAPTER 7

# Economic Evaluation of Mental Health Services and Treatment Initiatives

## Andrew Healey and Martin Knapp

*KEY ISSUES*

◆ Resource scarcity

◆ Efficiency

◆ Economic evaluation

◆ Costing interventions and treatment/service outcomes

◆ Valuation of outcomes

*INTRODUCTION*   Psychiatric morbidity imposes a heavy economic burden on society. Smith *et al.* (1995) estimated the social costs of a range of psychiatric disorders based on UK estimates of service use for different diagnostic categories and national expenditure figures. Looking only at the services provided by the NHS (hospital and community health services and primary care), local authority social services departments, and the voluntary and private care sectors, they calculated these costs to amount to £4.5 billion (1995/96 prices). This total cost does not cover all mental illnesses – it omits disorders in childhood and adolescence, for example – and it does not include all special housing costs, criminal justice service expenditures, family costs, the total value of lost earnings or general impairment to quality of life. The estimate is also based on 1986 service utilisation and costing estimates, and as such is rather dated. Nevertheless, Smith and colleagues' broad estimate – the first of its kind in the UK – serves to demonstrate the enormous costs attributable to mental illness.

Although these types of social burden indicators (akin to cost-of-illness estimates) often provide useful introductions to economic discussions of mental illness, they cannot address the central policy questions that concern decision makers. Are there effective interventions or methods of organising services that can increase social welfare by improving health-related quality of life in the event of illness and/or prevent episodes of illness and/or offset any other economic costs arising from morbidity? If so, do these effects justify the costs which the interventions impose by diverting scarce resources away from other valued uses?

Economists working in the field of health and social care evaluation have developed, and are still developing and improving, various evaluative tools that address these questions. These tools seek to inform policy makers as to the costs and consequences of different health and social care interventions and policies. The purpose of this chapter is to introduce these tools – the main modes of economic evaluation – offering a brief discussion of the decision-making problems they address, with examples of their application. The chapter concludes by discussing some of the methodological developments that are seen as necessary if economic evaluations are to be more extensively applied in the mental health care area.

## RATIONALES FOR ECONOMIC EVALUATION

During the twentieth century, public and private expenditures on mental health services rose quite substantially in real terms (Raftery, 1995). Apart from a brief downturn during the First World War, spending rose steadily but surely up to the mid 1940s and the advent of the National Health Service. Since the 1940s gross current expenditure (excluding capital finance) on hospital and community mental health services has grown to around £2.4 billion (in 1993/94), and gross expenditure on mental illness-specific personal social services (day care and residential care) increased from £90 million to £109.5 million (House of Commons Health Committee, 1995; all figures inflated to 1995/96 prices).

How much of the UK economy's resources should be spent on providing health and social care services for people with mental illness is, like any other public finance issue, a controversial and value-laden question. There is no simple right or wrong answer. Different stakeholders in the mental health care system and in the wider society – the government, NHS purchasers, provider agencies, the general public, patients, their families and others – hold their own, and often quite different, views on the adequacies or otherwise of current spending. Economics can be a source of guidance on these and related thorny issues. It provides a widely tested conceptual framework within which to examine alternative levels of funding for health and social care interventions. More pragmatically, it addresses policy and practice issues of an incremental nature: should a new service be provided or the scale of funding for an existing intervention be increased? Should existing services have their funding reduced or withdrawn? The economic approach is built on the fundamental premise that society's needs and wants outstrip the resources available to meet them. Scarcity is endemic. Choices are unavoidable as to how scarce resources are to be allocated to activities that produce goods and services valued by individuals within society. If more resources are allocated to mental health care, the opportunities for pursuing other valued activities elsewhere in the economy are given up.

For some types of goods and services it is accepted that market forces can be relied on to allocate resources reasonably well; that is, the market will ensure their most highly valued utilisation. When this occurs, competitive markets are said to allocate resources efficiently. In reality, however, and for various well-known reasons, market forces generally fail to allocate resources efficiently or appropriately: they will not be used to maximum social advantage, or the burdens and benefits may be thought to be distributed inequitably (see Box 7.1). Consequently, the allocation of resources to mental health services, and their allocation to individual people, is in part decided by government (or its agents), and ought then to be influenced by evidence from economic evaluations. Decision makers might then be better informed regarding efficient policy or practice options.

To avoid confusion, it is worth noting that the so-called 'internal market' that has developed over recent years in the provision of health and social care in the UK does not fully conform with the textbook notion of a market where consumers (i.e. patients) would express their demands for health care via their willingness to pay a market price. Although market forces now play a role in health and social care resource allocation, the financing of services remains largely the responsibility of the government. The needs for economic evaluation consequently stem from the financing decisions governments and their agents (and the equivalent decisions of insurance companies and other purchasers in other health care systems) are required to make, and the treatment decisions to be taken by providers. Market forces cannot be relied on to guide all (or perhaps even many) such decisions.

In these circumstances, it is the purpose of economic appraisal to provide decision makers and other system stakeholders with information on the costs and benefits of different options for resource investment. Different types of economic evaluation aim to inform resource allocation in different contexts, and the following section gives an overview of the three most useful methods.

**Box 7.1** Market failure
and health care
financing systems

A primary reason why there is market failure in the health
care sector is because of the inherent uncertainty surrounding people's demands for health care and the considerable
(and in many cases prohibitive) expense associated with
many types of treatment. In consequence, private insurance
markets prevail in some health care systems – most notably
in the US – in which individuals (or their employers) pay a
premium to protect themselves against the risk of illness.
Unfortunately, private insurance can lead to further ineffi-
ciencies and inequities: insurance markets can eventually
collapse because individuals with higher health risks which
are unobservable to insurers charging premiums based on
average population risks push people with lower health risks
out of the market due to rising premiums. In response to
this, insurers will screen potential policy holders for their
respective health risks. Although this will improve market
efficiency (people who are willing to pay the premium related
to their own risk category can obtain insurance) there will be
a pool of high risk individuals (typically the poor and chronically sick) who will remain uninsured.

   This inequity is put forward as a key justification for universal health coverage either in the form of public insurance
schemes (e.g. the Netherlands and Germany) or tax-based
systems of finance as in the UK. A problem shared by both
private insurance and universal coverage systems is that
health care is provided free at the point of consumption.
Although this may satisfy specific equity criteria (i.e. that
access to care should not depend on ability to pay) it can
lead to an inefficient level of use given that people have no
incentive to take into account the full costs of provision. This
is compounded even further by lack of efficiency incentives
faced by health and social care providers.

*MODES OF*
*EVALUATION*

*Cost-effectiveness*
*analysis*

Cost-effectiveness analysis (CEA) has been the most commonly
used evaluative technique, not just in the appraisal of mental health
services, but in health and social care more generally. Primarily,
CEA is concerned with ensuring that health and social care
resources are used to maximum effect (in terms of health gain or
some other predefined objective). More often than not, CEA is
employed to help in choices between alternative interventions
available to or aimed at specific patient groups. It can address two
main types of question.

1. If two treatment options are of equal cost, which provides the
   greater health-related benefits from a given budget?

2. If two options have been found to be equally beneficial in terms of patient or population impact, which is less costly?

CEAs traditionally formulate decision making rules using cost-effectiveness ratios based on unidimensional measures of outcome, for example 'cost per life-year saved' or 'cost per successfully treated case', and the intervention with the lowest cost per unit of effect is recommended. However, outcome measures such as 'life-years gained' offer convenience but little else in the evaluation of most mental health interventions: saving or extending lives is not irrelevant, but it is rarely the primary treatment concern. Consequently, most mental health care CEAs concurrently use a range of instruments measuring symptomology, functioning and general quality of life (Bowling, 1991; Thornicroft and Tansella, 1996), alongside the cost consequences of each alternative.

As a source of information for purchasers drawing up health and social care contracts, multiple effectiveness indicators can often pose more questions than they can answer; ambiguities are bound to arise where the success of treatment and service alternatives varies depending on which effectiveness measure is chosen. Purchasers who use economic data in their contracting arrangements might have to make a series of complex trade-offs involving value judgements that often remain hidden. This problem will be compounded where interventions also differ in terms of their cost. In fact, most completed CEAs in mental health care have not generated too many trade-off difficulties to date, but this does not remove the potential difficulty.

More significantly, in the broader scheme of things, many of the outcome scales employed in evaluations of mental health care are condition-specific, or at least applicable to psychiatric morbidity only, which immediately precludes the use of CEA for making cross-programme comparisons of costs and outcomes. For example, how does the development of a new community-based psychiatric service fare on cost and outcome grounds when compared with the expansion of a methadone maintenance programme for drug misusers or the introduction of a breast cancer screening service? When health and social care decision makers seek guidance from economists on these kinds of choices, alternative methods of evaluation are required.

*Cost–utility analysis*    A newer approach to economic evaluation, cost–utility analysis (CUA), is similar to CEA with the important exception that it measures and then values the impact of an intervention on a patient's health-related quality of life alongside the cost of achieving that improvement. The value of health improvement from a treatment is measured in conflated units of utility. CUAs avoid the potential ambiguities and hidden value judgements that arise with multidimensional outcomes in CEA, and in principle CUAs can be

**Box 7.2** Quality
adjusted life-years
(QALYs)

QALYs are founded on the assumption that people, whether they are patients involved in the clinical decision making process or healthy members of the general public asked to make hypothetical trade-offs, would be willing to give up survival duration in a health state characterising a physical or psychiatric disorder in return for fewer years in full health. In order to estimate the 'rate of exchange' between improved quality of life and length of life, researchers are faced with the difficult task of determining what subjective level of unpleasantness people attach to different health states, i.e. what utility they attach to being in a given state of ill-health relative to being in full health and being dead.

The three most widely applied techniques used to elicit individuals' preferences for health states are: rating scales; the standard gamble; and the time trade-off. Each of these methods places a given health state on a scale of zero (death) to one (full health). Allowance is also made for the fact that some extreme states of ill-health might be valued at worse than death. QALYs are then calculated as the number of years spent in a given health state weighted by the utility score attached to that health state. For example, if the health state associated with the neuroleptic treatment of schizophrenia is valued at 0.6, two years spent on maintenance therapy equates to 1.2 QALYs.

applied to choices across a range of health and social care programmes.

The most common value-based measure of health outcomes used in CUAs is the quality-adjusted life-year (QALY) (Williams, 1985; Torrance, 1986, see Box 7.2). A variant on the same theme is the Healthy-Life-Year-Equivalent (HYE; Mehrez and Gafni, 1989) which tries to overcome some of the restrictive assumptions arguably incorporated in the QALY. QALYs are not only convenient summary measures of outcome, but also recognise the inadequacy of using life expectancy data as generic measures of effectiveness. They are constructed on the premise that people value quality as well as length of life, as reflected in the willingness of some individuals to trade off better life expectancy against a shorter life in better health. The results of a recent study by Dolan *et al.* (1996), for example, suggested that when faced with a hypothetical choice, a sample of the general public were willing to trade life expectancy in states of mild, moderate and severe ill-health for fewer years in full health.

Despite its attractive features and its growing use across a wide span of health care contexts, CUA has rarely been applied in mental

**Box 7.3** Some
assumptions
underlying the
construction of QALYs

As currently formulated, QALYs reflect varying assumptions regarding people's preferences for making trade-offs over quality and length of life. One such assumption is that people will be willing to trade-off the same proportion of their remaining life years in a given state of ill-health for fewer years in better health irrespective of the number of life years remaining. So, for example, a patient who regards 12 years in full health as equivalent to 15 years in their current health state would also regard 4 years in full health as equivalent to 5 years in their current health state. There are a number of reasons why actual preferences may violate this assumption, not least that expected duration in a given health state may impact on the proportion of life years people would be willing to give up in return for fewer years in better health (Sutherland et al., 1982). Mehrez and Gafni (1989) have developed an alternative preference-based measure of health-related quality of life known as the Healthy Life Year Equivalent (HYE) which they claim does not impose the same restrictive assumptions as the QALY. However, in a recent debate in the health economics literature Loomes (1995) demonstrates that QALYs and HYEs are in fact no different from each other.

health evaluations, partly because of concerns regarding the insensitivity of current QALY measures to changes in mental health-related well-being (Chisholm et al., 1997). More generally, the methodological assumptions underlying the construction of QALYs have been criticised (Loomes and McKenzie, 1989; Carr-Hill, 1989, see Box 7.3).

The explicit policy goal behind the application of CUA to cross-programme prioritisation is to ensure that the mix of health and social care provision produces maximum gains in health-related quality of life from available resources. To facilitate this, UK advocates of QALYs have been compiling interventions into 'QALY league tables' – rankings of QALYs gained from specific interventions over and above their immediate alternative, combined with the additional costs involved (Williams, 1985; Bryan et al., 1991). By these standards the higher the cost per QALY gained the lower the priority that might be attached to a given programme. Birch and Gafni (1992) provide a detailed exposition and critique of current CUA applications.

*Cost-benefit*
*analysis*

Cost–benefit analysis (CBA) is unique among economic evaluations in that it seeks to determine from an economy-wide, or societal, perspective whether investments in given programmes of care should take place. If a mental health intervention offers positive net benefits to society (benefits exceed costs) it represents a worthwhile investment. If information were available on all costs and benefits associated with the range of mental health services that could be provided, it would in principle be possible to determine, in efficiency terms, how much overall should be spent on programmes of mental health care. However, the funding realities faced by health and local authorities may prevent all interventions with positive net benefits from being implemented. Moreover, it is conceivable that a small number of expensive programmes targeted at specific mental disorders may use up most of the funds allocated for mental health programmes. The resultant mix of services across different patient groups might be rejected on the grounds of an unequal or unfair distribution of benefits.

The primary requirement of CBA that distinguishes it from other forms of evaluation is that all outcomes or consequences are valued in money terms. This ensures that opportunity costs of directing scarce resources from other valued uses – as approximated by the competitive market price for resource inputs – can be traded-off explicitly against the non-resource consequences (whether positive or negative) resulting from programme implementation. The main outcome from effective mental health programmes is the direct improvement in well-being enjoyed by people experiencing psychiatric morbidity. Valuing these programme effects should be based on individuals' willingness to pay for the expected improvements in health-related well-being (Mishan, 1988).

It should be stressed that a CBA which aims to take a societal perspective should avoid using willingness-to-pay valuations based exclusively on the preferences of current service users or people with a history of psychiatric morbidity. Most people in the general population who would value the availability of mental health interventions, and any other type of health care, do so because they face a risk of experiencing a mental illness. Valuations should therefore be representative of the preferences of the general population who face a statistical chance of experiencing an episode of any given type of illness (Gafni, 1991).

Beyond people's private valuations of outcomes, allowance should also be made for individuals' preferences for the well-being of others. These preferences might arise both from paternalism directed at other family members or more generally from what Culyer (1980) describes as 'the caring externality': people have inherent concerns that others should have access to health and social care if needed, and are prepared to back this concern with a payment into a collectively resourced health care arrangement. Although no research has yet been carried out to assess the extent of these altruistic valuations in health and social care policy settings, work in the area of public health and safety suggests that people are willing to pay a premium over and above the valuation placed on improvements in their own well-being for health and safety improvements affecting others living in their community (Viscusi *et al.*, 1987).

Beyond the private and altruistic valuations attached to health and social care outcomes there are, of course, broader social consequences associated with mental health care provision that should be identified and valued in a full CBA. For example, there may be positive or negative effects on the well-being of carers, or effects on public safety: policies aimed at providing more independent living might impose more responsibilities on families or compromise public safety. Quantification of these broader programme effects should again be made with reference to the willingness-to-pay valuations of those sections of society affected.

The use of CBA in health care evaluation, for some years regarded as infeasible or reductionist, has recently enjoyed a resurgence with the development of survey instrumentation that can, in principle, allow individuals' willingness to pay for health care benefits to be directly determined (usually referred to as contingent valuation or the stated preference approach; Johannesson and Jönsson, 1991; Tolley *et al.*, 1994). Critics typically point to distributional problems of interpretation (willingness to pay is limited by ability to pay), and to the questionable validity of survey valuations based on the presentation of hypothetical scenarios to respondents (see Box 7.4). In its favour, the willingness-to-pay approach is the only means of valuation consistent with the economic theory that underpins CBA, and it provides an explicit means of assessing the importance of public policy that might otherwise be left to the hidden value judgements of decision makers. It also provides a means by which to value in monetary terms those treatment outcomes – improvements in functioning and health, broadly defined – that have previously tended to be labelled 'intangible'. The willingness-to-pay approach to benefit valuation is still grappling to gain acceptance with both researchers and policy makers and has therefore had only limited application not only in the evaluation of mental health interventions, but of health and social care services more generally.

*ECONOMIC EVALUATION AND MENTAL HEALTH INTERVENTIONS: APPLICATIONS*

There are not vast numbers of completed economic evaluations in the mental health field, but enough to make it impossible for us to provide a comprehensive review in this chapter. Our aim here is to show how the evaluative modes outlined above can be applied in the appraisal of mental health interventions in the UK. It is important to bear in mind that the quality of the data and conclusions reached are in turn dependent on the scientific rigour of the design and the correct application of economic principles. It is beyond the scope of this chapter to review in detail the

**Box 7.4** Deriving
willingness-to-pay-
based valuations

Ideally economists would prefer to rely on market-based values as measures of people's willingness to pay, thereby reflecting actual as opposed to hypothetical trade-offs. For example, a number of studies have used multivariate statistical analysis to examine the relationship between wages across industries with varying levels of occupational risk of injury and death – the theory being that people with riskier jobs will demand higher wages (Viscusi, 1993). The compensating wage differentials estimated from these analyses are taken as being a reflection of the value that people place on their own safety and as such have been used in the appraisal of public interventions that improve individuals' level of safety in a variety of policy settings.

However, we would be hard pushed to find market-based trade-offs that could be used to estimate the value of mental health and social care interventions. Even though a small fraction of the population will pay directly for their own treatment (for example, private sessions of psychotherapy) it is unlikely that their preferences and valuations of therapy will be representative of the rest of society. Moreover, the role of health and social care practitioners as agents acting on behalf (and hopefully in the interest) of their patients suggests a degree of ambiguity regarding the extent to which prices determined in private markets are a reflection of patient rather than practitioner preferences. For these reasons the use of survey instrumentation for valuation purposes becomes unavoidable.

robustness of each study's conclusions, and the interested reader is referred to Drummond *et al.* (1987) for an expert 'quality-control' checklist.

Most economic evaluations reviewed here are built on existing prospective (clinical) evaluations of services and treatments. In such instances the health economist has traditionally had a limited input into the choice of design, which emphasises the old adage that an economic evaluation can only be as good as the broader evaluation upon which it is based. What constitutes a 'good study design' is a controversial issue, with one school of thought advocating the randomised controlled trial (RCT) as an appropriate gold standard. A more pragmatic line favoured by some other researchers is that the RCT is neither practicable nor necessarily desirable due to its reliance on highly experimental circumstances as a means of generating scientifically defensible results that are difficult to replicate in the real world (Black, 1996). A couple of the studies outlined below are not based on prospective designs, but combine retrospective analysis of clinical data with expert opinion to generate decision analytic models of costs and treatment outcomes.

***CEAs in mental health care evaluation***   Most cost-effectiveness studies of mental health interventions have been concerned with appraising service initiatives for replacing hospital with home-based acute care, or comparing alternative service configurations for providing community-based support.

Considerable interest has been shown over the last 20 years in examining the relative cost-effectiveness of community and hospital-based care. One of the broadest economic evaluations is being carried out by the Centre for the Economics of Mental Health as part of the Team for the Assessment of Psychiatric Services (TAPS), looking at the cost-effectiveness of people with long-term mental health problems moving from hospital to community settings in North London (Leff, 1997). Results to date from the economic evaluation are based on a sample of 751 long-stay patients without dementia who were transferred from hospital over a period of 8 years, who have been in the community for a year. Initially, cost and outcome comparisons were made subsequent to the matching of community and hospital patients, but appropriate 'matches' were later not available and before–after comparisons were made. Although community care was on average probably no less costly than hospital, patient well-being was generally shown not to be adversely affected and improvements were registered along some outcome dimensions. Consequently, community-based care was more cost-effective than hospital for these people after one year in the community (Beecham *et al.*, 1997).

For people going through an acute phase of their illness, an economic evaluation integrated with an existing randomised controlled trial found that a home-based intervention for people facing emergency hospital admission (the Maudsley Daily Living Programme, DLP) offered short-term cost-effectiveness advantages over hospital-based acute care. Patient outcomes for the DLP were superior over the first 20 months (Marks *et al.*, 1994; Audini *et al.*, 1994), whereas the cost advantage in the first period had disappeared by the fourth year (Knapp *et al.*, 1994; Knapp, 1997). Another randomised controlled trial, this time of an experimental home-based outreach initiative for psychiatric referrals, demonstrated that a more multidisciplinary approach to the management of patients was equally effective but less costly than standard care (Burns *et al.*, 1993a, b).

A third study examining a new approach to organising community care assessed the cost-effectiveness of a service based on outpatient consultations and standard psychiatric nursing input compared to a community support team where nursing staff provided generic support for people with mental illness organised around a form of care management (Muijen *et al.*, 1994; McCrone *et al.*, 1994). Patients were randomly allocated between the experimental and control arrangements, and the new approach to community psychiatric nursing was found to be more cost-effective in the short term, although not over a longer period.

Other CEAs in the UK have evaluated pharmacological interventions in the treatment of psychiatric morbidity in primary care. Davies and Drummond (1993), using clinical decision analysis, used the expert opinion of psychiatrists and a retrospective analysis of US data to determine the cost-effectiveness of clozapine versus standard neuroleptic therapy. Clozapine was found to be less costly overall and afforded a net gain in life years with either mild or no disabling effects. Jönsson and Bebbington (1994), using similar methods, found lower costs per successfully treated patient with paraoxetine compared to its more established alternative, imipramine. Scott and Freeman (1992) conducted an evaluation of the costs and treatment outcomes associated with routine care delivered by GPs or specialist psychological therapy, finding no additional gains in clinical outcome associated with specialist care but significant additional costs.

We are aware of a great many CEAs now underway for mental health care treatments and practices. Many of these manage to overcome methodological and practical difficulties encountered by previous studies and will be able to offer decision makers much useful information.

*CUAs in mental health care evaluation*    In the absence of an appropriate system of valuation scores for health states relevant to psychiatric morbidity, it should not be surprising that there are very few mental health CUAs either completed or underway.

Wilkinson *et al.* (1992) examined the costs and effects of care for people with functional psychiatric disorders in an uncontrolled study, deriving a cost per QALY gained for treating schizophrenia of £10 934. The valuations were based on the Charing Cross Health Indicator (Rosser and Kind, 1978), which is now rarely used. Cost per QALY estimates for treating affective psychoses or neurotic disorders were not computed as the changes in quality of life scores were not significant. A rather different study was conducted by Drummond *et al.* (1991) who offered a CUA using the Care Giver Quality of Life Instrument (CQLI) within an RCT that examined the effect of targeting support for caregivers of people with dementia in Canada. The CQLI score differential between control (standard patient care) and experimental groups was not statistically significant.

Hatziandreu *et al.* (1994) compared maintenance treatment for depression using sertraline (Lustral, an SSRI) with episodic treatment using dothiepin (a tricyclic). Utility scores derived from two expert panels (one of GPs, one of psychiatrists) were used to rate various health states salient to the treatment of depression. Together with estimates of the duration and pattern of episodes of major depression and treatment, annual QALY values were derived. The baseline lifetime cost per additional QALY gained using maintenance treatment with sertraline was estimated to be £21 172 at 1988/89 prices (for women aged 35).

*CBAs in mental health care evaluation*

The classic mental health CBA was conducted by Weisbrod *et al.* (1980) for the well-known Assertive Community Treatment model developed in Madison, Wisconsin. The authors concluded that the additional costs per patient incurred by the experimental intervention over long-stay hospital treatment were outweighed by the additional benefits. Jones *et al.* (1980), in a study conducted in the North of England, evaluated the costs and benefits of treating patients with schizophrenia on first admission in either a district general hospital or an area mental hospital. After taking account of the consequences for public agencies and changes in clinical outcomes the latter was found to be the favourable policy option. Ginsberg *et al.* (1984) concluded that there was a positive net benefit to society of using a nurse psychotherapy service for people with neuroses over the standard GP care given to the control group. Both these studies attempted to be comprehensive in their valuation in money terms of the effects of each alternative.

In all of these CBAs the cost implications were assessed, not just in terms of the direct costs of delivering interventions but also the resource implications for other agencies. Weisbrod *et al.* (1980), for example, examined the cost consequences of assertive community treatment for the criminal justice system. However, none of these studies adopted copy-book CBA models as they all emphasised the value of productivity gains at the workplace rather than societal willingness-to-pay for health improvements as the measure of the value attached to the outcomes. The use of productivity gains valued at market wages has been a commonly employed technique for benefit valuation in CBAs of health and social care programmes. However, this implies that the level of societal welfare can be measured with reference to economic indicators like the Gross National Product (GNP) – an approach that does not have any basis in the theoretical underpinnings of CBA (see Box 7.5).

*FUTURE DEVELOPMENTS IN MENTAL HEALTH ECONOMIC EVALUATIONS*

We are firmly of the view that there should be more economic evaluations of mental health policies and practices. But it is equally imperative that those evaluations should be designed well, conducted carefully and interpreted appropriately.

What methodological developments are therefore required for economic evaluation to play a more informative role in resource allocation decisions in mental health care? It is clear that, although the role of the economist in evaluative work has become more

**Box 7.5** Combining the QALY and willingness-to-pay approach to measure health-related welfare improvements

The correct approach to measuring changes in a person's well-being (whether this relates to their health or otherwise) is to establish the amount of variation in their money income that would leave them indifferent between their post- and pre-change circumstances. Depending on whether we are dealing with potential increments (which is usually the case with health and social care) or reductions in welfare, the income variation required will either relate to their maximum willingness to pay (for an increment) or the minimum compensation they would accept (for a decrement).

The key point to make here is that a properly conducted CBA seeks to inform decision making based on the preferences of individuals affected by policy interventions as expressed via their willingness to pay or to accept compensation. This contrasts with the approach taken by many CBAs in health care evaluation in which social benefits from health care are couched in terms of productivity gains to the economy. One obvious reason for rejecting this approach is that non-productive individuals (the unemployed, children, the retired) are immediately excluded from the cost–benefit calculus. In addition, no account is taken of the impact of illness on people's ability to enjoy activities outside the work place. As already noted in the text, willingness-to-pay valuations for health and social care outcomes are not widely available. However, where relevant, the impact of interventions on people's earnings can be used as a partial estimate of the value they attach to mental health services and treatments.

extensive, particularly in the appraisal of community-based initiatives, there remains a sizeable methodological gap preventing economists from providing policy makers with information that allows explicit trade-offs of costs against the beneficial outcomes of services. Whereas costing methods for mental health services based on sound economic principles have developed in leaps and bounds over the past decade, the design of instrumentation for the measurement and valuation of mental health-related outcomes has remained comparatively static.

*Costing developments: principles*

Setting up or expanding existing mental health services requires an investment in physical and human resource inputs. New building space will need to be acquired, appropriately equipped and powered; staff will have to be employed and trained in specific tasks; there will need to be administration arrangements; and, of course, medications and other specific treatment resources will be required. A successful treatment service also relies on other factors such as the quality and enthusiasm of staff, the motivations of clients and the therapeutic relationships formed between staff and users. Although these latter factors do not have a cost in any immediate or intuitive sense, they can be identified as so-called non-resource inputs which potentially influence the outcomes produced by an intervention, and as such should be recognised in a full economic appraisal (Knapp, 1995).

The economic cost of delivering mental health services measures the opportunities forgone from diverting scarce resources from other beneficial uses. Even where resources are apparently provided free of charge (for example, volunteer carers) there will often still be an opportunity cost – a volunteer might be employed in other valued activities elsewhere in the economy, for instance. The costs of resource inputs might be reflected in their market prices, for example a psychiatric nurse's salary could approximate the value of their skills outside the NHS; but these market prices are often poor reflections of opportunity costs. Market distortions may arise where institutional arrangements (such as wage bargaining between trade unions and employers, or BMA reimbursement guidelines) keep salaries above their market clearing levels; or the development of specialist skills that become scarce relative to demand can lead to salaries in excess of the amount needed to keep resources in their current uses – what economists refer to as rent or 'producer surplus'. Where market price is thought to be significantly different from the cost of a resource input, adjustments should be made for appropriate evaluative costing, although most health and social care evaluations rely on market wages and other prices as reasonably fair indicators of opportunity cost.

Ideally, an economic evaluation should attempt to value the long-run marginal cost of providing care. The long-run perspective takes into account the capital financing implications that will invariably arise with a major service development, as well as the possible need to employ additional staff. The cost of capital is calculated to reflect the discounted annual financial returns that could have been yielded over the lifetime of an investment (in buildings and/or equipment) if the money needed for a capital development had been invested on the financial markets or elsewhere.

Many people with chronic mental health problems living independently in the community utilise a range of services provided by many statutory and non-statutory agencies. A comprehensive approach to service costing will therefore be required. Comprehensiveness is vital for making like-with-like comparisons between long-stay hospital care (where everything is provided 'in-house') and care in community settings (Weisbrod *et al.*, 1980; Knapp *et al.*, 1993), and for estimating fully any cost-offsetting effects from services and treatments. Comprehensiveness is also important in order to guard against any changes in the balance of health and social service use that might generate incentives to pass the buck between agencies. Many policy initiatives not only affect the total costs of care but also their distribution between those agencies financing mental health services (Kavanagh and Knapp, 1995).

*Costing developments: practice*
In practice, the costs of mental health services are estimated from the financial accounts of statutory and non-statutory agencies, making allowances for capital invested based either on NHS capital charges or recent valuations of specific plots of land or buildings. To assess marginal cost implications, costs should be presented with reference to the nature of the discrete units of services used by patients. Thus, for example, unit costs for residential facilities are usually expressed in terms of cost per day or cost per week, whereas use of peripatetic services (GPs, CPNs, social workers) is usually expressed as a cost per minute or visit.

Considerable progress has been made in recent years in developing instrumentation for measuring comprehensive service use (McCrone and Weich, 1996). The Client Service Receipt Inventory (CSRI: Beecham and Knapp, 1992; Beecham, 1995) is one instrument developed specifically for social care and mental health evaluations, although it is now being used more widely. A similar form of instrument, the Economic Questionnaire, was developed by Weisbrod *et al.* (1980) for the economic appraisal of the assertive community treatment programme. The CSRI primarily identifies frequency and intensity of service contact over a retrospective period for specific individuals, collected via interviews with patients and/or carers and key workers (and occasionally via postal questionnaire), and supplemented where possible with case-record material. Data collected from the CSRI can be combined with unit cost information to estimate the marginal costs of episodes of care.

The collection of patient-level data within the context of prospective evaluative work usually generates information on variability in patient resource use and costs. There is now growing recognition that standard economic evaluations should be supplemented with multivariate statistical analyses of these variations. The primary goal would be to understand the reasons for cost variations and to provide policy makers with insights into the predicted costs of care for individuals or groups of patients with specific characteristics. Analyses of variations can also reveal the expected costs of achieving service outcomes (Knapp, 1997).

The statistical exploration of covariance between costs, outcomes, needs and other patient characteristics has already been a feature of some UK evaluations (Knapp, 1995). Siegal *et al.* (forthcoming) outline a number of statistical approaches that might be adopted in clinical and economic evaluations examining cost, effect and other covered linkages. They suggest, for example, that probabilistic statistical models could be used to estimate the 'success' or 'failure' of given treatments for given levels of cost. Functional relationships between costs and outcomes are important considerations in areas like psychotherapy, for example, where analysis of dose–response relationships have demonstrated that therapist involvement with patients – and, by implication, levels of resource use and cost – can have a significant influence on patient outcomes (Howard *et al.*, 1986; Orlinsky and Howard, 1986; Healey and Knapp, 1996).

*The valuation of mental health service outcomes*

We have already emphasised the importance of valuing the health-related outcomes from interventions. Deriving a preference or valuation-based summary index of outcomes allows broad cost–benefit comparisons to be made across disparate programmes using either the cost–utility method, with its current emphasis on the use of QALYs, or the more orthodox approach based on willingness-to-pay and cost–benefit analysis. Although both modes of evaluation are gaining popularity in the broader health economics field (Gerard, 1991; Johannesson and Jönsson, 1991), there has been little UK research looking at the development of preference-based outcome measures applicable to mental illness.

In a UK and European context, QALY scores are now quite regularly derived from the recently developed EuroQoL which covers a range of health-related quality of life dimensions, with societal valuations attached to each health state included in its descriptive system (EuroQoL, 1990). The EuroQol identifies a possible 245 states of health (including death and full health), covering six components of health-related quality of life: mobility, self-care, usual activities, social relationships, pain and mood. In the development of the instrument two methods of eliciting community valuations have been used – the visual analogue scale and the time trade-off method – and both forms of instrumentation were used to elicit health state values from samples of the general population within the UK and other European countries.

The EuroQol represents an advancement on the original Charing Cross (Rosser–Kind) valuation matrix (Rosser and Kind, 1978), which covered states of health relating only to disability and distress. Other quality of life instruments used to derive valuation scores include the Index of Health Related Quality of Life (developed by Rosser and colleagues but not published) and an adaptation of the Short Form 36 (SF-36) for valuation purposes which is currently under development (Brazier, 1993). Neither the EuroQol nor the SF-36 have been tested as valid, reliable and sensitive instruments with psychiatric populations. There would be considerable merit in carrying out feasibility exercises on one or both instruments to allow preference-based approaches to measuring the success of interventions to take hold in the mental health field. If the EuroQol and SF-36 prove to be inadequate, then existing mental health-related quality of life instruments could perhaps be adapted or new descriptive systems developed for these purposes.

Good economic evaluations need good effectiveness measures, based on the conventional instrumentation of clinical and social evaluations in mental health care. We will not discuss these instruments here, as they are covered elsewhere (see Chapter 6). It is important to emphasise that good CUAs and CBAs, although relying on summary measures of outcome (utility and money values, respectively), should also ensure that they examine the finer detail of effectiveness measurement picked up by these other and more familiar instruments.

The future of CBA in mental health care depends on the ability of economists to generate willingness-to-pay based valuations for treatment outcomes. As explained earlier, contingent valuation surveys are one recommended approach to eliciting how much people would be prepared to pay for specific types of health care. Although at face value the contingent valuation approach is seen as an ideal way forward for providing a theoretically consistent means of assessing the benefits of health care interventions, there remain grave concerns among some commentators regarding the validity of the approach as a tool for measuring what it purports to measure – people's preferences and values over outcomes from public policies (Hausman, 1993; O'Reilly *et al.*, 1994). On a more practical note, these surveys are expensive to conduct given the size of population samples required to generate representative societal values and the research time required to develop appropriate survey instrumentation (Mitchell and Carson, 1988). These practical problems are compounded by the need to conduct the surveys across many mental health interventions, or at least those recommended for expansion or contraction, if willingness-to-pay values are used to rank different programmes. (This issue is pertinent not just to mental health care but health care evaluation generally.) If anything, this highlights one advantage of the QALY approach to outcome valuation, using instruments like the EuroQoL, in which a set of valuation scores are derived that are, in principle, transferable across settings.

Advocates of the willingness-to-pay method have suggested that the QALY and willingness-to-pay approaches can be integrated as a means of placing money valuations on avoided morbidity or improvements in health (French and Mauskopf, 1992; Tolley *et al.*, 1994). This involves 'pegging' utility scores derived for states of health, currently used to formulate QALYs, to estimates of the value of a statistical life year (see Box 7.6). In principle these valuations would be transferable and applicable to a variety of health and social care evaluations where an assessment is required of their costs and benefits.

**Box 7.6** The value of a statistical life year

The value of statistical life is calculated as the mean amount that individuals would be willing to pay (or accept in compensation) for a small reduction (increase) in their own risk of death, multiplied by the population at risk. For example, if on average people were willing to pay £30 for a policy that reduced their risk of death by 1/100 000 (i.e. one life will on average be saved per one hundred thousand population at risk), then the value of the statistical life saved is equal to £3 000 000 (30 × 100 000). On its own this approach offers policy makers a means of determining the value of mental health interventions that save lives either through preventing suicide among those suffering from acute illness or through improving the safety of their families and the community in general. Two further stages are required in order that the value of life be used to assess the value placed on morbidity-related outcomes from health and social care interventions by the population at risk of experiencing episodes of psychiatric illness.

1. Utility scores are attached to relevant health states reflecting their undesirability with reference to full/normal health (=1) and being dead (=0). This enables the loss of functioning associated with a period of illness to be assessed in utility terms. For example, if 3 months of depression treated with antidepressants is valued at 0.7, this implies a loss of functioning of 0.3 relative to full health.

2. This loss of functioning is converted into a monetary equivalent by combining utility scores and the value of a life year (or the value of any period of time relevant to the episode of morbidity, e.g. life months). The value of a life year is estimated by dividing the statistical value of life by the discounted expected remaining life years for the average age of the population at risk. Remaining life years are discounted to reflect the commonly held belief that people place more importance on life years in the near rather than distant future. If the value of a life month was estimated to be £15 000, then the monetary equivalent of lost functioning from an episode of depression lasting three months (using the above utility scores) is £4500 (£15 000 × 0.3). This monetary equivalent is analogous to the value of life in that it represents the value of avoiding a statistical episode of depression.

*(continued)*

**Box 7.6** *(continued)*

> The approach outlined here can in principle enable the benefits of psychiatric interventions to be assessed in terms of the value of their relative health outcomes, either with regard to interventions that directly improve quality of life or prevent psychiatric relapse. It is important to recognise that valuations produced should be made with reference to the preferences of the general at-risk population, and not exclusively people with a history of a given disorder or those currently experiencing an episode of illness.

Pursuing mental health-related outcome valuation will present economists and psychometricians with all the challenges already being faced in non-mental health areas and public policy in general. If valuation, either of a QALY or willingness-to-pay nature is to gain broad acceptance and application in mental health care appraisal, valid and reliable tools for health status measurements applicable to mental illness will be required to provide a base on which to generate individual preferences which themselves should have proven validity and reliability.

## *CONCLUSION*

The resource implications of mental illness can be considerable, and the attention given to developing better modes of treatment and more effective systems of care is raising many new demands for economic evaluation. As we have described, few such evaluations have been completed to date, although we know of quite a number now in train. Many are now underway, for example, at the Centre for the Economics of Mental Health, between them addressing a wide range of treatment modes as utilised by a variety of patient groups. In five years time there should thus be a much larger body of UK-specific economic evaluative evidence to guide policy and practice decisions and to inform associated discussions. Included in this new body of evidence will be research findings for areas of mental health intervention hitherto relatively neglected, including child and adolescent mental health care, services for people with addictions, forensic psychiatry and psychotherapy.

With government and health and social care agencies expressing growing demands for cost and outcome data but in the absence of appropriate channels of dissemination, the impact of economic evaluation on mental health and social care policy could remain rather limited. For this reason it is encouraging that formal means of disseminating review data have now been established, like the Cochrane Collaboration which includes groups with a specific interest in generating data on the effectiveness and efficiency of interventions in the treatment of disorders like schizophrenia

(Cochrane Collaboration Schizophrenia Review Group, 1994). The establishment of central information systems of evaluative evidence is part of a general push towards evidence-based medicine at both a policy and clinical decision making level (Sackett and Rosenberg, 1995). Although this is to be welcomed, it is vital that effectiveness data on specific interventions are reported alongside evidence on the resource and cost consequences of services and treatments. This is a concern regarding evidence-based medicine expressed by other commentators, for example Maynard (1996).

The lack of first-hand data on the costs and outcomes of specific interventions provides one obvious reason why systematic reviews of economic evidence in the mental health field have been lacking. Where reviews have been conducted they usually reveal a paucity of information on which policy makers can rely. For example, we ourselves have recently conducted a review of economic evaluations of psychotherapeutic interventions on behalf of the Department of Health in England (Healey and Knapp, 1994). Out of 12 studies loosely identified as being economic appraisals, only a handful that were based on well-designed clinical evaluations provide useful estimates of the effectiveness and cost consequences of short-term interventions. No economic evaluations have yet been carried out on longer-term psychodynamic forms of therapy.

To take a second example, Hotopf *et al.* (1996) recently conducted a review of evidence on both the effectiveness and cost-effectiveness of prescribing selective serotonin re-uptake inhibitors and tricyclic antidepressants in the pharmacological treatment of depression. They concluded that the cost-effectiveness studies based on decision-analytic modelling procedures adopt assumptions that overestimate the costs of treatment failure. As such they argue that no conclusions can be drawn on the economic viability of either drug regime and advocate the need for a large-scale cost-effectiveness study based on a prospective clinical trial. Although the current position regarding economic evaluative evidence may seem rather frustrating, it is at least encouraging that practitioners and policy makers alike are beginning to recognise the reality of resource scarcity and that no service or treatment can have an automatic claim over available economic resources.

We have given particular emphasis to the development of better outcome measures in economic evaluations, and especially the need to explore the development and application of utility and/or willingness-to-pay approaches to outcome valuation so that cost–utility and cost–benefit comparisons can be made. These would allow a broader range of questions to be addressed and thus would offer decision makers further insights and guidance. The present generation of evaluations should provide very helpful evidence on the comparative costs of alternative treatments or modes of care for particular groups of people with mental health problems (and their distribution across agencies or stakeholders), as well as the comparative effectiveness along a number of dimensions. But these evaluations do not give decision makers the data-informed facility to make comparisons across different patient groups or diagnostic areas, nor ultimately to determine, at least in economic terms, how much should be spent on programmes of mental health care.

Economic evaluations should be seen as highly desirable components of mental health care reviews and discussions. There is no doubt that there are many constituencies of support for more such evaluative work, nor that the findings of such research should be integrated into policy and practice discussions. Perhaps a growing concern – which may seem churlish in the context of such a large unmet need for economics evidence – should be the limitations of some of the methodological approaches now employed. With the accumulating weight of evidence should come increasing sophistication and discernment in the employment of appropriate evaluative modes and constituent techniques.

*DISCUSSION*
*QUESTIONS*

1. How can health economics inform the difficult choices that have to be made about the allocation of resources to people with serious mental health problems?
2. What other criteria, apart from efficient resource allocation, should be used to ensure that minimum levels of need are met?
3. What are the shortcomings of using cost-effectiveness analysis (CEA) to guide priority setting across health and social care programmes?
4. What are the main features of cost–utility analysis (CUA) and cost–benefit analysis (CBA)? How advanced is the use of such strategies in a mental health service context?

*FURTHER READING*

The following texts will provide the reader with a general introduction to the pertinent issues concerning the economics of health and social care financing and provision. Most of these texts will provide an overview of economic evaluation in health and social care policy, but will also cover broader ranging discussions including: market failure and the financing and provision of health and social care; agency relationships in health and social care; efficiency versus equity in the financing and delivery of services; the organisation of health and social care.

♦ Culyer, A.J. (1989) The normative economics of health care finance and provision. In: McGuire, A., Fenn, P. and Mayhew, K. (Eds) *Providing Health Care: The Economics of Alternative*

*Systems of Finance and Delivery.* Oxford: Oxford University Press.

♦ Donaldson, C. and Gerrard, G. (1993) *Economics of Health Care Financing: The Visible Hand.* London: Macmillan.

♦ Knapp, M.R.J. (1984) *The Economics of Social Care.* London: Macmillan.

♦ McGuire, A., Henderson, J. and Mooney, G. (1988) *The Economics of Health Care: An Introductory Text.* London: Routledge and Kegan Paul.

♦ Mooney, G. (1992) *Economics Medicine and Health Care,* 2nd edn. Hemel Hempstead: Harvester Wheatsheaf.

Economic evaluation of health and social care interventions.

♦ Drummond, M., Stoddart, G. and Torrance, G.W. (1987) *Methods for the Economic Evaluation of Health Care Programmes.* Oxford: Oxford University Press.

This widely used text provides an essential and practical overview of the economic evaluation of health care.

♦ Knapp, M.R.J. (Ed) (1995) *The Economic Evaluation of Mental Health Care.* Aldershot: Ashgate.

Sets out the modes of economic evaluation and their application in mental health contexts.

♦ Netten, A. and Beecham, J. (Eds) (1994) *Costing Community Care: Theory and Practice.* Aldershot: Ashgate.

Principles and applications of cost research in social care.

The three texts above provide detailed discussion of how to go about costing health and social care interventions (with the book by Knapp giving a particular emphasis to mental health interventions).

♦ Netten, A. and Dennett, J.H. (1996) *Unit Costs of Health and Social Care.* Personal Social Services Research Unit, University of Kent at Canterbury.

This has a detailed listing of current unit cost estimates for hospital and community based health and social care services updated annually.

♦ Tolley, G., Kenkel, D. and Fabian, R. (1994) *Valuing Health for Policy: an Economic Approach.* Chicago: The University of Chicago Press.

This book covers issues pertinent to the design and application contingent valuation surveys to health outcome valuation.

♦ Torrance, G.W. (1986) Measurement of health state utilities for economic appraisal. *Journal of Health Economics,* 5, 1–30.

This paper reviews methods for deriving health state utility scores for the construction of QALYs.

**REFERENCES**    Audini, B., Marks, I.M., Lawrence, R.E., Connolly, J. and Watts, V. (1994), Home-based versus outpatient/inpatient care for people with serious mental illness. Phase II of a controlled study. *British Journal of Psychiatry*, 165, 204–210.

Beecham, J.K. (1995), Collecting and estimating costs. In: Knapp, M.R.J. (Ed) *The Economic Evaluation of Mental Health Care*. Aldershot: Ashgate.

Beecham, J. and Knapp, M.R.J. (1992), Costing psychiatric options. In: Thornicroft, G., Brewin, C. and Wing, J. (Eds) *Measuring Mental Health Needs*. Oxford: Oxford University Press.

Beecham, J., Hallam, A. and Knapp, M. (1997), Costing care in the hospital and in the community. In: Leff, J. (Ed) *Caring in the Community: The Reality of Psychiatric Community Care*. Chichester: Wiley.

Birch, S. and Gafni, A. (1992), Cost-effectiveness/utility analyses: do current decision rules lead us to where we want to be? *Journal of Health Economics*, 11, 279–296.

Black, N. (1996), Why we need observational studies to evaluate the effectiveness of health care. *British Medical Journal*, 312, 1215–1218.

Bowling, A. (1991), *Measuring Health: a Review of Quality of Life Measurement Scales*. Open University Press.

Brazier, J. (1993), The SF-36 Health Survey Questionnaire – a tool for economists. *Health Economics*, 2, 213–215.

Bryan, S., Parkin D. and Donaldson, C. (1991), Chiropody and the QALY: A case in assigning categories of disability and distress to patients. *Health Policy*, 18, 169–186.

Burns, T., Beadsmoore, A., Bhat, A.V., Oliver, A. and Mathers, C. (1993a), A controlled trial of home based acute psychiatric services. I: Clinical and social outcome. *British Journal of Psychiatry*, 163, 49–54.

Burns, T., Raftery, J., Beadsmoore, A., McGuigan, S. and Dickson, M. (1993b), A controlled trial of home based acute psychiatric services. II: Treatment patterns and costs. *British Journal of Psychiatry*, 163, 55–61.

Carr-Hill, R. (1989), Background material for the workshop on QALYs; Assumptions of the QALY procedure. *Social Science and Medicine*, 28, 469–477.

Chisholm, D., Healey, A. and Knapp, M. (1997), QALYs and mental health care. *Social Psychiatry and Social Epidemiology*, 32, 68–75.

Cochrane Collaboration Schizophrenia Review Group (1994), Schizophrenia and the Cochrane Collaboration. *Schizophrenia Research*, 13, 185–188.

Culyer, A.J. (1980), *The Political Economy of Social Policy*. Oxford: Martin Robertson.

Davies, L.M. and Drummond, M.F. (1993), Assessment of the costs and benefits of drug therapy for treatment-resistant schizophrenia in the United Kingdom. *British Journal of Psychiatry*, 162, 38–42.

Dolan, P., Gudex, C., Kind, P. and Williams, A. (1996), The time trade-off method: results from a general population study. *Health Economics*, 5, 141–154.

Drummond, M., Stoddart, G. and Torrance, G.W. (1987), *Methods for the Economic Evaluation of Health Care Programmes*. Oxford: Oxford University Press.

Drummond, M.F., Mohide, E.A., Tew, M., Streiner, D.L., Pringle, D.M. and

Gilbert, R.J. (1991), Economic evaluation of a support program for caregivers of demented elderly. *International Journal of Technologically Assessed Health Care*, 7, 209-219.

EuroQoL Group (1990), EuroQoL – a new facility for the measurement of health related quality of life. *Health Policy*, 16, 199-208.

French, M.T. and Mauskopf, J.A. (1992), A quality of life method for estimating the value of avoided morbidity. *American Journal of Public Health*, 82, 1553-1555.

Gafni, A. (1991), Willingness-to-pay as a measure of benefits: relevant questions in the context of public decision making about health care programmes. *Medical Care*, 29, 1246-1252.

Gerard, K. (1991), *A review of cost-utility studies: Assessing their policy-making relevance*. Health Economics Research Unit Discussion Paper 11/91. Departments of Public Health and Economics, University of Aberdeen.

Gerard, K. and Mooney, G. (1992), *QALY league tables: three points for concern – goal difference counts*. Health Economics Research Unit Discussion Paper series, Number 04/92. University of Aberdeen.

Ginsberg, G., Marks, I. and Waters, H. (1984), Cost-benefit analysis of a controlled trial of nurse therapy for neuroses in primary care. *Psychological Medicine*, 15, 683-690.

Hatziandreu, E.J., Brown, R.E., Revicki, D.A. *et al.* (1994), Cost–utility of maintenance treatment of recurrent depression with sertraline versus episodic treatment with dothiepin. *PharmacoEconomics*, 5, 249-264.

Hausman, J.A. (Ed) (1993), *Contingent Valuation: A Critical Assessment*. Amsterdam: North-Holland.

Healey, A. and Knapp, M. (1994), Economic Evaluation and Psychotherapy: review for the Department of Health. *Centre for the Economics of Mental Health, Working Paper* 30.

Healey, A. and Knapp, M.R.J. (1996), Psychotherapy: individual differences in costs and outcomes. In: Miller, N., Magruder, K. and Rupp, A. (Eds) *The Cost Effectiveness of Psychotherapy: A Guide for Practitioners, Researchers and Policymakers*. New York and Chichester: Wiley.

Hotopf, M., Lewis, G. and Normand, C. (1996), Are SSRIs a cost-effective alternative to tricyclics? *British Journal of Psychiatry*, 168, 404-409.

House of Commons Health Committee (1995), *Public Expenditure on Health and Personal Social Services*, Memorandum received from the Department of Health containing replies to a written questionnaire from the committee. London: HMSO.

Howard, K., Kopta, S.M., Krause, M.S. and Orlinsky, D.E. (1986), The dose-effect relationship in psychotherapy. *American Psychologist*, 41, 159-164.

Johannesson, M. and Jönsson, B. (1991), Economic evaluation in health care: Is there a role for cost–benefit analysis? *Health Policy*, 17, 1-23.

Jones, R., Goldberg, D.P. and Hughes, H. (1980), A comparison of two different services treating schizophrenia: a cost–benefit approach. *Psychological Medicine*, 10, 493-505.

Jönsson, B. and Bebbington, P.E. (1994), What price depression? The cost of depression and the cost-effectiveness of pharmacological treatment. *British Journal of Psychiatry*, 164, 665-673.

Kavanagh, S. and Knapp, M.R.J. (1995), At the crossroads of health policy, health economics and family policy: whose interest to provide a family oriented service? In: Gopfert, M. and Webster, J. (Eds) *Disturbed Mentally Ill Parents and their Children*. Cambridge: Cambridge University Press.

Knapp, M.R.J. (1984), *The Economics of Social Care*. London: Macmillan.

Knapp, M.R.J. (Ed) (1995), *The Economic Evaluation of Mental Health Care*. Aldershot: Ashgate.

Knapp, M.R.J. (1997), Making music out of noise: understanding cost variations. *British Journal of Psychiatry*, supplement, forthcoming.

Knapp, M.R.J., Beecham, J., Hallam, A. and Fenyo, A. (1993), The costs of community care for former long-stay psychiatric hospital residents. *Health and Social Care in the Community*, 1, 193-201.

Knapp, M.R.J., Beecham, J., Koutsogeorgopoulou, V. *et al.* (1994), Service use and costs of home-based versus hospital based care for people with serious mental illness. *British Journal of Psychiatry*, 164, 195-203.

Knapp, M.R.J., Marks, I.M., Wolstenholme, J. *et al.* (1996), Home-based versus hospital-based care for serious mental illness: a controlled cost-effectiveness study over four years. *British Journal of Psychiatry*, in press.

Leff, J. (Ed) (1997), *Caring in the Community: The Reality of Psychiatric Community Care*. Chichester: John Wiley.

Loomes, G. (1995), The myth of the HYE. *Journal of Health Economics*, 14, 1-7.

Loomes, G. and McKenzie, L. (1989), The use of QALYs in health care decision making. *Social Science and Medicine*, 28, 299-308.

Marks, I.M., Connolly, J., Muijen, M., McNamee, G., Audini, B. and Laurence, R.E. (1994), Home-based versus in/outpatient care for serious mental illness: a controlled study. *British Journal of Psychiatry*, 157, 661-670.

Maynard, A. (1996), Cost effectiveness and equity are ignored, (letter). *British Medical Journal*, 313, 170.

McCrone, P. and Weich, S. (1996), Mental health care costs: paucity of measurement. *Social Psychiatry and Psychiatric Epidemiology*, 31, 70-77.

McCrone, P., Beecham, J. and Knapp, M.R.J. (1994), Community psychiatric nurse teams: cost-effectiveness of intensive support versus generic care. *British Journal of Psychiatry*, 165, 218-221.

Mehrez, A. and Gafni, A. (1989), Quality adjusted life years and healthy year equivalents. *Medical Decision Making*, 9, 142-149.

Mishan, E.J. (1988), *Cost Benefit Analysis*, 4th edn. London: Unwin Hyman.

Mitchell, R.C. and Carson, R.T. (1988), *Using Surveys to Value Public Goods: the Contingent Valuation Method, Resources for the Future*. Washington, DC.

Muijen, M., Cooney, M., Strathdee, G., Bell, R. and Hudson, A. (1994), Community psychiatric support teams: intensive support versus generic care. *British Journal of Psychiatry*, 165, 211-217.

Netten, A. and Dennett, J.H. (Ed) (1996), *Unit Costs of Health and Social Care*. Personal Social Services Research Unit, University of Kent at Canterbury.

Oliver, J.P.J. (1992), The social care directive: development of a quality of life profile for use in community services for the mentally ill. *Social Work and Social Sciences Review*, 3, 5-45.

O'Reilly, D., Hopkin, J., Loomes, G. *et al.* (1994), The value of road safety: UK research on the valuation of preventing non-fatal injuries. *Journal of Transport Economics and Policy*, January, 45-59.

Orlinksy, D.E. and Howard, K.J. (1986), Process and outcome in psychotherapy. In: Garfield, S.L. and Bergin, A.G. (Eds) *Handbook of Psychotherapy and Behaviour Change*, 3rd edn. New York: John Wiley and Sons.

Raftery, J. (1995), Have the 'lunatics taken over the asylums'? The rising cost of psychiatric services in England and Wales, 1860-1986. In: Knapp, M.R.J. (Ed) *The Economic Evaluation of Mental Health Care*. Aldershot: Ashgate.

Rosser, R. and Kind, P. (1978), A scale of valuation of states of illness: is there a social consensus? *International Journal of Epidemiology*, 7, 347-357.

Sackett, D.L. and Rosenberg, W.N. (1995), The need for evidence-based medicine. *Journal of the Royal Society of Medicine*, 88, 624-680.

Scott, A.I.F. and Freeman, C.P.L. (1992), Edinburgh primary care depression study: treatment outcome, patient satisfaction, and cost after 16 weeks. *British Medical Journal*, 304, 883-887.

Siegal, C., Laska, E. and Meisner, M. (forthcoming), Statistical methods for cost-effectiveness analyses. *Controlled Clinical Trials*.

Smith, K., Shah, A., Wright, K. and Lewis, G. (1995), The prevalence and costs of psychiatric disorders and learning disabilities. *British Journal of Psychiatry*, 166, 9-18.

Sutherland, H.J., Llewellyn-Thomas, H., Boyd, N.F. and Till, J.E. (1982), Attitudes towards quality of survival: the concept of maximal endurable time. *Medical Decision Making*, 2, 299-309.

Thornicroft, G. and Tansella, M. (Eds) (1996), *Mental Health Outcome Measures*. New York: Springer.

Tolley, G., Kenkel, D. and Fabian, R. (1994), *Valuing Health for Policy: an Economic Approach*. Chicago: The University of Chicago Press.

Torrance, G.W. (1986), Measurement of health state utilities for economic appraisal. *Journal of Health Economics*, 5, 1-30.

Viscusi, W.K. (1993), The value of risks to life and health. *Journal of Economic Literature*, December, 1912-1946.

Viscusi, W.K., Magat, W.A. and Forrest, A. (1987), Altruistic consumer valuations of multiple health risks. *Journal of Policy Analysis and Management*, 7, 227-245.

Weisbrod, B.A., Test, M.A. and Stein, L.I. (1980), Alternative to mental hospital treatment: economic benefit cost analysis. *Archives of General Psychiatry*, 37, 400-405.

Wilkinson, G., Williams, B., Krekorian, H., McLees, S. and Falloon, I. (1992), QALYs in mental health: a case study. *Psychological Medicine*, 22, 725-731.

Williams, A. (1985), The economics of coronary bypass grafting. *British Medical Journal*, 291, 326-329.

Zung, W.W.K. (1965), A self-rating depression scale. *Archives of General Psychiatry*, 12, 63-70.

# SECTION II

# SPECIFIC INTERVENTION STRATEGIES

# CHAPTER 8

# Family Intervention

## Gráinne Fadden

**KEY ISSUES**

- ◆ Evidence of the effectiveness of family interventions
- ◆ Training clinical staff in the skills needed to apply family interventions
- ◆ Systems of supervision that will ensure that skills, once acquired, are maintained
- ◆ Ensuring that the range of different family interventions which have been shown to be effective are provided in routine clinical practices

**INTRODUCTION**  A number of studies published in the 1980s demonstrated the effectiveness of providing family interventions in schizophrenia. The effective interventions were educational in nature, focusing on practical problems and the development of coping skills. When combined with psychopharmacological treatments, these family approaches consistently resulted in dramatic decreases in relapse rates. Later studies attempted to replicate and extend the earlier research by applying the interventions in different settings, and with different target groups. Recent reviews and a meta-analysis of published studies conclude that there is no doubt about the effectiveness of family interventions in reducing relapse. The interventions have also been found to be culturally robust, applicable to routine clinical settings, and to result in reduced costs for the care of people with schizophrenia. In spite of the evidence of their effectiveness, these approaches are not being applied routinely, and the majority of people with schizophrenia do not receive family intervention.

The present chapter traces the development of these family approaches, and describes the common components of effective interventions. The present state of knowledge regarding what interventions work with what types of family and in what setting is summarised. Questions which remain unanswered are identified in addition to areas which require further research. The main challenges in relation to this area are how clinicians can be trained effectively to use these interventions, and how the interventions can be implemented in routine clinical settings.

**BACKGROUND**   In the 1950s with the advent of neuroleptic medication as a treatment for schizophrenia, and the introduction of deinstitution-alisation policies, there was optimism about the outcome that could be achieved for people suffering from this disabling disorder. Before this there were problems in managing the positive symptoms of schizophrenia in community settings because of the disruptive and disturbing nature of these symptoms. Management took place for the most part in institutional settings, mainly in large psychiatric hospitals, and it was thought that negative symptoms such as apathy and lack of motivation resulted from the unstimulating nature of these environments. It was hoped, therefore, that if positive symptoms were controlled by medication, people with schizophrenia could live in more natural environments in the community where they would not develop the negative symptomatology which had been attributed to the effects of institution-alisation.

By the 1970s, the picture was far less optimistic. Unpleasant side-effects caused problems with compliance with neuroleptic medication, and even with full compliance it became clear that for a large proportion of those treated, the prophylactic effects of medication were limited. Relapse rates of 30–40% within the first 1–2 years of treatment were reported (Leff and Wing, 1971; Johnson, 1976), and these figures were confirmed by later studies (Hogarty, 1984; Hogarty *et al.*, 1979; Schooler *et al.*, 1980). Furthermore, about 7% of those treated with neuroleptics showed no improvement at all in acute symptomatology (Leff and Wing, 1971). It was apparent that although medication was helpful, many people continued to experience psychotic symptoms, and between a quarter and a half of those on medication relapsed within 1–2 years.

The work of Brown *et al.* (1972), Vaughn and Leff (1976) and others, and the development of the concept of Expressed Emotion (EE) suggested that stressful factors in the person's natural environment and particularly within the family were also associated with higher levels of relapse. Relapse in schizophrenia was found to be higher when people returned to live with families where there were high levels of criticism and/or overinvolvement (Leff and Vaughn, 1981).

It became apparent that simple theories regarding the aetiology of schizophrenia were insufficient. Zubin and Spring (1977) proposed a vulnerability-stress model to explain how episodes of schizophrenia are triggered, a model further described by Nuechterlein and Dawson (1984). In simple terms the model proposed that each person with schizophrenia has a vulnerability to developing episodes of the disorder, and has a particular stress threshold. Episodes result from an interaction of stressful events in the environment and the particular individual's inherent vulnerability. The adoption of the vulnerability-stress model for schizophrenia and its consequent implications for treatment, and the knowledge gained from research on Expressed Emotion (EE) were two of the factors which influenced a number of researchers to study the effects of offering a combination of pharmacological and family interventions to people with schizophrenia from the late 1970s onwards.

A number of additional factors added to the popularity of this type of research at that time. Community care policies and the closure of several large institutions resulted in more people with mental health problems remaining in the family home than previously. This led to the development of research studies examining family burden – the effects on other family members when one person in the family has a serious mental health problem. The family burden research provided a useful balance to the research on Expressed Emotion and demonstrated the stressful effects of caring for a mentally ill relative at home (Creer and Wing, 1974; Fadden et al., 1987a). Theories regarding the role of the family in the aetiology of schizophrenia (Bateson et al., 1956; Laing, 1960; Lidz, 1975), although not supported by research evidence, further added to the stress in families by suggesting that they had in some way played a causative role in their relative's illness. It became clear that family members had needs in their own right. The growth of user movements and advocacy groups allowed carers to articulate these needs and their desire to be involved actively in their relative's treatment (Hatfield, 1983). For several reasons, therefore, the time was right to examine the effectiveness of offering family interventions which it was hoped would reduce relapse rates in the schizophrenia sufferer, and reduce stress and burden in all family members.

**FAMILY INTERVENTION STUDIES**

Interest in evaluating various family interventions has increased dramatically from the early 1980s to the mid 1990s. A good indication of this growth in interest is the number of studies included in major reviews of the area. Thus the review by Strachan (1986) concentrated on four studies, Lam's (1991) review included six major studies, and the most recent review by Dixon and Lehman (1995) describes 15 groups of studies. The latter review excluded a number of studies which did not meet their inclusion criteria, and even since this review was prepared, further studies evaluating various aspects of family interventions have been published. For mental health professionals new to this area, the picture can appear confusing and complicated. The purpose of this chapter is to help the reader to make sense of these studies, to summarise what we can say with certainty with regard to family interventions, and to identify those questions to which the answers remain unclear. It is helpful to separate the first generation studies – those published up to 1990 – from those which have been published from 1991 onwards.

*Early studies of psychoeducational interventions with families*

The earliest controlled studies of family interventions are listed in Box 8.1. These studies were conducted by enthusiastic teams of researchers who were developing the particular interventions in question, and in general family intervention was compared with 'routine' or individual treatment. In all eight studies, the family intervention was provided in addition to neuroleptic medication.

The studies by Kottgen *et al.* (1984), Goldstein *et al.* (1978), Leff *et al.* (1989, 1990) and the study variously reported by Haas *et al.* (1988), Spencer *et al.* (1988) and Glick *et al.* (1990), differ from the other four studies in important respects either in relation to the nature of the intervention, location in which therapy was carried out or the selection criteria used. Goldstein *et al.* (1978) did not preselect families rated as high EE. The intervention was brief (six sessions) and was aimed at helping the patient and family to accept the psychosis, to identify stresses and to plan how to minimise or avoid stresses in the future. The participants in the study were young, and two-thirds were experiencing their first episode of schizophrenia. Apart from outcome data at six months post-intervention, no longer-term outcome data have been reported.

The Hamburg study (Kottgen *et al.*, 1984; Dulz and Hand, 1986) also focused on young people experiencing their first or second episode of schizophrenia. The therapeutic orientation was psycho-dynamic, and patients and their relatives received group therapy separately. The study has also been criticised on methodological grounds (Vaughn, 1986). The study by Leff *et al.* (1989, 1990) rather than comparing family treatment with some kind of indivi-dual treatment, compared two types of family intervention, family sessions in the home (including patients) versus a relative's group (excluding patients).

The study reported by Haas *et al.* (1988), Spencer *et al.* (1988) and Glick *et al.* (1990) differed from the others in that it described a short-term inpatient family intervention with a group who were not preselected for high EE. Unlike the study by Goldstein *et al.*, however, the group studied were not young first episode patients. Their mean age was 30 years, and the level of disability was high. It is difficult to separate out if the results were attributable to the inpatient treatment itself or to the fact that those who received this treatment were more likely to engage in additional outpatient treatment.

**Box 8.1** Results of early family intervention studies

| Study | Location | 9/12 month relapse rates | 2 year relapse rates |
|---|---|---|---|
| Falloon et al. (1982, 1985) | California, USA | | |
| Family intervention | | 6 | 17 |
| Individual treatment | | 44 | 83 |
| Hogarty et al. (1986, 1991) | Pittsburg, USA | | |
| Family intervention | | 23 | 32 |
| Control group | | 41 | 66 |
| Leff et al. (1982, 1985) | Camberwell, London, UK | | |
| Family intervention | | 8 | 40 |
| Control group | | 50 | 78 |
| Tarrier et al. (1988, 1989) | Salford, UK | | |
| Family intervention | | 12 | 33 |
| Routine treatment | | 53 | 59 |
| Goldstein et al. (1978) | California, USA | | |
| Family intervention | | 0 | — |
| Routine treatment | | 48 | — |
| | | (6 mth follow-up) | |
| Kottgen et al. (1984) | Hamburg, Germany | | |
| Family intervention | | 33 | — |
| Control group (High EE) | | 50 | — |
| Leff et al. (1989, 1990) | Camberwell, London, UK | | |
| Family intervention | | 8 | 33 |
| Relatives group | | 36 | 36 |
| Haas et al. (1988), Glick et al. (1990) | New York, USA | Family intervention superior to control | Family intervention superior for female patients |

The other four studies (Falloon *et al.*, 1982, 1985; Hogarty *et al.*, 1986, 1991; Leff *et al.*, 1982, 1985; Tarrier *et al.*, 1988, 1989), although differing in terms of the stated goals, the exact content, and the method of intervention employed, nonetheless have several key features in common. These are summarised in Box 8.2.

It is not possible in the present review to describe these four approaches in detail. Readers interested in the differences and

**Box 8.2** Common features of successful psychosocial interventions in schizophrenia

◆ Acceptance of a vulnerability – stress model of schizophrenia.

◆ Person with schizophrenia is maintained on medication.

◆ Intervention begins during or soon after an acute episode when family motivation is high.

◆ Development of a positive working alliance between family and therapist.

◆ Patient and family seen together for at least some of the intervention sessions.

◆ Some if not all of the intervention sessions conducted in the family home.

◆ Emphasis on family education and provision of information about the disorder in order to enhance understanding.

◆ Behavioural or cognitive–behavioural orientation with emphasis on practical day to day issues.

◆ Enhancement of family problem-solving skills.

◆ Changes in communication patterns in the family resulting in greater clarity of expression and less emotive exchanges between family members.

◆ Reduction of unpleasant family atmosphere because of reduced stress and enhanced coping strategies.

◆ Maintenance of realistic expectations for patient and other family members.

◆ Encouragement of interests outside the family for all family members through a process of goal-setting, expansion of social network or participation in family group or support meetings.

◆ Interventions are maintained over a period of time with follow-up, or take place in the context of on-going service.

commonalties in these interventions are referred to the original journal articles or the 'Further Reading' section of this chapter which describes in detail how these family approaches work in practice. The key elements would appear to be the here-and-now focus of the interventions, the emphasis on skills acquisition by family members, the provision of information about the disorder, and the positive non-blaming attitude of the therapists. At some point in the intervention, the family and the person with the disorder must be seen together. The families in these studies were also selected on the basis of being rated as high EE and the patients had long-standing problems.

What conclusions can be drawn from the outcome of these first eight studies? The outcome data on patient relapse are presented in Box 8.1. The results of the studies show quite clearly that for people with schizophrenia who have had a number of episodes with a range of symptoms, disabilities and handicaps, and whose families are classified as high EE, the interventions which are most effective are those with the characteristics described in Box 8.2. The results are consistent and dramatic. In those families who received the psychoeducational interventions, relapse rates at 9 months or one year post-intervention ranged from 6 to 12%, whereas in the routine treatment control groups, the relapse rates ranged from 41 to 53%. At 2-year follow-up, relapse rates in the intervention groups ranged from 17 to 40% whereas those in the control groups ranged from 66 to 83%.

In summary, family interventions have been shown to result in at least a fourfold reduction in relapse rates at one year post-intervention, and even though relapse increases in the second year, the rates are still only half what they are when no such intervention is provided. It is clear that relapse rates in schizophrenia remain high if treatment consists of medication and routine monitoring only (Tarrier *et al.*, 1994; Scottish Schizophrenia Research Group, 1992). Critics of family interventions have sometimes argued that these approaches succeed only in delaying relapse, not in preventing it. However, what is also now clear is that delaying relapse has a positive effect (Hogarty and Ulrich, 1977). In a review of the treatment literature, Wyatt (1991) noted the important prognostic value of preventing or delaying psychotic exacerbation. In other words, the longer relapse is delayed or prevented, the better the eventual outcome in schizophrenia.

It is of course important not to focus solely on relapse rates when evaluating the success of these interventions. The studies which measured the patients' social functioning reported improvements in those patients where family intervention had been provided (Falloon *et al.*, 1987; Barrowclough and Tarrier, 1990). The Falloon study also reported reduction in family burden in the group who received the family intervention. This is important given the evidence that the burden on families of those with schizophrenia increases over time (Fadden *et al.*, 1987a). The longest published follow-up of a cohort of relatives of patients identified during their first episode of schizophrenia indicated that 43% of relatives continued to display case level of disturbance after 5 years (Scottish Schizophrenia Research Group, 1992). This is significantly higher than would be expected in a sample drawn from the general population. The family intervention studies which included an economic analysis found that the costs of the family approach were less than those of the control condition, 20% less in the Falloon study (Cardin *et al.*, 1985) and 27% less in the Tarrier study (Tarrier *et al.*, 1988). The family interventions have, therefore, been shown to provide a range of positive effects for both patients, families and those responsible for service provision.

Having gleaned a clear picture of what is effective with high EE families in schizophrenia, it is important to look at what can be learned from the other four 'first generation' studies referred to at the beginning of this section. Once again, constraints of space permit only a summary of lessons learned from these studies, but the studies provided some important pieces of information regarding effective components of family intervention:

♦ Interventions which adopt a psychodynamic approach are not effective (Kottgen *et al.*, 1984).
♦ Young people with schizophrenia (recent onset or first episode) may benefit from brief educational and crisis-oriented family approaches (Goldstein *et al.*, 1978).
♦ Relatives' groups where families must attend meetings outside the home and relatives are seen without the patient, experience major problems because of non-engagement or non-attendance. Although they can result in reasonable success rates for those who attend, they cannot be recommended overall because of non-acceptance levels of up to 50% (Leff *et al.*, 1989, 1990).
♦ For those with long-standing problems, brief inpatient family treatment may only be effective for females who have poor pre-hospital functioning. As the positive results do not become apparent for 18 months post-admission, the inpatient family intervention may serve only to improve engagement with out-patient family treatment. For males with long-standing problems, brief inpatient family intervention either has no effect or moderately negative effect (Glick *et al.*, 1990).

### *The role of family education*

Some of the studies referred to in the previous section tried to separate out the specific effects of the educational component of the family intervention and other groups of researchers have also addressed this topic (Smith and Birchwood, 1987). For those particularly interested in this aspect of family interventions or the effects of providing relatives with information, readers will find the article by Lam (1991) and further articles by Tarrier and Barrow-clough (1986) and Birchwood *et al.* (1992) particularly informative.

The results from this aspect of family intervention seem clear and consistent. The provision of information would appear to play an important role in engagement of the family. Information is best provided early on when the person first develops schizophrenia, otherwise families may develop inaccurate rigid views which are later hard to shift. Brief educational packages are not effective in reducing relapse rates though they may be helpful for low EE families (Tarrier *et al.*, 1988) or for those where the psychotic illness is of recent onset (Goldstein *et al.*, 1978; Linszen *et al.*, 1996). They can also result in benefits for relatives such as reduction in stress levels and family burden and increased optimism about the outcome of their relative's disorder.

*'Second generation' family intervention studies*

Once it became clear that offering a psychosocial/psychoeducational intervention to families of those with schizophrenia resulted in such unquestionably superior results to offering medication and undefined or non-targeted 'routine follow-up' alone, there were calls for the introduction of these methods into ordinary services and routine clinical practice (Kuipers and Bebbington, 1985). Leff *et al.* (1982) recommended that professional mental health staff should be systematically trained in psychosocial intervention techniques. Tarrier *et al.* (1988) predicted that this may not be a simple task as minimal contact with relatives of those with schizophrenia was not standard practice let alone attempts to offer anything more intensive to family members. Smith and Birchwood (1990) highlighted the issues that needed to be considered in developing routine clinical services for families, and proposed a family service model to deal with potential difficulties which might be encountered. In addition to the question of whether these approaches could be incorporated into routine clinical settings, there was curiosity about a number of issues: could they have an impact on people with other diagnoses or patterns of symptomatology; could a range of professionals be trained to implement those approaches?

The 'second generation' family intervention studies aimed to examine these questions. Although the results of the later studies do not appear to be as clear cut as those of earlier studies, each is valuable in that it further defines what type of family intervention is most appropriate for what group of patients and their families. Readers are referred to articles by Dixon and Lehman (1995), Goldstein and Miklowitz (1995) and Mari and Streiner (1994, 1995) for the most up-to-date reviews of all studies which have been published to date. Because the more recent studies differ from the earlier studies in terms of control groups used, the nature of the interventions, and the settings in which they are delivered, it can be difficult to compare the studies and the results obtained.

The following section outlines what common results appear to be emerging from recent studies, and refers back to the first 'generation' studies where appropriate.

*RESEARCH UNDERPINNING FAMILY INTERVENTIONS*

*Family interventions decrease the frequency of relapse in schizophrenia*

There is no longer any doubt about the effectiveness of family interventions in schizophrenia. Studies have consistently shown that offering psychoeducational/psychosocial interventions to the family results in a significantly better outcome when compared with medication and routine follow-up only. This is the conclusion drawn by all major reviews of the research. Dixon and Lehman (1995) conclude 'there is an impressive body of evidence suggesting that family interventions are efficacious at delaying, if not preventing relapse for persons with schizophrenia who have significant family contact'.

The meta-analysis of research findings of family intervention studies conducted by Mari and Streiner (1994) made arguable assumptions in that they classified all cases lost to follow-up as relapses in the experimental group and free from relapse in the control group. In spite of this conservative approach, they concluded that family intervention proved to be an efficacious treatment when relapse was taken as the primary outcome. They further noted that these interventions were effective in decreasing hospitalisations and in improving compliance with medication. In an updated report where the results of further studies were added to the meta-analysis, Mari and Streiner (1995) once again concluded that in schizophrenia 'family intervention as part of a multi-faceted approach decreases the frequency of relapse over a period of 6 months to 2 years'. They noted that in those studies which had conducted an economic analysis, the costs of care in the group receiving the family intervention were always lower than in the routine treatment control groups. They commented on the cost–benefit balance, i.e. the costs in time and resources of family therapy compared with the costs of a single relapse and concluded that the cost–benefit ratio was acceptable to the families of those with schizophrenia as well as to most providers and managers of care. The effect of these family interventions is robust across cultures (Xiong *et al.*, 1994; Zhang *et al.*, 1994).

As most of the studies conducted so far limit the follow-up period to 2 years, and relapse typically increases in the second year, there is agreement that time-limited interventions which are not provided as part of an on-going service delay rather than prevent relapse. However, the recently reported 5- and 8-year follow-up relapse rates in the original Salford study (Tarrier *et al.*, 1994) suggest that the reduction in relapse rates is sustainable over time.

To conclude, therefore, those offering services to people with schizophrenia should without doubt be offering family intervention as part of the treatment package. The more difficult question is what types of family intervention should be offered to which families?

*Psychodynamic family interventions are not effective*

The dynamic group approach used in the study by Kottgen *et al.* (1984) did not produce significantly better outcomes than standard care. The study by McFarlane (1994) included a multifamily comparison group with a dynamic orientation. Because the group had unacceptably high relapse rates (47%) at one year, people were no longer randomised to that treatment condition. The counselling approach used by Vaughan *et al.* (1992) did not prove to be effective. The only types of approach which have first been shown to be effective are those which are psychoeducational in nature, characterised by those elements outlined in Box 8.2.

*What works for people with schizophrenia with long-standing problems whose families are rated as high EE?*

Where studies have selected high EE families and the patients are not experiencing their first episode of schizophrenia but rather have a range of disabilities, no approach other than individual family therapy where the patient is included in some if not all of the sessions has been shown to be effective. Those who have offered support groups to relatives (excluding the patient) have had major problems with high refusal or non-compliance rates (Leff *et al.*, 1989, 1990; McCarthy *et al.*, 1989; McCreadie *et al.*, 1991). The family group counselling approach used by Vaughan *et al.* (1992) was not successful. The brief crisis-oriented psychoeducational inpatient intervention offered by Glick *et al.* (1990), although possibly showing some effectiveness for women with schizophrenia, either had no effect or possibly a detrimental effect on males. Those reporting successes for other types of interventions either did not preselect for high EE (Bellack, 1995; Goldstein *et al.*, 1978; McFarlane *et al.*, 1995) or the patients had schizophrenia of recent onset (Goldstein *et al.*, 1978; Linszen *et al.*, 1996). For this group which Hogarty *et al.* (1986) describe as often being characterised as male, young, never married and living with parents, it would appear that the most effective type of family intervention is one of the successful 'first generation' interventions (Falloon *et al.*, 1982; Leff *et al.*, 1982; Hogarty *et al.*, 1986; Tarrier *et al.*, 1988).

*What do low EE families need?*

Mari and Streiner (1995) commented that the needs of low EE families have been neglected. There are indications that low EE families do need some level of intervention, and that it may be unwise in the long-term to assume that they do not have any difficulties. Tarrier *et al.* (1988) report a considerable though not significant change from low to high EE in the group who did not receive any intervention. This was not evident in the low EE group who received a brief educational intervention. They point to the risk of relatives in low EE families developing critical or hostile attitudes if they do not receive any specialist intervention. There are suggestions in the literature that detailed, lengthy interventions may not be acceptable to low EE families or may not produce the most effective results. In the Leff *et al*. (1982) study, low EE families tended to drop out of treatment. Linszen *et al*. (1996) reported slightly higher relapse rates in low EE families who were offered a full psychoeducational family intervention compared with those who received some brief educational sessions. It would appear, therefore, that low EE families need some type of intervention, but that possibly a brief number of sessions with an emphasis on education may be sufficient. It would seem sensible to add to this some system of on-going monitoring to assess if their needs have changed. This area requires further research.

*What is effective with young people experiencing a first episode of schizophrenia, or where their psychotic illness is of recent onset?*

There are indications in the literature that it is beneficial if families receive some intervention as soon as possible after the onset of a psychotic illness. Tarrier and Barrowclough (1986) note that in the absence of information from professionals, families are likely to develop their own lay views about the illness. These views may be inaccurate and may lead to behaviour and coping strategies which are unhelpful. Once established, these views can become entrenched and difficult to shift later on. Tarrier and Barrowclough (1986) therefore advise that information should be provided as soon as possible after the illness begins.

The Goldstein *et al*. (1978) study produced significant results when young people with recent onset psychotic illnesses were offered a brief crisis-oriented family intervention. Linszen *et al*. (1996) with a similar group of patients offered an inpatient brief educational treatment emphasising stress management. Those who received an intensive outpatient family intervention in addition did not have a significantly better outcome than those receiving individual treatment, and in some cases the outcome was worse. This would suggest that the brief family intervention may have been sufficient for those with psychosis of recent onset.

More research is needed into what is most beneficial to families at the onset of a psychotic illness. Even if brief educational intervention seems sufficient, as with low EE families, it would seem to be important to have an on-going monitoring system to assess changing needs.

*Continuity of care or separate family interventions*

Because for many people schizophrenia has long-term effects, there would appear to be a consensus of opinion that family intervention should be provided in the context of on-going service provision. In most studies where family intervention was effective, the family therapists were either case managers for the patients or had close liaison with the established services (McFarlane *et al*., 1995; Falloon *et al*., 1982; Tarrier *et al*., 1988; Brooker *et al*., 1994). Linszen *et al*. (1996) emphasise the importance of continuity of care. The intervention in the unsuccessful Vaughan *et al*. (1992) study was offered by a separate research team, and this was identified by the authors as one of the reasons for the lack of success of the intervention. Vaughan *et al.* (1992) conclude that the use of an intervention that does not take responsibility for patient management or that does not liaise with the established services appears to be ineffective.

*Are multifamily groups as effective as individual family interventions?*

The question arises as to whether it would be more economic, in terms of staff time and finances, to provide interventions to groups of families rather than to individual families. The study by McFarlane *et al.* (1995) demonstrated superior results for multifamily group therapy over individual family therapy. Similar results were reported from the NIMH study (Keith *et al.*, 1989; Bellack, 1995; Schooler *et al.*, 1989) where no significant differences were found between those who received a Falloon style behavioural family therapy intervention and those who attended multifamily group meetings. Bellack (1995) reported relapse rates at 2 years of 29% for the individual family therapy group (Applied Family Management) and 35% for the multifamily group therapy (Supported Family Management). These studies were conducted with people with a range of psychotic disorders and the families were not assessed for EE status. It is not clear, therefore, for which groups of patients and relatives the intervention was most successful. Patients were included in the multifamily group sessions, and family group interventions which have not included the person with the disorder have not been shown to be effective or have very high non-compliance rates (Vaughan *et al.*, 1992; McCarthy *et al.*, 1989; McCreadie *et al.*, 1991; Leff *et al.*, 1989). The Leff *et al.* (1989) intervention was successful only for those highly motivated families who attended the groups.

The McFarlane *et al.* (1995) intervention proved to be particularly effective for those families where the patients had a preponderance of positive psychotic symptoms. There are indications that in families where positive symptoms are not the central issue, a more low key, supportive family group intervention may be helpful (McCarthy *et al.*, 1989; Kuipers *et al.*, 1989). More research needs to be conducted to clarify when multi-group family interventions are most effective. Box 8.3 summarises what is known to date with regard to multifamily group interventions.

*Should family interventions take place in the family home or in a clinic/ hospital setting?*

The study by Randolph *et al.* (1994) successfully replicated Falloon's Behavioural Family Therapy model in a clinic setting. However, caution must be advised against drawing conclusions on the basis of this one study. Dixon and Lehman (1995) commented that, in the light of the Randolph study, there did not appear to be any evidence that intervention at home was superior to clinic-based interventions. Their conclusion does not seem warranted in the light of the fact that interventions when provided at home have been particularly successful (Falloon *et al.*, 1982; Brooker *et*

**Box 8.3** Multifamily
group interventions

◆ Engagement and compliance can be major problems.

◆ Family group interventions which do not include the
patient have not been shown to be successful in reducing
patient relapse.

◆ Multifamily groups can be particularly beneficial when the
patient has severe positive symptomatology at discharge.

◆ Supportive family groups for relatives may be helpful for
relatives of those with long-term problems though they
may not significantly decrease patient relapse rates.

*al.*, 1994) and that non-attendance/compliance rates are usually
extremely high when families have to attend sessions outside the
home (McCreadie *et al.*, 1991; McCarthy *et al.*, 1989). Leff *et al.*
(1989) had a 50% refusal rate for the clinic-based family group
intervention, but only one family refused treatment at home. It
would appear therefore that interventions are more easily accepted
by families if they are provided in the family home.

*Can family*
*interventions be*
*applied in routine*
*clinical practice?*

The studies by Brooker *et al.* (1994) and McFarlane *et al.* (1995)
demonstrate that mental health professionals can be trained in
family intervention approaches, and that the interventions can be
delivered in routine clinical practice settings. These studies suggest
that careful training and supervision is needed if family interventions are to be successfully implemented.

*Training of mental*
*health staff*

It is clear that the training of staff is a very important factor in
relation to whether interventions are successful or not. Those
studies where clinicians delivering the interventions did not
receive specialised training were not successful (Vaughan *et al.*,
1992; McCreadie *et al.*, 1991) whereas those who received training, and in particular where close supervision monitored adherence to the treatment programme, were highly successful (Brooker
*et al.*, 1994; Randolph *et al.*, 1994; McFarlane *et al.*, 1995).

*Families who are*
*difficult to engage*

Very little attention has been paid to those families who are difficult
to engage in treatment, although there is clear evidence that those
who refuse treatment or who drop out of treatment have a higher
risk of relapse (Hogarty *et al.*, 1986; Tarrier *et al.*, 1988). Leff *et al.*
(1990) reported a relapse rate of 60% over two years for those who
were unwilling or unable to accept treatment. This group of
families needs urgent attention, and efforts must be made to
conduct research on how to improve engagement strategies.

There is some evidence to suggest that it may be easier to engage families when the patient is experiencing an acute episode. The first generation studies tended to engage families at that time, and some studies where an attempt has been made at other stages during the course of the illness have had very high refusal rates (McCarthy *et al.*, 1989; McCreadie *et al.*, 1991). However, in the study by Brooker *et al.* (1994) families were not specifically engaged during an episode, but the intervention produced successful results. This may have been because the families were already on the caseloads of the community psychiatric nurses who were trained in this study.

*THE ESSENTIAL INGREDIENTS FOR SUCCESSFUL IMPLEMENTATION OF FAMILY INTERVENTIONS*

The second generation studies have added useful information to what was already known about family interventions, and there are now some points about which there is no confusion. It is clear that psychodynamic approaches are not effective, that for interventions to be successful the patient and the family must be seen together at least for some sessions, that individual family therapy is indicated for those who are not experiencing their first episode and whose families are high EE. There are indications for specific treatments in the literature which need further investigation. These include the evidence that brief educational and crisis-oriented approaches may be most appropriate for those with recent onset psychosis, and that it may be beneficial to provide low EE families with brief educational interventions. There are other issues where there are differing findings. Some clinic-based interventions are successful and some are not, and there are also varying results in relation to whether the family was engaged when the patient was episodic. Is it possible to distil the essential ingredients for the successful implementation of family interventions?

Careful reading of the literature suggests that three factors (Box 8.4) emerge as being important in influencing whether or not the treatments are successfully implemented.

With regard to the successful 'first generation' studies, the issue of training did not arise as the interventions were delivered by

**Box 8.4** Factors influencing the success of treatments

1. Training and supervision of staff – *therapist variables.*
2. Whether or not the family is engaged during an acute episode – *family variables.*
3. Whether the intervention is home based or clinic based – *interaction between therapists and family* and ease of delivery/acceptance of therapy.

**Box 8.5** Factors influencing the successful implementation of family interventions

| Study | Staff[a] | Engaged during an episode of illness | Intervention provided in the family home | Outcome[b] |
|---|---|---|---|---|
| Vaughan et al. (1992) | No | Yes | No | No |
| McCreadie et al. (1991) | No | No | No | No |
| Brooker et al. (1994) | Yes | No | Yes | Yes |
| Kuipers et al. (1989), McCarthy et al. (1989) | Yes | No | No | No |
| Randolph et al. (1994) | Yes | Yes | No | Yes |
| Linszen et al. (1996) | No | Yes | No | No |

[a] Staff: trained and supervised throughout study to monitor adherence to family intervention.
[b] Outcome: family intervention significantly better in terms of patient relapse.

those developing the programmes in question. In these studies too, the families were all engaged when the patient was episodic and in most cases some of the intervention was conducted in the family home.

It is interesting to apply these criteria to second generation studies and to observe the pattern that emerges. Box 8.5 lists a number of the more recent studies and classifies them according to the variables in Box 8.4. The first point that is clear is that the training and supervision of staff is an extremely important factor. In those studies which showed successful outcomes (Brooker et al., 1994; Randolph et al., 1994), the therapists were trained by those who developed the particular interventions in question, and their colleagues who were highly experienced trainers and therapists. Supervision was intense. Randolph et al. (1994) report that therapists had weekly supervision sessions. In the Brooker et al. (1994) study therapists provided audio tapes of clinical sessions and were rated by the trainers as being competent in Behavioural Family Therapy skills. With this level of training and supervision, in spite of the fact that each study did not meet one of the other two criteria, the outcome was successful.

When there was no training or the training was conducted by less experienced trainers, or where the supervision was not so detailed, the outcome of the family interventions was not successful. The McCreadie *et al.* (1991) study reported very poor results using a Leff-style intervention, and met none of the three criteria listed. The therapists had received no training in family interventions in schizophrenia, and this was later quoted as a contributing factor to the poor outcome (Birch, 1991). In the Vaughan *et al.* (1992) study similarly, the therapists did not receive any training, and thus the intervention provided was not based on an assessment of need. They concluded that family interventions should only be carried out by suitably trained staff. In the Linszen *et al.* (1996) study, one of the therapists was trained by an experienced team of trainers and subsequently trained the other therapists in the study. Although supervision was regular at the beginning of the study, later on supervision was only held 'when needed ... as it appeared that the therapists adhered closely to the Falloon model'. The suggestion in the study that low EE families were offered training in skills which they apparently did not need, rather than an intervention based on assessment of their skills deficits which is how Behavioural Family Therapy should be used, raises issues about the familiarity of the therapists with the Falloon approach.

**Box 8.6** Effects of staff training and supervision

It would appear that staff training and supervision are critical factors, and the existing literature suggests the following.

♦ Where training and supervision are inadequate or non-existent, the family intervention will not be successful.

♦ If training and supervision are satisfactory, the outcome can still be successful if the therapy is clinic-based provided the family is engaged during an episode when they are highly motivated. Conversely, where there are no problems with therapist skill, families can be engaged at times other than during an episode, provided they are seen at home thereby making it easier for them to engage in therapy.

♦ Even where training/supervision is satisfactory, if there are problems both with the motivation of the family and the ease with which they can receive therapy, the outcome will not be successful.

*FAMILY INTERVENTIONS IN DISORDERS OTHER THAN SCHIZOPHRENIA*

Although there is evidence that families in which one member suffers from a long-term disorder other than schizophrenia can experience similar difficulties (Fadden *et al.*, 1987b), to date there have been few studies which have attempted to apply family intervention to people with other disorders. Goldstein and Miklowitz (1994) are conducting a study where Behavioural Family Therapy is being offered to families of those with bi-polar disorder. Although the trial is not yet complete, early results look promising. Glick *et al.* (1994) report positive results after a brief psychoeducational family intervention for people with major affective disorder, and there are suggestions that those with bi-polar disorder who are female may particularly benefit from this type of approach (Clarkin *et al.*, 1990). Similarly, Anderson *et al.* (1986) reported beneficial results for a multifamily group intervention for people with affective disorders. The application of family interventions to a range of mental disorders is an area requiring further research.

*IMPLEMENTATION OF FAMILY INTERVENTIONS INTO ROUTINE CLINICAL SETTINGS*

Even though the efficacy of family interventions for schizophrenia has been clearly demonstrated, the evidence suggests that most families are not offered any detailed help. The Clinical Standards Advisory Group on Schizophrenia (Department of Health, 1995), assessed the quality of service provision in eleven representative districts in Britain, and reported that 'the availability of family approaches was limited in all districts because of the lack of trained staff, or because trained staff did not target the severely mentally ill'. White (1991) and the recent report on mental health nursing in Britain (Department of Health, 1994) point to the fact that people with schizophrenia were not being represented on the caseloads of mental health nurses in the community. The lack of targeting of those with serious mental health problems is, therefore, the first issue which must be overcome before psychosocial family interventions can be more widely disseminated.

It had been hoped in the past that specialised training in family interventions would not be necessary for trained professional staff. Kuipers and Bebbington (1985) suggested that as availability of training is likely to be limited, professionals should use the expertise afforded by their general training. However, the studies by McCreadie *et al.* (1991) and Vaughan *et al.* (1992) demonstrate clearly that when staff do not have specific training in family approaches, the outcome of their intervention is likely to be unsuccessful. It would appear that intervening with families effectively requires a range of complex skills, knowledge and attitudes.

The studies by Brooker *et al.* (1994), Randolph *et al.* (1994) and McFarlane *et al.* (1995) demonstrate that clinicians can be taught the skills necessary to implement these approaches successfully, provided skilled and experienced trainers are involved. Careful supervision is required to ensure that skills are maintained but attendance by staff in routine clinical practice at supervision sessions can be a major problem (Fadden, 1997; Brennan and Gamble, 1995). Even when staff effectively acquire the necessary skills, there is evidence that they face major difficulties in implementing these approaches in their place of work. Kavanagh *et al.* (1993) in a survey of clinicians trained in family interventions found that the average number of families seen by each therapist was 1.4. In a similar survey, Fadden (1997) reported a similar figure of 1.7 families seen by each therapist. In both surveys the main difficulties in implementing the intervention were issues to do with the services in which they worked. Those most frequently reported were difficulties integrating this work with other demands at work, allowance of time by the service to carry out the work, and lack of availability of time-in-lieu or overtime for time spent on appointments with families. Clearly, service issues such as these must be addressed before clinicians will be able to intervene effectively with families.

There is no doubt that staff training and supervision, and the integration of family intervention into existing services are the main challenges which must be addressed if the present situation where families generally do not receive intervention is to change.

*CONCLUSION*

In the early 1980s, Beels and McFarlane (1982) talked about a Utopian-style service where a range of family interventions of proven effectiveness would be available to those with severe mental health problems – brief crisis-oriented intervention for those recently diagnosed as psychotic, individual family psycho-educational intervention where this was indicated, and multifamily groups for those who would benefit from interaction with others in a similar situation. In the late 1990s, the scenario which they painted still seems Utopian. The reality is that in most services, families of those with long-term disorders receive at best limited support from professionals and very few have available to them a range of interventions appropriate for different stages of their relative's illness. The fact that effective treatments are available but are not being offered is unjustifiable on moral or ethical grounds.

If the present situation is to change, the main focus must be on developing successful methods of disseminating these interventions into ordinary clinical services. The issues to be addressed are training of clinicians, on-going supervision and monitoring of skills acquired, and how service systems need to change to facilitate this type of work. Recent attempts to train clinicians to apply these interventions in routine practice settings have demonstrated that there are major obstacles to doing this because of the way in which service systems are organised, and because of conflicting demands on staff time

(Kavanagh *et al.*, 1993; Brennan and Gamble, 1995; Fadden, 1997). This problem appears to be widespread and is not culture-bound. Resources, both in terms of finance and also the expertise of those trainers and clinicians committed to this area of work, need to be directed at finding solutions to these challenges in order that those with major mental disorders can begin to receive effective treatment.

*DISCUSSION*
*QUESTIONS*

1. Given that there is no longer any doubt about the effectiveness of family interventions, how can clinicians, service users and service providers be made more aware of this fact so that the interventions are applied more broadly than is the case at present?
2. Evidence suggests that different types of family intervention are appropriate for different patients and their families. How can this be accommodated in ordinary clinical settings so that each family receives the most efficacious intervention?
3. What is the best system for training staff so that they acquire the skills necessary for the successful implementation of these interventions, and how can adequate supervision be ensured following training?
4. What changes need to take place in clinical services to enable staff who have been trained in the use of these interventions to be able to implement what they have learnt?
5. How can clinical staff deal with the conflicting demands of different purchasers of their services so that the needs of people with serious and enduring mental health problems are adequately met?

*FURTHER READING*

◆ Anderson, C., Reiss, R. and Hogarty, G. (1986) *Schizophrenia and the Family.* New York: Guilford Press.
Describes the interventions used in the Hogarty studies. Contains particularly useful sections on engaging families in therapy. Provides a detailed description of the psychoeducational approach.

◆ Barrowclough, C. and Tarrier, N. (1992) *Families of Schizophrenic Patients – Cognitive Behavioural Intervention.* London: Chapman & Hall.
A very useful description of how a range of psychological approaches can be used in family work with sections on management of violence and suicide risk.

◆ Falloon, I., Laporta, M., Fadden, G. and Graham-Hole, V. (1993) *Managing Stress in Families.* London: Routledge.
A practical guidebook for clinicians describing how behavioural and

cognitive approaches are applied in practice. Contains several illustrative case examples.

◆ Kuipers, L., Leff, J. and Lam, D. (1992) *Family Work for Schizophrenia - A Practical Guide*. London: Gaskell.
This is a detailed manual of instructions for family work covering the practical issues that can arise. There are sections on a range of topics such as: dealing with anger, overinvolvement and grief.

**REFERENCES**    Anderson, C.M., Griffin, S., Rossi, A., Pagonis, I., Holder, D.P. and Treiber, R. (1986), A comparative study of the impact of education vs process groups for families of patients with affective disorders. *Family Process*, 25, 185–205.

Barrowclough, C. and Tarrier, N. (1990). Social functioning in schizophrenic patients. I. The effects of expressed emotion and family intervention. *Social Psychiatry and Psychiatric Epidemiology*, 25, 125–130.

Bateson, G., Jackson, D., Haley, J. and Weakland, J. (1956), Toward a theory of schizophrenia. *Behavioural Science*, 1, 251–264.

Beels, C. and McFarlane, W.R. (1982), Family treatments of schizophrenia: background and state of the art. *Hospital and Community Psychiatry*, 33, 541–550.

Bellack, A.S. (1995), The NIMH treatment strategies in schizophrenia study. Paper presented at the 1995 World Congress of Cognitive and Behavioural Psychotherapies, Copenhagen.

Birch, J. (1991), Family intervention (correspondence). *British Journal of Psychiatry*, 158, 717–718.

Birchwood, M., Smith, J. and Cochrane, R. (1992), Specific and non-specific effects of educational intervention for families living with schizophrenia: a comparison of three methods. *British Journal of Psychiatry*, 160, 806–814.

Brennan, G. and Gamble, C. (1997), Schizophrenia family work and clinical practice. *Mental Health Nursing*, 17, 12–15.

Brooker, C., Falloon, I., Butterworth, A., Goldberg, D., Graham-Hole, V. and Hillier, V. (1994), The outcome of training community psychiatric nurses to deliver psychosocial intervention. *British Journal of Psychiatry*, 165, 222–230.

Brown, G.W., Birley, J.L.T. and Wing, J.K. (1972), Influence of family life on the course of schizophrenic disorder. *British Journal of Psychiatry*, 121, 241–258.

Cardin, V.A., McGill, C.W. and Falloon, I.R.H. (1985), An economic analysis: costs, benefits and effectiveness. In: Falloon, I. (Ed) *Family Management of Schizophrenia*. Baltimore: Johns Hopkins University Press.

Clarkin, J.F., Glick, I.D., Haas, G.L. *et al.* (1990), A randomised clinical trial of inpatient family intervention. V. Results for affective disorders. *Journal of Affective Disorders*, 18, 17–28.

Creer, C. and Wing, J.K. (1974), *Schizophrenia at Home*. Surbiton, Surrey: National Schizophrenia Fellowship.

Department of Health (1994), *Working in Partnership: A Collaborative Approach to Care*. London: HMSO.

Department of Health (1995), *Report of a Clinical Standards Advisory Group on Schizophrenia*, Volume 1. London: HMSO.

Dixon, L.B. and Lehman, A.F. (1995), Family interventions for schizophrenia. *Schizophrenia Bulletin*, 21, 631–643.

Dulz, B. and Hand, I. (1986), Short-term relapse in young schizophrenics: can it be predicted and affected by family (CFI), patient and treatment variables? An experimental study. In: Goldstein, M., Hand, I. and Hahlweg, K. (Eds) *Treatment of Schizophrenia: Family Assessment and Intervention*. Berlin: Springer-Verlag.

Fadden, G. (1997), Implementation of family interventions in routine clinical practice following staff training programs: a major cause for concern. *Journal of Mental Health*, 6, 599–612.

Fadden, G., Kuipers, L. and Bebbington, P. (1987a), The burden of care: the impact of functional psychiatric illness on the patient's family. *British Journal of Psychiatry*, 150, 285–292.

Fadden, G., Bebbington, P. and Kuipers, L. (1987b), Caring and its burdens: a study of the spouses of depressed patients. *British Journal of Psychiatry*, 151, 660–667.

Falloon, I.R.H., Boyd, J.L., McGill, C.W., Razani, J., Moss, M.B. and Gilderman, A.M. (1982), Family management in the prevention of exacerbations of schizophrenia: a controlled study. *New England Journal of Medicine*, 306, 1437–1440.

Falloon, I.R.H., Boyd, J.L., McGill, C.W. *et al.* (1985), Family management in the prevention of morbidity of schizophrenia: clinical outcome of a two year longitudinal study. *Archives of General Psychiatry*, 42, 887–896.

Falloon, I.R.H., McGill, C.W., Boyd, J.L. and Pederson, J. (1987), Family management in the prevention of morbidity of schizophrenia: social outcome of a two year longitudinal study. *Psychological Medicine*, 17, 59–66.

Glick, I.D., Burti, L., Okonogi, K. and Sacks, M. (1994), Effectiveness in psychiatric care. III Psychoeducation and outcome for patients with major affective disorder and their families. *British Journal of Psychiatry*, 164, 104–106.

Glick, I.D., Spencer, J.H., Clarkin, J.F. *et al.* (1990), A randomised clinical trial of inpatient family intervention. IV Follow-up results for subjects with schizophrenia. *Schizophrenia Research*, 3, 187–200.

Goldstein, M.J. and Miklowitz, D.J. (1994), Family intervention for persons with bi-polar disorder. *New Directions for Mental Health Services*, 62, 23–35.

Goldstein, M.J. and Miklowitz, D.J. (1995), The effectiveness of psychoeducational family therapy in the treatment of schizophrenia disorders. *Journal of Marital and Family Therapy*, 21, 361–376.

Goldstein, M.J., Rodnick, E.H., Evans, J.R., May, P.R.A. and Steinberg, M.R. (1978), Drug and family therapy in the aftercare of acute schizophrenia. *Archives of General Psychiatry*, 35, 1169–1177.

Haas, G.L., Glick, I.D., Clarkin, J.F. *et al.* (1988), Inpatient family intervention. II Results at hospital discharge. *Archives of General Psychiatry*, 45, 217–224.

Hatfield, A. (1983), What families want of family therapists. In: McFarlane, W.R. (Ed) *Family Therapy in Schizophrenia*. New York: Guilford Press.

Hogarty, G.E. (1984), Depot neuroleptics: the relevance of psycho-social factors. *Journal of Clinical Psychiatry*, 45, 36–42.

Hogarty, G.E. and Ulrich, R.F. (1977), Temporal effects of drug and placebo in delaying relapse in schizophrenic out-patients. *Archives of General Psychiatry*, 34, 297–301.

Hogarty, G.E., Schooler, N.R., Ulrich, R.F., Mussare, F., Herron, E. and Ferro, P. (1979), Fluphenazine and social therapy in the aftercare of schizophrenic patients: relapse analyses of a two year controlled study of fluphenazine decanoate and fluphenazine hydrochloride. *Archives of General Psychiatry*, 36, 1283–1294.

Hogarty, G.E., Anderson, C.M., Reiss, D.J. *et al*. (1986), Family psychoeducational, social skills training and maintenance chemotherapy in the aftercare treatment of schizophrenia. I One year effects of a controlled study on relapse and expressed emotion. *Archives of General Psychiatry*, 43, 633–642.

Hogarty, G.E., Anderson, C.M., Reiss, D.J. *et al*. (1991), Family psychoeducational, social skills training and maintenance chemotherapy in the aftercare treatment of schizophrenia. II Two year effects of a controlled study on relapse and adjustment. *Archives of General Psychiatry*, 48, 340–347.

Johnson, D.A.W. (1976), The duration of maintenance therapy in chronic schizophrenia. *Acta Psychiatrica Scandinavica*, 53, 298–301.

Kavanagh, D.J., Piatkowska, O., Clarke, D. *et al*. (1993), Application of cognitive-behavioural family intervention for schizophrenia in multidisciplinary teams: what can the matter be? *Australian Psychologist*, 28, 181–188.

Keith, S.J., Bellack, A., Frances, A., Mance, R. and Matthews, S. (1989), The Treatment Strategies in Schizophrenia Collaborative Study Group. The influence of diagnosis and family treatment on acute treatment response and short-term outcome in schizophrenia. *Psychopharmacology Bulletin*, 25, 336–339.

Kottgen, C., Sonnichsen, I., Mollenhauer, K. and Jurth, R. (1984), Group therapy with families of schizophrenic patients: results of the Hamburg Camberwell – Family Interview study III. *International Journal of Family Psychiatry*, 5, 83–94.

Kuipers, L. and Bebbington, P. (1985), Relatives as a resource in the management of functional illness. *British Journal of Psychiatry*, 147, 465–470.

Kuipers, L., McCarthy, B., Hurry, J. and Harper, R. (1989), Counselling the relatives of the long-term adult mentally ill. II A low cost supportive model. *British Journal of Psychiatry*, 154, 775–782.

Laing, R.D. (1960), *The Divided Self: An Existential Study in Sanity and Madness*. London: Penguin Books.

Lam, D. (1991), Psychosocial family intervention in schizophrenia. *Psychological Medicine*, 21, 423–441.

Leff, J., Kuipers, L., Berkowitz, R., Eberlein-Vries, R. and Sturgeon, D. (1982), A controlled trial of social intervention in the families of schizophrenic patients. *British Journal of Psychiatry*, 141, 121–134.

Leff, J., Kuipers, L., Berkowitz, R. and Sturgeon, D. (1985), A controlled trial of social intervention in the families of schizophrenic patients: two year follow-up. *British Journal of Psychiatry*, 146, 594–600.

Leff, J., Berkowitz, R., Shavit, N., Strachan, A., Glass, I. and Vaughn, C. (1989), A trial of family therapy v. a relatives' group for schizophrenia. *British Journal of Psychiatry*, 154, 58–66.

Leff, J., Berkowitz, R., Shavit, N., Strachan, A., Glass, I. and Vaughn, C. (1990), A trial of family therapy versus a relatives' group for schizophrenia: two year follow-up. *British Journal of Psychiatry*, 154, 571–577.

Leff, J.P. and Vaughn, C. (1981), The role of maintenance therapy and relatives' expressed emotion in relapse in schizophrenia: a two year follow-up. *British Journal of Psychiatry*, 139, 102–104.

Leff, J.P. and Wing, J.K. (1971), Trial of maintenance therapy in schizophrenia. *British Medical Journal*, iii, 599–604.

Lidz, T. (1975), *The Origin and Treatment of Schizophrenic Disorders*. London: Hutchinson.

Linszen, D., Dingemans, P., Van Der Does, J.M. *et al.* (1996), Treatment, expressed emotion and relapse in recent onset schizophrenic disorders. *Psychological Medicine*, 26, 333–342.

Mari, J.D. and Streiner, D.L. (1994), An overview of family interventions and relapse on schizophrenia: meta-analysis of research findings. *Psychological Medicine*, 24, 565–578.

Mari, J.D. and Streiner, D. (1995), Family intervention and schizophrenia. *The Cochrane Database of Systematic Reviews*, Issue 1.

McCarthy, B., Kuipers, L., Hurry, J., Harper, R. and LeSage, A. (1989), Counselling the relatives of the long-term adult mentally ill. I Evaluation of the impact on relatives and patients. *British Journal of Psychiatry*, 154, 768–775.

McCreadie, R.G., Phillips, K., Harvey, J.A., Waldron, G., Stewart, M. and Baird, D. (1991), The Nithsdale Schizophrenia Surveys. VIII Do relatives want family intervention – and does it help? *British Journal of Psychiatry*, 158, 110–113.

McFarlane, W.R. (1994), Multiple family groups and psychoeducation in the treatment of schizophrenia. *New Directions for Mental Health Services*, 62, 13–23.

McFarlane, W.R., Lukens, E., Link, B. *et al.* (1995), Multiple family groups and psychoeducation in the treatment of schizophrenia. *Archives of General Psychiatry*, 52, 679–687.

Nuechterlein, K.H. and Dawson, M.E. (1984), A heuristic vulnerability – stress model of schizophrenic episodes. *Schizophrenia Bulletin*, 10, 300–312.

Randolph, E.T., Eth, S., Glynn, S.M. *et al.* (1994), Behavioural family management in schizophrenia: outcome of a clinic-based intervention. *British Journal of Psychiatry*, 164, 501–506.

Schooler, N.R., Keith, S.J., Severe, J.B., Matthews, S. and the Treatment Strategies in Schizophrenia Collaborative Study Group (1989), Acute treatment response and short-term outcome in schizophrenia. *Psychopharmacology Bulletin*, 25, 331–335.

Schooler, N.R., Levine, J., Severe, J.B. *et al.* (1980), Prevention of relapse in schizophrenia: an evaluation of fluphenazine decanoate. *Archives of General Psychiatry*, 37, 16–24.

Scottish Schizophrenia Research Group (1992), The Scottish first episode schizophrenia study. VIII. Five year follow-up: clinical and psychosocial findings. *British Journal of Psychiatry*, 161, 496–500.

Smith J. and Birchwood, M. (1987), Education for families with schizophrenic relatives. *British Journal of Psychiatry*, 150, 645–652.

Smith, J. and Birchwood, M. (1990), Relatives and patients as partners in the management of schizophrenia: the development of a service model. *British Journal of Psychiatry*, 156, 654–660.

Spencer, J.H., Glick, I.D., Haas, G.L. *et al.* (1988), A randomised clinical trial of inpatient family intervention III: Effects at 6 month and 18 month follow-ups. *American Journal of Psychiatry*, 145, 1115–1121.

Strachan, A.M. (1986), Family intervention for the rehabilitation of schizophrenia: toward protection and coping. *Schizophrenia Bulletin*, 12, 678–698.

Tarrier, N. and Barrowclough, C. (1986), Providing information to relatives about schizophrenia: some comments. *British Journal of Psychiatry*, 149, 458–463.

Tarrier, N., Barrowclough, C., Porceddu, K. and Fitzpatrick, E. (1994), The Salford intervention project: relapse rates of schizophrenia at five and eight years. *British Journal of Psychiatry*, 165, 829–832.

Tarrier, N., Barrowclough, C., Vaughan, K. *et al.* (1988), The community management of schizophrenia: a controlled trial of behavioural intervention with families to reduce relapse. *British Journal of Psychiatry*, 153, 532–542.

Tarrier, N., Barrowclough, C., Vaughn, C. *et al.* (1989), Community management of schizophrenia: a two year follow-up of a behavioural intervention with families. *British Journal of Psychiatry*, 154, 625–628.

Vaughan, K., Doyle, M., McConahy, N., Blaszczynski, A., Fox, A. and Tarrier, N. (1992), The Sydney intervention trial: a controlled trial of relatives' counselling to reduce schizophrenic relapse. *Social Psychiatry and Psychiatric Epidemiology*, 27, 16–21.

Vaughn, C. (1986), Comments on Chapter 5. In: Goldstein, M., Hand, I. and Hahlweg, K. (Eds) *Treatment of Schizophrenia: Family Assessment and Intervention*. Berlin: Springer-Verlag.

Vaughn, C. and Leff, J.P. (1976), The influence of family and social factors on the course of psychiatric illness. *British Journal of Psychiatry*, 129, 125–137.

White, E. (1991), *The Third Quinquennial Survey of Community Psychiatric Nursing Services*. University of Manchester: Department of Nursing Monograph.

Wyatt, R. (1991), Neuroleptics and the natural course of schizophrenia. *Schizophrenia Bulletin*, 17, 325–352.

Xiong, W., Phillips, M.R., Hu, X. *et al.* (1994), Family-based intervention for schizophrenic patients in China: a randomised controlled trial. *British Journal of Psychiatry*, 165, 239–247.

Zhang, M., Wang, M., Li, J. and Philips, M. (1994), Randomised control trial of family intervention for 78 first episode male schizophrenic patients: an 18 month study in Suzhou, Jiangsu. *British Journal of Psychiatry*, 165 (Suppl. 24), 96–102.

Zubin, J. and Spring, B. (1977), Vulnerability – a new view of schizophrenia. *Journal of Abnormal Psychology*, 86, 103–126.

# CHAPTER 9

# Cognitive Behaviour Therapy for Severe Mental Illness

## Strategies and Techniques

## David G. Kingdon

**KEY ISSUES**

- ♦ How cognitive behaviour therapy (CBT) can be used for severe mental illness
- ♦ The application of CBT for different conditions
- ♦ The evidence for the efficacy of CBT

**INTRODUCTION**

Cognitive behaviour therapy (CBT) has been developing as a treatment for mental health problems over the past thirty to forty years. It has been commonly used for a wide range of mental health problems including depression and anxiety. More recently it has been developed for use in schizophrenia and personality disorder. Until relatively recently the emphasis has been on common but less severe disorders but there has been interest in using CBT with severe mental health problems since the early 1950s. Beck published a case study in 1952 (Beck, 1952) of the successful use of structured reasoning techniques and homework assignments with a patient who had paranoid psychosis, believing that the KGB were coming into his shop to check on him.

Unfortunately for those suffering from psychosis a change in job apparently led to Beck's attention being switched to research into depression. This chapter will review techniques used in severe mental illness and refer to relevant sources for further reading.

Cognitive behaviour therapy is based on a theory of the emotional disorders (Box 9.1). It is rooted in experimental and

**Box 9.1** Cognitive behaviour therapy

Based on:

♦ Beck and Ellis's theories of emotional disorders

♦ Experimental and research studies

♦ Defined therapy techniques
  problem-oriented
  aimed at changing errors or biases in cognitions
  involving appraisal of situations and stresses
  modifying assumptions about self, the world and the future.

Sources: Beck (1976) and Blackburn and Davidson (1990).

research studies and these continue to develop. Evaluation is fundamental not only in the evolution of CBT but also in terms of work with each individual. Controlled studies with independent evaluation are accepted as legitimate methods to demonstrate overall efficacy; and in individual therapy, checking out patients' responses and reactions to the therapy and therapist are an essential part of intervention. Cognitive behaviour therapy uses defined therapy techniques which tend to be problem-oriented; feelings are certainly not ignored but generally these are linked to thoughts or perceptions and that connection becomes the major focus of treatment. This means changing errors or biases in cognitions following appraisal of situations and stresses. It may also involve reviewing and where appropriate modifying assumptions about one's self, the world and the future.

The concept of automatic thoughts is very important in cognitive behaviour therapy but not always easy to understand or explain to patients. As you read this chapter, on occasion and for varying periods, you will be concentrating on the written word but you may also be thinking, for example, 'I'm getting bored, I think I'll make a cup of tea' or 'what does he mean?'. The thoughts occurring may even seem quite unrelated although often inspired by connection with a perception, e.g. the smell of cooking produces thoughts about meals, or the sound of someone speaking leads to thoughts about the person or what they are saying. It is this flow of automatic thoughts that is important to capture as such thoughts may be relevant to the continuation or even development of mental health problems in the patient. For example, when someone experiences a bereavement, their thoughts might be 'I'm sad that my mother has died', 'I will miss her', 'I'll never cope without her'. The latter thought is especially depressing and would be expected to interfere with the person's

**Box 9.2** The cognitive
therapy scale

♦ General therapeutic skills
    agenda-setting
    feedback
    understanding
    interpersonal effectiveness
    collaboration
    pacing and efficient use of time

♦ Conceptualisation, strategy and techniques
    guided discovery
    focusing on key cognitions and behaviours
    strategy for change
    application of C–B techniques
    homework

Sources: Young and Beck (1980) and Burns (1980).

life significantly if it persisted. However, once this thought has been identified, it can be discussed and different ways of coping with it can be examined.

There are certain characteristics which are a part of cognitive behaviour therapy and these are defined in the Cognitive Therapy Scale (Box 9.2). They are in two parts: general therapeutic skills and conceptualisation, strategy and techniques. General skills include agenda-setting, feedback, understanding, interpersonal effectiveness, collaboration, pacing and efficient use of time. Specific techniques might include: guided discovery, focusing on key cognitions and behaviours, strategy for change, application of cognitive-behavioural techniques and setting of homework.

Surprisingly there is little evidence that the competence of therapists correlates to how well a person responds to therapy. However, using this scale it has been possible to demonstrate the influence of therapist competence on outcome. In a study of the use of cognitive behaviour therapy in neurotic disorder, mental health nurses working as part of mental health teams and undertaking the research part-time, were given a basic training in cognitive behaviour therapy (see below: Tyrer *et al.*, 1988). Therapists were allocated according to their competence, as defined by attributes on the Cognitive Therapy Scale which were established during supervision and training. Those who were judged more competent had better outcomes (Kingdon *et al.*, 1996). There is therefore some empirical evidence that training and supervision are effective, which may seem obvious, but in many services there remains an ethos that 'it's all common-sense anyway' and staff simply muddle along. This seriously detracts from the potential effectiveness of a CBT service for patients with a serious mental illness.

The study cited above, which was part of the Nottingham study of neurotic disorder, is relevant to this chapter because it defined certain areas in which therapists with a basic knowledge of cognitive behaviour therapy were effective or otherwise (similar results have been found in the US (Elkin *et al.*, 1989)). The patients had diagnoses of generalised anxiety disorder, panic disorder and dysthymia and were allocated at random to treatment with dothiepin (28 patients), diazepam (28), placebo (28), a self-help treatment programme (42) and cognitive behaviour therapy (84). They received either six weeks of drug treatment, five one-hour sessions of cognitive behaviour therapy, five 15-minute sessions introducing the self-help treatment programme (which basically consisted of a relaxation exercise cassette with advice on how to use it and how to make contact with local self-help groups) or placebo. The outcome of the study was that those in the 'diazepam' group had particularly poor outcomes and sought extra treatments most frequently. Both cognitive behaviour therapy and antidepressant medication seemed equally effective especially in the group who were also found to have personality disorder (as defined using the Personality Assessment Schedule). Patients who did not have a personality disorder also responded well to the self-help treatment. About 36% of the group had a personality disorder and their symptoms were rated as more severe both subjectively and objectively. Those with personality disorder made improvements but did less well than those without personality disorder; they did less well in placebo, self-help and diazepam groups, but as well with cognitive behaviour therapy and dothiepin. This has implications for the management of minor neurotic disorder and personality disorder, suggesting that those who will have enduring problems are those who have not responded to antidepressants, self-help or basic CBT, but that these interventions ought to be attempted first (possibly in the order presented above). People with a diagnosis of personality disorder are especially likely to be among this group and are discussed further below.

## PERSONALITY DISORDER

It might seem strange for a chapter on the use of CBT in severe mental health problems to discuss personality disorder before other mental health problems, nonetheless the appropriate assessment and management of personality disorder is becoming recognised increasingly as an important area. Personality disorder is very common among those with enduring problems but is often missed or poorly managed. It can even be argued that the hallmark of success for a community mental health team is the manner in which it offers intervention for this group of people. This is because there is such potential for conflict with other agencies, the local community and, of course, within the team itself. A clear understanding and consistent management of personality disorder cannot resolve all these difficulties but can help to improve relationships both for the individuals concerned and between the agencies involved.

If assessment of the individual's personality prior to illness onset is not undertaken in a competent manner, the goals and objectives of therapy may be unrealistic in terms of the time allowed for change and inappropriate in the intervention techniques used. This can be profoundly dispiriting for patient and therapist alike. If a person has developed characteristics over many years, the likelihood is that they will find change and adaptation of them difficult, perhaps even more than of their symptoms which may have been present for shorter periods.

There are many classifications of personality disorder available and a small number of instruments available to measure it. In clinical practice, use of such instruments is cumbersome and usually impractical, but a simple classification of disorder is essential so that appropriate management strategies can be developed. Tyrer *et al.* (1988) have used a personality assessment schedule to derive five categories which encompass the common groupings relevant to mental health practice: obsessional, dependent, schizoid, antisocial and no personality disorder.

Beck *et al.* (1990) include others such as borderline, avoidant, paranoid, histrionic, passive–aggressive and narcissistic. Unfortunately there are few controlled studies of management of personality disorder and this includes the use of CBT in personality disorder. The notable exception is the study by Linehan *et al.* (1993) with borderline personality disorder, and also the research led by Tyrer cited above. Linehan *et al.*'s work is practical and a pilot study has shown that the approach has potential. She used the rather intimidating term 'dialectical behaviour therapy' to describe a development of cognitive behaviour therapy.

Assessment of personality involves reviewing patterns of relationships before mental health problems presented. The personal history provides a standard model to use and can be very effective in determining nature, stability or the pattern of breakdown in relationships (past and current: with parents or other carers in childhood, siblings, schoolfriends, teachers, and later with employers, friends, police and partners). After assessment, an early step is collaboration on negotiating agreed and realistic objectives which are subscribed to by all involved – informal and formal carers and the individual themselves. These objectives need to be flexible and to develop as earlier ones are achieved. They may be very simple but may need to be regularly discussed and reviewed and only changed by mutual consent. In the early stages, frequent regular sessions are necessary to reduce crisis responses.

There will often be demands for immediate assistance to deal with ongoing anxiety and depressive symptoms. Measures to reduce such distress are necessary but so is patience to allow them to work. Dependency can develop rapidly and initially may need to be accepted by a service if it is a pre-existing component of the disorder. This may mean initial support in residential settings, e.g. hospital wards and therapeutic communities, followed by a gradual reduction in contact as coping strategies develop in more independent settings. For example, we have found that initial admission in crisis to a ward may be inevitable but gradual attendance at a day hospital or day centre from the ward enables controlled discharge – usually after a period of a few weeks – to day care. This breaks the cycle of repeated crisis calls to GPs or mental health workers, admissions to medical wards with overdoses of medication or substance abuse, or visits to accident and emergency departments with self-inflicted lacerations. Linehan *et al.* (1993) describe forming a contract with the patients to abstain from self-harming behaviour for a specified period. This can be a very difficult negotiation, but it can often be successfully established if it is made clear that the contract is for a time-limited period. This allows other interventions to be introduced which are more likely to be effective in dealing with the distressing symptoms the person is experiencing. The development of assertiveness and anxiety management skills can then begin.

Individuals with personality disorder tend to be very sensitive to any negative comment about themselves and respond either with hopelessness or hostility so it can be difficult to look at the pattern their relationships have taken. It may be more productive to concentrate first on current relationships, close ones if they have any or more superficial ones, e.g. with ward staff. When such associations are not satisfactory, using a gentle questioning approach to enable people to understand where they might have been misunderstood or misunderstood another's intentions, can be productive. For example, 'What do you think he meant by that? Could he have meant something else?'. It is tempting to interpret schemata (see below) to individuals (as is essentially done in psychoanalysis) but possibly counterproductive. These are such fundamental beliefs that there is a great deal to be gained from letting the person draw their own conclusions and, most importantly, learn that alternative ways of behaving are associated with improvements in their relationships. This can require courage as it means taking risks with new ways of responding and support may be needed from the therapist over such periods as well as for the relapses to previous ways of behaving. Continuity and consistency can be difficult to give but necessary. Positive reinforcement of small gains and patience with slow progress or relapse, while being clear about boundaries, can reap rewards. The principles for management of personality disorder emphasise being and appearing to be explicitly non-judgemental but limit-setting in a flexible and fair way. The need to avoid being engulfed while being collaborative, is a difficult balance to achieve, but including the individual and others involved in their care is important. The aim is for people with a personality disorder to develop coping strategies and to learn how their actions have both positive and negative consequences for themselves and others (see example in Box 9.3).

Other approaches using cognitive behaviour therapy have focused on the importance of detection and modification of the individual's maladaptive schemata (Beck *et al.*, 1990). Our minds make sense of the world around us and our relationships with other people by organising what we perceive, i.e. see and hear, into recognisable forms, which can be defined as 'schemata'. For the most part, this is not simply useful but is essential, e.g. black, furry creatures with green eyes which meow are necessarily perceived as cats with implications for our behaviour towards them. However, these schemata may be maladaptive and doctors, social workers or nurses, for example, may be viewed as threatening authority figures who are unlikely to be sympathetic. This may be appropriate to a person's experience but for it to be generalised to all doctors, social workers and nurses and for the person to act as if this were so, is likely to seriously interfere in the person's ability to receive assistance from them. Schemata can fundamentally affect relationships, e.g. they may take the form of 'I am needy and weak' (dependent personality disorder) or 'If I don't push people, they'll push me around' (antisocial personality disorder). Beck *et al.* (1990) provide a very useful list of such schemata. Understanding and recognising them can assist the therapist in developing a management plan to work with the maladaptive schemata that the person is using, thus eventually assisting the person themselves.

Probably most important of all in working with people with personality disorder is not to do so alone. It is very important to work as part of a team with appropriate supervision – Linehan specifically puts this in place for all those trained by her.

***AFFECTIVE DISORDER***

Affective disorder occurring as a severe and enduring mental illness is quite common in most populations. The use of the techniques developed in the management of anxiety and depression by Ellis and Beck has been very well described by many authors (see especially Blackburn and Davidson, 1990). There is emerging evidence that the use of CBT can reduce relapse and be effective in depression which is unresponsive to other measures (Scott, 1995, 1996).

When long-standing affective disorder is experienced two factors seem to be of particular importance: personality and social circumstances (especially dysfunctional relationships). If unrecognised, dependent personality disorder can significantly confuse treat-

**Box 9.3** Case study 1

Peter, aged 29, had self-lacerated since the age of 14. This self-injurious behaviour had begun after a period where he had been bullied repeatedly at school. Parental support was absent and he was alienated from his peers. His arms and legs revealed multiple overlapping scars and other areas of his body had a variety of tattoos. He had formed a relationship with a supportive young woman but this was theatened by his impulsive behaviour and irritable mood.

He was seen by the therapist first while in the local accident and emergency department awaiting suturing of wounds. It was agreed that a collaborative approach to understanding his 'need' to self-lacerate and the development of alternative strategies was worth pursuing. He was assisted in isolating the thoughts which led up to him self-lacerating. These consisted of angry cognitions that generalised to 'everybody' accompanied by increasing agitation. The origin of these thoughts in past incidents was traced and his over-generalisation to current situations explored. Laceration gave him an overwhelming sense of relief but it was agreed that there were negative aspects to it in relation to its effect on his girlfriend and others. Over the next eighteen months, these thoughts and underlying beliefs were pursued and alternative coping strategies developed which included anxiety and anger management training, day care and pharmacotherapy. This was successful in reducing his impulsiveness, abolishing the self-lacerating and preserving the relationship with his girlfriend.

ment, which may be directed at the treatment of depression when the focus may need to shift to the development of coping strategies and family interventions (Box 9.4). Specific dysfunctional relationships, particularly marital relations, can produce continuing problems.

Manic episodes may prove particularly amenable to relapse prevention techniques when these occur in patients despite the use of lithium carbonate. Such techniques may be an alternative to the drug when patients are not prepared to accept such a prescription. Perry *et al.* (1995) have recently described a patient with whom they collaboratively developed an understanding of the early signs of hypomania (impaired judgement, over-excitement or disturbed sleep), and prepared a strategy to deal with them to abort episodes. This could involve techniques to reduce stress, control substance abuse or simply to restrain exuberance, and also early use of medication. The nature of hypomania is such that

**Box 9.4** Case study 2

> Jean, aged 51, had been persistently depressed for over four years. This had commenced when her mother died. Over the period, her husband had been working long hours and her daughters, now aged 22, 24 and 25, had got boyfriends and one had married. Her relationship with her own mother had been a very close one, such that they had effectively been 'best friends'. Exploring with Jean her assumptions about mother–daughter relationships, it emerged that she assumed that her relationship with her daughters would replicate that of her own with her mother. This had not happened and left her demoralised, depressed and isolated after her mother died, compounding the distress of the bereavement. Establishing this as a factor in the persistence of her depressive symptoms has allowed her to look at alternative ways of reducing her isolation.

insight may be impaired but in the early stages can be sufficiently preserved to enable the patient to appreciate both the onset of problems (or accept the judgement of friends and relatives that they may be developing) and the potential negative effects that such episodes can have. The implementation of this strategy appeared to be successful with the patient described and is now the subject of a controlled study.

## SCHIZOPHRENIA

Research into the use of CBT in schizophrenia has increased significantly over the past five years and research studies have suggested that it is an effective treatment to complement family intervention and pharmacology. These interventions are based, therefore, on evidence but further research is needed before they can be described as an essential component in the management of patients with schizophrenia. However, it could be said that current methods for working with patients, such as the use of supportive techniques concentrating on symptoms and signs, are backed by even less empirical validation. The techniques which are now described are being used by an increasing number of therapists and seem to be proving effective in clinical practice. Experience of using cognitive behaviour therapy in depression and anxiety, working with patients with schizophrenia, and an understanding of the theoretical basis for the use of these techniques are invaluable when working in this manner (Haddock and Slade, 1996; Fowler *et al.*, 1995; Kingdon and Turkington, 1994). Supervision by an experienced therapist is important, although peer supervision by other therapists can be an alternative where the former is not possible. Working alone can be very strenuous and at times dispiriting. Discussion with others assists in learning the techniques and gives support in using them.

***Getting started***  With any new patient it is necessary to assemble available information before seeing them, but this is particularly important in patients with schizophrenia. Such data collection is, at worst, omitted or undertaken half-heartedly either because the onset of the illness was years before or the patient is unable to remember or describe the circumstances fully themselves. When this is the case, casenotes (medical, nursing, social work or psychology), the referrer or family may be able to supplement available information. The large bulging file can often contain invaluable information and, however daunting it may seem, it is usually worth reading in a selective manner. Where case notes are missing or the person has moved around a lot, the family doctor's 'Lloyd George' file may have information going back to the start of problems and may provide relevant data. This is important because apparently unintelligible speech and delusions often become meaningful once the past history is understood.

However, to balance this, it is essential not to make assumptions and as far as possible to confirm information found elsewhere with the patient to establish accuracy. A common information base should be established so that when patient and clinician come to differ about the conclusions arising from this information, both can see clearly where such differences lie and then begin to explore and eventually understand reasons for the discrepancies.

It is important to have an agenda in mind before the first session, e.g.:

♦ introduction – who you are; why you're seeing them: '... to talk about the problems you've been having ...'
♦ inquire into major current concerns
♦ trace the history of the problems
♦ take a personal history
♦ review current needs
♦ finally, check with patient whether they have any concerns about your conversation.

Any agenda needs to be flexible and to be checked with the patient at a reasonably early stage in the session as there may be other matters they want to discuss. A start will usually be made on most agenda items in the first session with someone who is presenting with a first episode of schizophrenia, but this may not be the case with someone with longer-term problems. Completion of discussion of any of the items is unlikely as each will usually need to be returned to over subsequent sessions. However, where agenda items have not been sufficiently explored they need to be noted for return and completion later. Early omissions are sometimes easily forgotten and assumptions can then be made at a later stage on insufficient evidence. You may think you know more about the patient's early teenage years and family background, for example, than may actually be the case.

*Inquiry into major concerns*

After a brief introduction, 'Maybe you could tell me about what's been happening' is a very simple statement to start with. Taking a non-directive stance quickly establishes how free the patient feels, or is able, to talk. A general exploration of their concerns avoiding any judgemental statements or even opinions – even when these are asked for – allows information to be gathered and a rapport to be built up. If the patient is unresponsive, it may be necessary to prompt from anything factual known from their history. If they are thought-disordered, initially allowing them to flow can help to establish contact but then it becomes very important to start to focus on one problem at a time. There is some debate about whether the most central delusional belief should be avoided until less emotionally important ones have been explored, but in practice beliefs are usually intertwined and that which the patient most wants to discuss usually becomes the focus.

*Trace antecedents of onset*

Fairly early on in the assessment determine when the problems began: 'When did this all start?' or, if they have difficulty determining a precise starting point, 'When did you last feel well?'. Most patients will have some idea of when their problems began and some will have a clear view of their circumstances at the time. On the other hand, a few with longer histories may have little memory of events or have had such a gradual onset that they are quite uncertain of its beginning. Others may resist any implication that they have had any problems, in which case switch the discussion to when others first started showing concern, e.g. 'When did other people start telling you they thought something was wrong?' or 'When did you first see a psychiatrist or come into hospital?'. If there are still problems it may be appropriate to use their delusional beliefs or hallucinations as the object of inquiry, e.g. 'When do you think that the government started sending agents to follow you?' (if such beliefs have been expressed), or 'When did you first hear these voices/people swearing at you?'. There is a fine line between colluding with the patient and retaining a detached, sceptical but sympathetic viewpoint and it is important not to cross it. The emphasis on 'do you think/did you hear' allows the latter line to be taken without colluding.

The aim is to build a picture of the period preceding the onset of symptoms. Questions like 'What had been happening to you?', 'What was happening to you at the time?', 'Where were you living?', 'What were you doing?', 'Who were you seeing?' and 'Where were you working?' allow you to begin to construct a view with the patient of how things were before they went wrong. Using assessment of the personal history to build up a biography from birth through childhood to adulthood, including details of family, schooling, jobs and relationships, can allow the problem period to be approached in a non-threatening way. If they ask why you want to know about these personal matters, the explanation is that you need to understand their background to understand the problems they are having now; but you then need to make clear that they are quite free to tell you just what they want you to know. If they are hesitant, reiterate that they can move onto something else if they wish. Gentle inquiry ('guided discovery') is much more successful than probing questions, especially in the patient with paranoia.

*Developing explanations*

### *The vulnerability-stress model of schizophrenia*

The 'vulnerability-stress' model of schizophrenia has been increasingly accepted as the most useful in understanding this diagnosis. It is also one which can be explained reasonably easily to lay people. Basically the theory proposes that individuals have various characteristics which make them vulnerable to schizophrenia when they are subject to stress. The personal history will give information on these vulnerabilities, specifically any family history of mental health problems, birth difficulties, brain injury or relevant personality types (schizoid and paranoid). Tracing the antecedents of problems allows isolation of relevant stressors, e.g. work, school, university, family, sexuality or isolation. Drug or alcohol abuse may also be stressors in their own right. There remains some controversy about the role of stress in bringing on schizophrenia but it certainly seems to play a part in provoking relapse.

Explanations for patients involve suggesting that they may have been particularly vulnerable to becoming ill because of, e.g. a family history coupled with specific or excessive stress. Recovery becomes more likely as the stress reduces or is coped with more successfully. However, there may be secondary factors maintaining their illness, for example becoming unemployed, relatives' and friends' attitudes, or likely loss of self-esteem. Dealing with these perpetuating factors is a particularly important part of any intervention.

The stress-vulnerability model of schizophrenia also implies a continuum between schizophrenia and 'normality' rather than there being neat distinctions between the two. There is some evidence to confirm this view inasmuch as the symptoms of schizophrenia do vary such that normal perceptions can blend into 'pseudohallucinations' and these in turn can translate to hallucinations; similarly normal ideas can become 'overvalued' and lead to delusions which can vary in how strongly they are held. It is probably important for patients to know that, because of their symptoms, they are not distinctly different from others although this is not, in any way, intended to suggest that these experiences are not often both severely disabling and distressing.

### Normalising rationale for individual symptoms

The symptoms that patients experience may be very confusing to them and to the therapist. Developing a common language is necessary in order to make progress and to understand the factors that might precipitate or exacerbate them. There are a number of states in which symptoms similar and, at times, identical to schizophrenia can occur (summarised in Kingdon and Turkington, 1994). For example, people deprived of sleep may gradually develop paranoid delusions and hallucinations; similarly people who experience sensory deprivation or hostage situations can do the same. Such 'altered states of consciousness' may also lead to heightened suggestibility. Explaining to patients that the symptoms they have can be experienced by people in these sorts of stressful situations may open up ways of discussing any relevance to their own situation. For example, many patients experience sleeping problems prior to the onset of symptoms or relapse so it may be helpful to ask 'Were you sleeping properly at the time?'. If not, try 'Do you think that might have had an effect? what sort of effect?' and explaining that often when people don't sleep properly there can be a range of effects which include tiredness, confusion, depression, anxiety, even ideas of reference, paranoia and hearing voices. Although states of deprivation can be relevant, more often it is the stress caused by isolation that is most relevant, such as changing work circumstances or moving house. It may be worth asking 'Were you on your own a lot?' and, if so, explaining that 'What can happen is that things can get you down or confuse you when there is nobody around to help you work them out and stop them getting out of proportion'.

### Reframing as cultural beliefs

A particular problem with the way in which symptoms of schizophrenia are approached is that they are often 'mystified' by being given technical terms such as 'thought broadcasting' or 'passivity phenomena', although readily available terminology exists. For example, 'thought broadcasting and insertion' is often referred to by patients as 'telepathy'. Inquiring 'Do you think people read your thoughts?' or asking whether they believe that they can read others' thoughts establishes whether these phenomena are present. Then asking 'What is it that makes you believe your thoughts are being read?' establishes the evidence which supports this belief. Often, however, there is little that they can cite specifically. Some patients believe that close members of their family or nursing staff are involved, and here it is reasonable to ask 'Why not check out with the nurses/your family if they can read your thoughts?'.

Establish the mechanisms that might be at work within the context of a patient's belief system. Many patients simply jump to the conclusion that such phenomena are occurring without any or much consideration of how they might be taking place. 'Do you mean something like telepathy?' begins to provide a common language to use. 'Do you know much about telepathy?' allows a discussion about the phenomena to develop: 'There have been some experiments to find out if telepathy actually exists; but the most that has ever been shown is that, at best, people were able to guess colours or shapes more often than you'd expect by chance but even that's disputed. They have never shown that more complex thoughts can be transmitted.' After seeing whether the patient has at least heard this, an alternative explanation can be suggested, 'Do you think you might just be very sensitive to the way people are feeling – and they to you …?', i.e. 'Could it be that people are quite sensitive to how you are, and responding to that?'. It might be worth at this stage, talking a bit about non-verbal communication – how somebody can be sensitive to another's feelings and even guess what they are thinking about from their expression, posture and previous discussions about important material.

Passivity phenomena are similar; the patient believes that his actions, feelings or thoughts are being controlled by someone or some unknown force. Eliciting this involves asking 'Do you think people are making you do/think/feel things against your will?'. Again the next step is an inquiry about 'How do you think they can do that?'. If the patient has no clear mechanism in mind, it may be reasonable to prompt, e.g. 'Do you mean some sort of hypnotism?' to provide a common language again. Discussion about hypnotism may allow debate of the phenomena the patient seems to be describing, 'Hypnotism is a well-demonstrated phenomenon but I understand that you need to agree to it for it to work and, to my knowledge, it couldn't make you do things against your will.' Alternatively the patient may not believe that an equivalent phenomenon is hypnotism, in which case, 'Do you mean some sort of magnetism or waves?' may help elicit an alternative and then, e.g. 'I don't know of any way it could affect people like that … perhaps we should find out more about these phenomena'. Finally discuss the practical implications of such beliefs; how is it interfering with the patient's life. It may be that even while these beliefs are present he is prepared to start to deal with the limitations he feels imposed on his life and experiment or learn coping strategies.

*Paranoid delusions*    Paranoid and other delusions are common and most distressing and disabling. They may not be discussed or described directly to the therapist because he or she is seen as part of those who are against the patient, or at least, he may not be sure of your allegiances. Building up trust is essential and so is, most importantly, listening to and hearing what the patient says, and assembling the evidence that the patient views as relevant before drawing any conclusion or attempting to provide any alternative explanation. Patients can readily dismiss clinicians for assuming they are mad without giving them a chance to explain their position. Only once the bulk of the evidence has been assembled do you start to debate it. Tracing the development of a delusion is crucially important.

Setting up hypotheses to test out beliefs can be useful but these need to be developed collaboratively, so that, were the delusions true, the patient would not feel they were being put in any danger. For example, if a patient believed that men in black cars were following him, the first step would be to elicit the precise meaning of the belief, i.e. men not women, in black cars, not any other colour. Would they be alone or with others? Is any make of car relevant or one specific type? How old would the car be? Would they expect the car to be reasonably new, completely new or older? On the basis of this clear and agreed understanding the patient would be asked to make a note of every car he saw over a period of time which met these criteria, and further to state whether he believed the person inside the car intended him harm. The reasoning processes involved could be explored – why exclude one person rather than another?

***Grandiose delusions***   Establishing evidence for grandiose delusions and then weighing that evidence is necessary but often rather frustrating as the beliefs can be difficult to counter directly. Often inference chaining is essential; this involves following through the implications of the belief with the patient.

For example, one patient was convinced that she belonged to Royalty and that there was a 'special person' in government looking after her needs. This belief was supported by a link in her family history with a royal family in France; however, there was no current link with any member of a royal family. She would not accept this but when asked 'Although you know I have not come to the same conclusion as you about this evidence, what if your beliefs were true? Why would that be important to you? What would it mean to you?'. Her response was that she would be 'regarded properly'; she was then asked if there was anyone in particular by whom she wanted to be regarded properly. She stated this was her daughter, who was not letting her see her grandchildren while she was expressing these beliefs, and her husband who she felt, with good reason, looked down on her. It was agreed that although the issue of whether she was royal or not was contentious, it was possible for the therapist to work with her and her family about this concern that she was not regarded properly. This discussion was valuable in improving the therapeutic relationship and refocusing it on an area that could be fruitfully explored. The delusional ideas became much less prominent as a result and have gradually withered away.

Inference chaining therefore involves asking, 'If your beliefs were true, what would that mean to you?' and following this through. There is a danger of colluding with the patient but this can be avoided if clear statements about not accepting the belief but wanting to look at the meaning to the patient are used. Inference chaining needs to be negotiated, led rather than driven, and discontinued if resisted or causing distress or agitation. It is also important to avoid putting meanings into the person's mouth – this is not an exercise in providing an interpretation of a symptom for them.

*Hallucinations*  Auditory hallucinations are very common in schizophrenia and frequently are the most distressing symptoms experienced. Somatic hallucinations, where for example the patient describes feeling themselves touched, hurt or interfered with sexually, are less common but will be dealt with later. Visual hallucinations also seem to present relatively rarely as clinically significant problems. All hallucinations can have their good and bad effects – sometimes, for example, patients find that the voices are good company. In these circumstances, the only problem they may cause is that discussion with family and especially strangers can cause social stigmatisation and ostracisation, in which case it can simply be worth discussing with whom and when to talk about them and when not. It may also be important to bear in mind that behaviour such as talking to the voices may make the individual appear bizarre and reinforce a perception of him as 'mad'.

Distressing hallucinations particularly need to be focused upon. A full assessment of their nature, content and how circumstances affect them is vital. Mechanisms by which they might be produced and their connection with delusional beliefs need to be explored. Coping strategies can be identified and often involve distraction, e.g. going for a walk, listening to music, taking a warm bath.

They may take the form of voices talking about the patient. Who is speaking? What are they saying? Is there any truth in what is said? Does the person understand what they mean? When did they start? Was it related to anything happening to them?

Command hallucinations – telling the person what to do – are particularly distressing as often the things described are violent or sexual and repugnant to the person concerned or at least frightening to them. The fear that they may act on them and the belief that they have to do so – the omnipotence of the voices – can be devastatingly tormenting. Reality testing, reviewing whether self-harm, abuse and guilt are relevant, are important steps. Asking 'What have you done to deserve this?' 'When did it start? What events were related?' 'What could you have done?' If an event is elicited, working it through in a similar way to grief counselling, may be appropriate. It is essential to establish that voices – thoughts – cannot directly make you act in any way despite the feeling of strength and conviction. Elicit inconsistencies and all-or-nothing thinking such as 'They always make me do things'. Review the commands and resultant actions, discuss methods of resistance

**Box 9.5** Case study 3

Paul, aged 18, had taken amphetamines with friends at a club one night and developed a psychotic reaction. This resolved rapidly but then after one similar episode involving amphetamines, the symptoms developed into a persisting schizophrenic illness. He believed that drug dealers were pursuing him and persecuting him through the television. He refused to leave the house and heard voices telling him to kill himself. His symptoms responded only partially to anti-psychotics to which he developed disabling side-effects.

Therapy involved tracing the development of the symptoms and direct linking of them to his current state. The persistence of the symptoms in the absence of amphetamines was related to the way in which bad experiences, e.g. road traffic accidents, can be etched on the memory and be revived easily with the accompanying emotions by simple triggers. A collaborative analysis of the voices was used to assist him in recognising their origin in his own mind. The reasons why dealers should be after him were explored – 'Had he paid them? Had he stolen from them? – Why then should they be after him?'. This approach gradually improved his confidence, helped him develop insight and coping strategies to deal with the voices and false beliefs. Over a period of six months he returned to college and resumed his social life with minimal disruption from symptoms.

and coping strategies. Most importantly, work through a process of critical analysis of the hallucinatory experience (see Box 9.5).

Somatic hallucinations can be very distressing and the feeling of physical interference, especially sexual, as real as if an assault were occurring. Assess their presence, nature and frequency, then discuss the feelings involved and any possible source or mechanism: 'Who do you think is doing this? How are they doing it?'. It may then be worth inference chaining, e.g. 'If you were being touched/assaulted, would you expect someone to see this happening?', 'Has anybody seen this?', 'Why do you think they have not?'. 'Is there some other method than direct physical touch – rays, electricity or magnetism?'. Sensitively explore other explanations, e.g. sexual feelings which are disowned, and especially somatic symptoms of anxiety. Get the patient to check out, e.g. If they feel they are being touched, they should look to see if someone is touching them.

*Negative symptoms*    Poor motivation and drive are seriously disabling and often frustrating for the patient, carer and staff. This can be particularly prominent after an acute episode and in these circumstances, it may be appropriate to think of the period as convalescence. It is certainly not helpful to unduly pressurise at that and later stages. Any change needs to be gradual and in small steps with appropriate appreciation given when gains are made and sustained.

*Suicide prevention*    Suicide occurs in up to 15% of people with severe mental illness and so any methods used need to take this into account. Cognitive behaviour therapy stresses the importance of checking with the patient how they are feeling, coping and thinking at regular intervals within and at the end of sessions. This is important in eliciting suicidal thoughts but direct questioning is necessary whenever there is a hint of risk, e.g. because of the content of hallucinations or the presence of depressive ideas especially hopelessness. Open access to services, at least for selected individuals, and available telephone contacts, can reduce risk. CBT aims at sustaining hope and decatastrophises situations by explaining and normalising, which may assist in reducing risk. Early identification and treatment of depression with cognitive behaviour therapy or other appropriate interventions, e.g. interpersonal therapies and medication, can also reduce risk. Involvement of relatives can mean that early signs of risk are picked up. Management of command hallucinations may be particularly important (see Chapter 12 for a fuller discussion of risk management).

*CONCLUSION*    Services for people with severe mental illness should emphasise the importance of developing techniques which are collaborative, needs-related and effective. The care programme approach was introduced with these principles in mind. Multidisciplinary working is central to the achievement of these aims and therapeutic techniques need to be accessible to all those who become key-workers for people with mental health problems as far as possible. Cognitive behaviour therapy can therefore have an important complementary place in collaborative management of severe mental illness alongside other methods of treatment. There is a need for further evaluation in personality disorder, resistant affective disorder and schizophrenia but the techniques being developed are relatively straightforward and seem to have clinical validity. They are becoming indispensable as part of every mental health worker's therapeutic armamentaria.

*DISCUSSION QUESTIONS*

1. What are the key characteristics of cognitive behaviour therapy?
2. What evidence is there to suggest that CBT can be useful for people diagnosed with a personality disorder?
3. What are the stages involved in the assessment of a client with schizophrenia when using CBT?
4. Which specific CBT strategies could be employed to intervene with a person experiencing hallucinations?

*FURTHER READING*

♦ Beck, A., Freeman, A. and associates (1990) *Cognitive Therapy of Personality Disorders*. New York: Guilford.
This is quite a weighty tome but can be useful for reference and has a very good list of the type of schemas used by different patient groups.

♦ Blackburn, I. and Davidson, K. (1990) *Cognitive Therapy for Depression and Anxiety*. Oxford: Blackwell.
Excellent book, now in paperback. Well-written and designed: invaluable for novices and pretty good for others.

♦ Fowler, D., Garety, P. and Kuipers, E. (1995) *Cognitive Behaviour Therapy of Psychosis: Theory and Practice*. London: Wiley.
Very useful and well-written book exploring areas such as engagement and schema.

♦ Kingdon, D. and Turkington, D. (1994) *Cognitive-Behavioural Therapy of Schizophrenia*. New York: Guilford Press; London: Lawrence-Ehrlbaum.
Basic theory and practice of cognitive behaviour therapy in schizophrenia.

♦ Linehan, M. (1993) *Cognitive-behavioural Treatment of Borderline Personality Disorder*. New York: Guilford Press.
Detailed description of very innovative techniques which have been subject successfully to controlled evaluation but not the easiest book to read.

♦ Scott, J. (1996) The role of cognitive behaviour therapy in bipolar disorder. *Behavioural and Cognitive Psychotherapy*, 24, 195–208.
Good brief reviews with useful references.

*REFERENCES*

Beck, A. (1952), Successful outpatient psychotherapy of a chronic schizophrenic with a delusion based on borrowed guilt. *Psychiatry*, 15, 305–312.

Beck, A. (1976), *Cognitive Therapy of the Emotional Disorders*. Chichester: Penguin.

Beck, A., Freeman, A. and associates (1990), *Cognitive Therapy of Personality Disorders*. New York: Guilford.

Blackburn, I. and Davidson, K. (1990), *Cognitive Therapy for Depression and Anxiety*. Oxford: Blackwell.

Burns, D. (1980), *Feeling Good: The New Mood Therapy*. New York: William Morrow.

Elkin, I., Shea, M., Watkins, J. *et al.* (1989), National Institute of Mental Health Treatment of Depression Collaborative Treatment Programme. *Archives of General Psychiatry*, 46, 971–982.

Fowler, D., Garety, P. and Kuipers, E. (1995), *Cognitive Behaviour Therapy of Psychosis: Theory and Practice*. London: Wiley.

Haddock, G. and Slade, P. (Eds) (1996), *Cognitive-behavioural Interventions in Psychotic Disorders*. London: Routledge.

Kingdon, D. and Turkington, D. (1994), *Cognitive-behavioural Therapy of Schizophrenia*. New York: Guilford Press; London: Lawrence-Ehrlbaum.

Kingdon, D. G., Tyrer, P., Murphy, S. *et al.* (1996), The Nottingham Study of Neurotic Disorder: influence of cognitive therapists on outcome. *British Journal of Psychiatry*, 169, 93–97.

Linehan, M. (1993), *Cognitive-behavioural Treatment of Borderline Personality Disorder*. New York: Guilford Press.

Perry, A., Tarrier, N. and Morriss, R. (1995), Identification of prodromal signs and symptoms and early intervention in manic depressive psychosis patients. *Behavioural and Cognitive Psychotherapy*, 23, 399–409.

Scott, J. (1995), Psychological treatments for depression. An update. *British Journal of Psychiatry*, 167, 289–292.

Scott, J. (1996), The role of cognitive behaviour therapy in bipolar disorder. *Behavioural and Cognitive Psychotherapy*, 24, 195–208.

Tyrer, P., Sievewright, N., Kingdon, D. *et al.* (1998), The Nottingham study of neurotic disorder: comparison of drug and psychological treatments. *Lancet*, 2, 235–240.

Young, J. and Beck, A. (1980), *The Cognitive Therapy Rating Scale*. Pennsylvania Centre for Cognitive Therapy.

# CHAPTER 10

# Early Intervention in Psychotic Relapse

## Max Birchwood, Jo Smith, Fiona Macmillan and Dermot McGovern

*KEY ISSUES*

♦ The concept of the prodrome

♦ Relapse signatures

♦ Cognitive approaches to early intervention

♦ Clinical and empirical validity of cognitive approaches

*INTRODUCTION*    The control of relapse is among many of the needs of people with psychosis. It is important, however, as each relapse brings with it an increased probability of future relapse and residual symptoms (McGlashan, 1988) as well as accelerating social disablement (Hogarty *et al.*, 1991). Even an ideal combination of pharmacological and psychosocial intervention does not eliminate the potential for relapse (Hogarty *et al.*, 1991).

These facts are not lost on those who themselves experience recurring psychotic symptoms. A survey by Meuser *et al.* (1992) found that patients expressed a strong interest in learning about 'early warning signs of the illness and relapse' and this was ranked second in importance out of an agenda of over forty topics. Their thirst for knowledge and understanding of this matter would seem to be driven by a perceived need for control rather than mere curiosity. In a study of 'secondary depression in schizophrenia' (Birchwood *et al.*, 1993) it was found that 'perceived control over illness' was the variable most closely linked to depression, more so than illness variables, locus of control or self-evaluative beliefs derived from culture bound beliefs about mental illness (Box

**Box 10.1** Items from the scale perceived control of psychotic illness

- ◆ If I am going to relapse there's nothing I can do about it.
- ◆ I cannot cope with my current symptoms.
- ◆ My illness frightens me.
- ◆ I am powerless to influence or control my illness.

10.1). The propensity of individuals to seek control of psychotic disorder is now well understood (Breier and Strauss, 1983; Kumar et al., 1989) and the question is raised as to the possibility of empowering individuals with real control over an event they fear most: relapse.

DSM-III-R (American Psychiatric Association, 1994) recognised that relapse, when defined as the re-emergence or exacerbation of positive symptoms, tends to be preceded by subtle changes in mental functioning up to four weeks before the event. Not only is this perceived as a loss of well-being by the individual but it appears to trigger a set of restorative manoeuvres, as shown by McCandless-Glincher et al. (1986).

McCandless-Glincher et al. (1986) studied 62 individuals attending for maintenance therapy, and inquired about their recognition of, and response to, reduced well-being. The patients were drawn from those routinely attending two medical centres; their age range (20–75 years), with an average illness duration of 28 years, suggests that such a group would be well represented in ordinary clinical practice. 61 said they could recognise reduced well-being; of these only 16 relied entirely upon others to identify symptoms for them. 9 were assisted by others and 36 identified the problems themselves. The majority (50 out of 61) of patients initiated some change in their behaviour when they recognised reduced well-being, including engaging in diversionary activities, seeking professional help and resuming or increasing their neuroleptic medication. Only 3 of this group had even been encouraged to self-monitor by mental health professionals, and a further 7 had received encouragement from relatives. Thus, these schizophrenic patients had initiated symptom monitoring and a range of responses almost entirely on their own initiative. The study by Kumar et al. (1989) comes to rather similar conclusions.

In essence there may be a relatively untapped pool of information which is not accessed adequately enough to initiate early intervention, except perhaps by individuals themselves. If individuals can recognise and act on symptoms suggestive of reduced well-being, then it is possible that patterns of early ('prodromal') symptoms heralding relapse may be apparent and identifiable, and may offer further avenues for relapse management in partnership with the individual with psychosis. In this chapter, the scientific data on the predictive validity of early symptoms is reviewed and a process of collaborative early intervention is described with case examples. The main thrust of this chapter, however, is to explore theoretically, and with case examples, the basis for a cognitive approach to early intervention based on the appraisal of early symptoms and its direct and indirect impact on relapse and delusion formation.

## DOES A PRODROME HERALD PSYCHOTIC RELAPSE?

Clinical, retrospective and prospective studies have addressed and continue to address this question. In this section we shall concentrate on the last two and consider the implications of the clinical studies in trying to interpret the empirical investigations.

Psychiatric services are, by and large, organised to respond to crises such as relapse; this constrains our ability to develop clinical experience of prodromal changes. Thus, the first systematic studies of the prodrome adopted the simple expedient of asking the patient and his relative or carer.

The interview study by Herz and Melville (1980) in the USA attempted systematically to collect data retrospectively from patients and relatives in this manner. It was widely regarded as definitive since they interviewed 145 schizophrenic sufferers (46 following a recent episode) as well as 80 of their family members. The main question 'Could you tell that there were any changes in your thoughts, feelings or behaviours that might have led you to believe you were becoming ill and might have to go into hospital?', was answered affirmatively by 70% of patients and 93% of families. These, and the results of a similar British study (Birchwood *et al.*, 1989), are shown in Box 10.2.

Generally the symptoms most frequently mentioned by patients and family members were dysphoric in nature: eating less, concentration problems, troubled sleep, depressed mood and withdrawal. The most common 'early psychotic' symptoms were 'hearing voices talking in a nonsensical way', 'increased religious thinking' and 'thinking someone else was controlling them'.

There is considerable agreement about the nature of these 'early signs' although somewhat less about their relative importance. Both studies concur in finding 'dysphoric' symptoms the most commonly prevalent. In the Herz and Melville study, although more families than patients reported the presence of early signs, there was considerable concordance between patients and families in the content and relative significance of early symptoms. There was substantial agreement between patients that non-psychotic symptoms persisted between episodes of illness – an important issue which is returned to below.

Both studies carefully questioned respondents about the timing of the onset of the prodrome. Most of the patients (52%) and their

**Box 10.2** Percentages of relatives reporting early signs

| Category | Birchwood et al. (1989) (n=42) | | Herz and Melville (1980) (n=80) | |
|---|---|---|---|---|
| | % | Rank[a] | % | Rank[a] |
| **Anxiety/agitation** | | | | |
| Irritable, quick tempered | 62 | 2(eq) | – | – |
| Sleep problems | 67 | 1 | 69 | 7 |
| Tense, afraid, anxious | 62 | 2(eq) | 83 | 1 |
| **Depression/withdrawal** | | | | |
| Quiet, withdrawn | 60 | 4 | 50 | 18 |
| Depressed, low | 57 | 5 | 76 | 3 |
| Poor appetite | 48 | 9 | 53 | 17 |
| **Disinhibition** | | | | |
| Aggression | 50 | 7(eq) | 79 | 2 |
| Restless | 55 | 6 | 40 | 20 |
| Stubborn | 35 | 10(eq) | – | – |
| **Incipient psychosis** | | | | |
| Behaves as if hallucinated | 50 | 7(eq) | 60 | 10 |
| Being laughed at or talked about | 36 | 10(eq) | 14 | 53.8 |
| Odd behaviour | 36 | 10(eq) | – | – |

[a] There were many other symptoms assessed. Percentage reporting only shown for parallel data.

families (68%) in the Herz and Melville study felt that more than a week elapsed between the onset of the prodrome and a full relapse. Similarly, Birchwood et al. (1989) found that 59% observed the onset of the prodrome one month or more prior to relapse, and 75% two weeks or more; 19% were unable to specify a time scale.

The clinical implications of this research will largely depend on the degree of specificity which early signs information affords. In particular a high false positive rate will tend to undermine the use of an early intervention strategy, in particular that which uses a raised dose of neuroleptic medication. Marder et al. (1984) assessed 41 patients on a range of psychiatric symptoms at baseline, two weeks later, monthly for three months and then every three months. Relapse was defined as the failure of an increase in medication to manage symptoms following a minor exacerbation of psychosis or paranoia. Thus, under this definition it is not known how many genuine prodromes were aborted with medication and whether those that responded to medication were similar to those that did not. Patients were assessed using a standard psychiatric

**Box 10.3** Prediction of prodromal signs

> The true prediction of prodromal signs can be clearly established only with prospective investigations. Such studies need to examine three issues:
>
> 1. Whether prodromes of psychotic relapse exist;
> 2. Their timing in relation to full relapse;
> 3. How often the prodromes fail as well as succeed to predict relapse (i.e. 'sensitivity' and 'specificity').

interview scale (Brief Psychiatric Rating Scale BPRS; Overall and Gorham, 1962) and a self-report measure of psychiatric symptoms (SCL90; Derogatis *et al.*, 1973). Changes in scores 'just prior to relapse' were compared with the average ('spontaneous') change for a given scale during the course of the follow-up period. Marder *et al.* found increases in BPRS depression, thought disturbance and paranoia and SCL90 scores for interpersonal sensitivity, anxiety, depression and paranoid ideation prior to relapse. They note that the changes they observed were very small (equating 2 points on a 21 point range) and probably not recognisable by most clinicians. A discriminant function analysis found the most discriminating ratings were paranoia and depression (BPRS) and psychotiscm (SCL90). They suggest: 'such a formula if used in a clinic would probably predict most relapses although there would be a considerable number of ... false positives' (Marder *et al.*, 1984, p. 46). Although this study strongly supported the presence of the relapse prodrome, it was unable to control for timing. The last assessment before relapse varied from between one and twelve weeks, weakening the observed effects. One would anticipate the prodrome to be at its maximum in the week or two prior to relapse; assessments carried out before this would measure an earlier, weaker stage of the prodrome, or miss it entirely.

A subsequent report from the same laboratory (Marder *et al.*, 1991) studied 50 schizophrenic patients monitored weekly for nonpsychotic prodromal episodes. This study compared different methods of monitoring for prodromes using experimenter administered scales (Brief Psychiatric Rating Scale, anxiety depression cluster and their Individualised Prodromal Scale), systematically varying the sensitivity of their instruments and observing the impact on their predictive efficacy. Thus, Figure 10.1 plots the hit rate against the rate of false positives under varying degrees of change in BPRS anxiety and depression from one to five points. This shows that using a change score of three, 50% of relapses are accurately predicted with a 20% false-positive rate; this was achieved only when patients with a relatively stable mental state were included.

**Figure 10.1** The relationship between sensitivity and error rates using various BPRS thresholds to define prodromes (from Marder *et al.*, 1991)

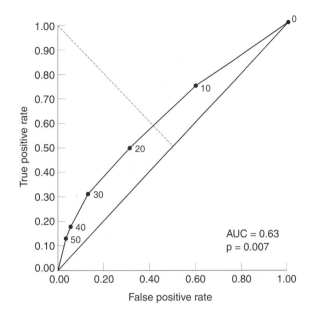

Subotnik and Neuchterlein (1988) considerably improved upon the Marder *et al.* studies by administering the BPRS fortnightly to 50 young recent onset schizophrenic patients diagnosed by RDC criteria. A total of 23 patients relapsed and their BPRS scores two, four and six weeks prior to the relapse were compared with their scores in another six-week period not associated with relapse, and with scores of a non-relapse group ($n = 27$) over a similar period. This research found that BPRS anxiety–depression (which includes depression, guilt and somatic concern) and thought disturbance (hallucinations and delusions) were raised prior to relapse. The contrast with the non-relapsed patients revealed a rise in low-level 'psychotic' symptoms as part of the prodrome, but not of the non-psychotic items (depression, somatic concern, guilt, etc.). This suggests that relapse is more probable. It was noted that 'mean elevations in prodromal symptoms were small ... 0.5–1.00 on a 7 point scale ... but in three patients no prodromal symptons were present ... in several others they did not begin to show any symptomatic change until 2–4 weeks prior to relapse ... thus lowering the magnitude of the means' (Subotnik and Neuchterlein, 1988, p. 411). These results support clinical observations that the nature and timing of prodromal signs are, like relapse itself, not universal, but include several between-subject variabilities. Nevertheless, Subotnik and Neuchterlein reported that a discriminant function analysis, using two BPRS 'psychotic' state scales, correctly classified 59% of relapses and 7% of non-relapse periods, suggesting a false-positive rate of 26%.

Hirsch and Jolley (1989), in the course of an early intervention study, measured putative prodromes ('neurotic or dysphoric episodes') in a group of 54 patients with DSM-III-R schizophrenia using SCL90 and Herz's Early Signs Questionnaire (ESQ; Herz *et al.*, 1982). Patients and their key workers received a one-hour teaching session about schizophrenia, particularly concerning the significance of the 'dysphoric' syndrome as a prodrome for relapse. It was hoped that this would enable them to recognise 'dysphoric' episodes. All subjects were symptom free at the onset of the trial. At each dysphoric episode, the SCL90 and the ESQ were administered and then weekly for two further weeks; otherwise each was rated monthly. Relapse was defined as the re-emergence of florid symptoms, including delusions and hallucinations. About 73% of relapses were preceded by a prodromal period of dysphoric and neurotic symptoms within one month of relapse. These prodromes were defined clinically, but confirmed by SCL90 scores, which were similar to those reported by the other two prospective studies, and included depression, anxiety, interpersonal sensitivity and paranoid thinking. Interpretation of this study is complicated by the design, in which half the subjects received active medication (haloperidol, 10 mg/day). Dysphoric episodes were much more common in the placebo (76%) than in the active group (27%) but the prompt pharmacological intervention does not allow us to ascertain whether these dysphoric episodes were part of a reactivation of psychosis (i.e. true prodromes) aborted by medication and to what extent these included 'false positives' related, perhaps, to the use of placebo.

Malla and Norman (1994) report a prospective study of 55 DSM-III-R schizophrenic patients in which monthly recordings of positive symptoms, thought disorder and putative prodromal 'dysphoric' symptoms were taken, using standard self-support scales (including the Beck Depression Inventory and the Scale for the Assessment of Positive Symptoms). They found that minor undulations in psychotic symptoms were not linked to dysphoric symptoms recorded one month previously. However, major exacerbations of positive symptoms were nearly always preceded by elevations (less than one standard deviation) of prodromal symptoms above baseline (specificity: 90%). 'Prodromes' anticipated only 50% of relapses, but this may have increased with fortnightly monitoring as adopted by Subotnik and Neuchterlein (1988) and Birchwood *et al.* (1989). Indeed, Gaebel *et al.* (1993), in an analysis based on an early intervention design, found greater predictive efficacy of prodromal symptoms two weeks prior to relapse.

A further prospective study (Birchwood *et al.*, 1989) used a scale designed to tap the specific characteristics of the prodrome, rather than that of general psychopathology. Construction of the scale was informed by the retrospective study reported in the same paper. Two versions of the scale were used for completion by both the patient and a chosen observer (e.g. relative, carer, hostel worker). It was reasoned that the behavioural observations by the observers might provide additional information if the individual under-reported or lost insight. Changes in baseline levels were readily apparent which is particularly important if the individual experiences persisting symptoms.

The authors reported an investigation of 19 young schizophrenic patients diagnosed according to the broad CATEGO 'S' class (Wing *et al.*, 1974). All except one were on maintenance medication, monitored in the context of a routine clinical service and were not involved in a drug trial. Eight of the 19 relapsed in the course of nine months, and, of these, 50% showed elevations on the scales between two and four weeks prior to relapse. A *post-hoc* defined threshold on their scale (less than or more than 30) led to a sensitivity of 63%, specificity of 82% and an 11% rate of false positives. This study was recently replicated by Jorgensen (in press) in Denmark using a large sample of patients (N=60) monitored using the same scale.

Figure 10.2 shows some of the results of individual prodromes. Figure 10.2a is that of a young male who relapsed 16 weeks after discharge. In this case, the first change was that of dysphoria/ withdrawal which was apparent five weeks prior to relapse. One to two weeks later he became steadily more agitated and within two weeks of relapse, low level ('incipient') psychotic symptoms appeared. Disinhibition and anxiety/agitation did not peak until somewhat later. It is noteworthy that the observer's behavioural observations showed striking concordance with self-report in respect of dysphoria but lagged behind up to two weeks in respect of the behavioural concomitants of incipient psychosis. This example also reveals an apparent improvement in well-being just prior to the onset of the prodromes. The second case (Figure 10.2b) is a young male, in whose case the rise in anxiety/agitation, dysphoria and incipient psychosis were noted by the observer, but the individual reported a slight rise in symptoms followed immediately by a sharp fall, presumably due to lack of insight. Case three (Figure 10.2c) demonstrates a definite rise in the scales which returned to baseline four weeks later and was not followed by a relapse. Although the increase in scores did not lead to a relapse, this individual had learnt that he had secured employment which seemed to be associated with a feeling of well-being noted by the individual and his mother; as the start of his job approached his symptoms increased then returned to baseline a few weeks after the start of the job. What was witnessed there was probably the impact of a stressful life event which on this occasion did not culminate in relapse.

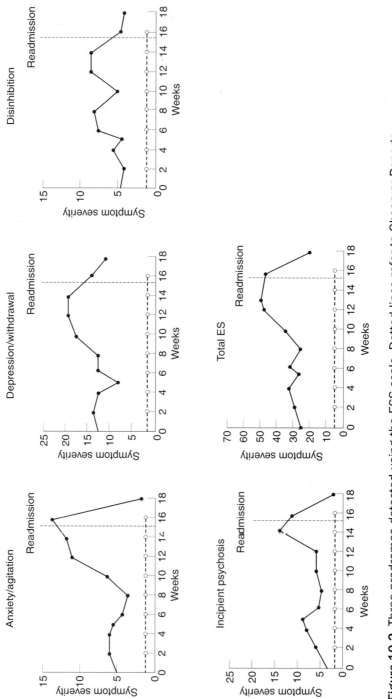

**Figure 10.2** Three prodromes detected using the ESS scale. Dotted lines refer to Observer Reports

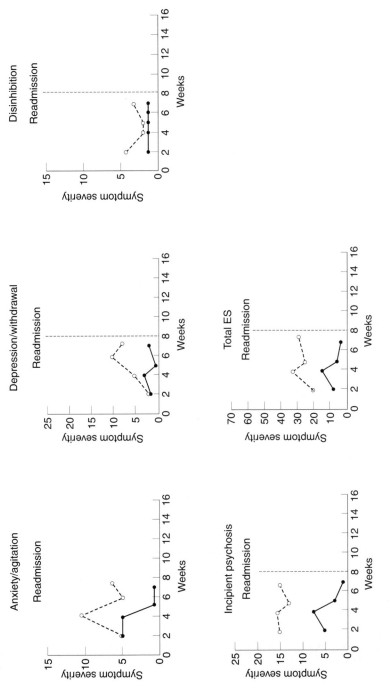

**Figure 10.2** *(continued)*

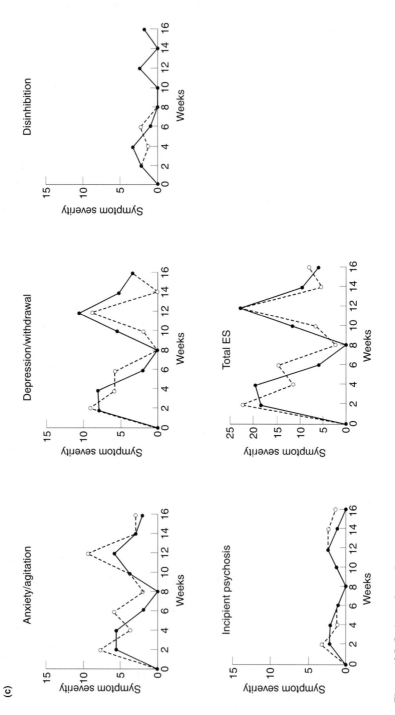

**Figure 10.2** (continued)

*CONTINUING QUESTIONS*

*Sensitivity and specificity*

The results of the five prospective studies are consistent with the clinical and retrospective studies, particularly supporting Herz and Melville's (1980) seminal investigation. The studies all found that the psychotic relapse is nearly always preceded by non-psychotic 'dysphoric' symptoms including anxiety, dysphoria, interpersonal sensitivity/withdrawal and low-level psychotic thinking, including ideas of reference and paranoid thoughts. In two of these studies (Marder *et al.* 1984; Hirsch and Jolley, 1989), the observations were confounded by a targeted medication strategy, so it was not clear how many of their putative prodromes were actually false positives. It is also possible that the use of an early intervention strategy exaggerated the magnitude of the recorded prodromes. Under normal conditions, the baseline levels of psychopathology would be increased in the non-relapsed patients by transient fluctuations in dysphoric symptoms which were not part of a relapse (i.e. the false positives), which might respond to medication, thus reducing the contrast between relapsed and non-relapsed groups.

The possibility of between-subject variability in the nature and timing of the prodromes will, however, act to reduce their apparent amplitude in group studies. Subotnik and Neuchterlein (1988) reported that some patients showed no prodromal symptoms. Among the patients who did show prodromal signs, some were elevated six weeks before relapse whereas in others this occurred a full month later, thus lowering the mean value for the whole group within the time frames (six, four or two weeks before relapse). The study by Birchwood *et al.* (1989) raises further potential complications, as not only does it reveal differences in the amplitude and timing of symptoms, but also that the pattern of prodromal symptoms showed subject variability – some may 'peak' on anxiety symptoms, others on disinhibition, and so forth.

*Prodromes: discrete or continuous?*

The prospective studies rather assume that prodromal and psychotic symptoms are discrete, dichotomous stages that may each be scored as present or absent. Each study uses slightly different definitions of prodrome and relapse that may well contribute to differences in figures for sensitivity and specificity (Malla and Norman, 1994). As Norman and Malla (1995) indicate, the notion of 'prodrome' is of course taken from general medicine where non-specific symptoms (e.g. malaise) precede the illness proper (e.g. AIDS). In fact, most of the prospective studies do not maintain such a clear distinction. Tarrier *et al.* (1991) included hallucinations in the prodrome, as did Herz and Melville (1980); Birchwood *et al.* (1989) included a scale of 'incipient psychosis' with items indicating low level psychotic signs ('something odd is going on which cannot be explained; feeling people are taking unusual notice of me'). Subotnik and Neuchterlein (1988) included BPRS 'thought disturbance' in their prodrome which is, of course, not strictly a non-psychotic symptom. Malla and Norman (1994), using only non-psychotic symptom measures, found no link between prodromes and psychosis, where both are viewed as continuous, but they did find that major increases in psychosis were preceded by non-psychotic signs, although the sensitivity was lower than that found in other prospective studies. Even the status of dysphoria as a non-specific prodromal symptom is contentious since there is sound evidence that depressed mood is a concomitant of acute psychosis and also depression emerges as a dimension of psychopathology in some of the studies of the structure of psychotic symptoms. Also, in some formulations, dysphoria is regarded as a reaction to a developing psychosis rather than a prodrome proper (Birchwood *et al.*, 1992).

It is probably of little consequence whether the 'prodromal' symptoms, in the formal medical sense, truly precede psychosis: what is clear is that relapse in most instances builds up over a period of between two and four weeks. As in psychosis itself, there is likely to be a considerable between-subject variability in the timing and nature of early symptoms. Identifying this individual information is the key to early intervention and is considered below. Also, there is now a well-established relationship between the duration of psychosis and susceptibility to treatment (Loebel *et al.*, 1992); thus even if early intervention fails to prevent the breakdown of severe hallucinations and delusions, it can, theoretically, at least shorten their duration.

## The concept of the relapse signature

The prospective studies have raised a number of questions. They have confirmed the existence of prodromes of psychotic relapse and found a true positive rate in the region of 50–60% with a false positive rate of up to 25%; however, their limitations have not enabled a clear picture to emerge of the true predictive significance of apparent early warning signs. If the concept of the relapse signature is borne out, then group studies in the mould of those of Subotnik and Neuchterlein (1988) would be inherently limited as they could not capture the apparent qualitative differences between patients in their early signs or symptoms. This is supported by Subotnik and Neuchterlein's finding that greater prediction success came when patients were compared against their own baseline, rather than that of other patients. It may be more appropriate to think of each patient's syndrome as a personalised relapse signature which includes core or common symptoms together with features unique to each patient. If an individual's relapse signature can be identified, then it might be expected that the overall predictive power of 'prodromal' symptoms will be increased. Identifying the unique characteristics of a relapse signature can be achieved only once a relapse has taken place; with each successive relapse further information becomes available to build a more accurate image of the signature. This kind of learning process had been acknowledged by patients (Breier and Strauss, 1983) and could be adapted and developed by professionals and carers, and forms the basis of our (Birchwood *et al.*, 1992) approach to early intervention.

*The relapse signature as an 'at risk' mental state*

The quasi-medical concept of the prodrome also carries with it the assumption that once the process of relapse has been embarked on, the progression to full relapse is irreversible (Herz and Lamberti, 1995); hence the invocation of the concept of sensitivity where anything less than 100% represents a limitation of 'early signs' information. We know from the work of McCandless-Glincher *et al.* (1986) and Breier and Strauss (1983) that patients are actively involved in attempting to regulate their own symptoms and believe they can halt a relapse, for example by taking medication or employing stress management. The stress vulnerability concept of psychosis suggests that relapse is an interaction of vulnerability, psychosocial stress and protective factors (such as personal coping); within this framework it is possible that their combined effect in some instances is to self-limit the process of relapse. The presence of a clear relapse signature should be viewed as placing the individual 'at risk' for relapse, not as a guarantee of it, and other factors may combine to influence the appearance of symptoms. The concept of the 'at risk mental state' was first coined by Yung *et al.* (1996) in relation to first episode prodromes. This framework indicates the need to define operationally the relapse signature *a priori*, which is considered below.

*COLLABORATIVE EARLY INTERVENTION*

*Engagement and education*

Early intervention rests on a close collaboration between patient, carer/relative and professionals. In common with many interventions, an ethos of trust and 'informed partnership' between these groups must be developed (Smith and Birchwood, 1990). Education about prodromes and early intervention opportunities needs to be provided, which might be given in the context of general educational intervention about psychosis (Birchwood *et al.*, 1992; Smith and Birchwood, 1990). Education must emphasise that some responsibility is being placed on the individual and relative to recognise a potential relapse and to initiate treatment. Engagement and compliance will be enhanced where the client has a stable, trusting relationship with individuals in the mental health services. As the experience of Jolley *et al.* (1990) illustrates, this requires psychoeducation to be a continuous feature of this relationship. The continuity of care inherent in the case management approach provides an appropriate support structure.

*Suitable clients*

Individuals with a history of repeated relapse or who are at high risk of relapse for reasons of non-adherence to a maintenance medication regime, or who are recovering from a recent relapse, living alone or in a high Expressed Emotion family environment, may be appropriate subjects to participate in an early intervention programme, as will those who fear relapse and are demoralised by their apparent inability to control it. For those with severe drug-refractory positive symptoms, discriminating a prodrome against such a background is likely to prove extremely difficult (indeed its very existence is questionable) and early intervention becomes less meaningful in this context. The absence of insight may preclude an individual's acceptance of an early intervention strategy; indeed the ultimate test will be the individual's acceptance of the approach, which in our experience has much to do with his or her dislike of the trauma which relapse/readmission can cause, as well as fear of the experience itself. The availability of a close relative or carer, to maximise information about prodromal signs and provide support, can be helpful but they must be selected in collaboration with the individual.

*Identifying the time window and relapse signature for early intervention*

Four problems need to be overcome if our knowledge about the process of relapse is to have clinical application. First, the identification of 'early signs' by a clinician would require intensive, regular monitoring of mental state at least fortnightly which is rarely possible in clinical practice. Second, some patients choose to conceal their symptoms as relapse approaches and insight declines (Heinrichs *et al.*, 1985). Third, many patients experience persisting symptoms, cognitive defects or drug side-effects which may obscure the visibility of the prodromes. Indeed, the nature of a prodrome in patients with residual symptoms (in contrast to those who are symptom-free) has not been studied, and is important, since in clinical practice the presence of residual symptoms is extremely common. Fourth, the possibility is raised that the characteristics of prodromes might vary from individual to individual and this information may be lost in scales of general psychopathology.

With regard to the latter, precise information about the nature and duration of an individual's prodrome or 'relapse signature' may be obtained through careful interviewing of the patient (and if possible, relatives and other close associates) about the changes in thinking and behaviour leading up to a recent episode. Where this is fed back, it may enable a more accurate discrimination of a future prodrome.

Such an interview is shown in Box 10.4. This involves five stages. The first establishes the date of onset of the episode and the time between this and any admission. The second establishes the date when a change in behaviour was first noticed, and in the third and fourth stages the sequence of subsequent changes is established using specific prompts if necessary. Finally, the prodrome is

**Box 10.4** Early signs interview: relatives version

**Stage One**: Establish date of onset, admission to hospital and behaviour at height of episode.
'On what date was X admitted to hospital?'
   Prompt:    Date, day, time: contemporary events to aid recall
'When did you decide he needed help?'
   Prompt:    Date
'What was X's behaviour like at this time?'

**Stage Two**: Establish date when change in X was first noticed.
'So X was admitted to hospital ... weeks after you decided he needed help ... '
'Think back carefully to the days and weeks before then.
When did you first notice a change in X's unusual behaviour or anything out of the ordinary?'
   Prompt:    Nature, time of change
'Were there any changes before then, even ones which might not seem important?'

**Stage Three**: Establish sequence of changes up to relapse.
'I'd like to establish the changes that took place after that up to (date) when you decided X needed help ... '
'What happened next (after last change)?'
   Prompt:    Was this a marked change?
               When did this happen?
               Can you give me some examples?
               Repeat question until point of relapse is reached.

**Stage Four**: Prompting for ideas not already elicited.
'During this build up to his relapse/admission to hospital ... was he anxious or on edge?'
   Prompt:    When did you notice this?
               Prompt items from relevant Early Signs checklist.
'Did he seem low in his/her spirits?'
   Prompt:    As above
'Did he seem disinhibited (excitable, restless, aggressive, drinking etc.)?'
   Prompt:    As above
'Did he seem suspicious or say/do strange things?'
   Prompt:    As above

**Stage Five**: Summary.
'Let me see if I'm clear on what happened before X's admission.'
'X was admitted on (date), (number) of weeks after you decided he needed help: he was (describe presentation).'
'You first noticed something was wrong on (date) when he (describe behaviour) ... then he began to ... ' (complete description of prodrome).
'Have I missed anything out?'

**Figure 10.3** Early
signs: KF

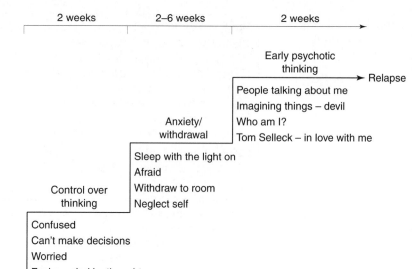

summarised. Figure 10.3 represents the outcome of one such
interview which was drawn by the client herself.

*Monitoring and*
*intervention*

In our work, individuals engage in a process of monitoring using
the 'Early Signs' scale described above. There are four objectives as
shown in Box 10.5. Thus, monitoring is conceived not as a lifetime
activity but as a relatively short-term manoeuvre to learn about the
process of relapse, to engage patient and professional in meaningful activity and to demonstrate that control can be achieved.

In the next stage, decision rules are agreed to define the onset of
a prodrome operationally; these may include a quantitative change
on the ESS scales and/or the appearance of individualised prodromal signs. This, then, is an entirely client driven and controlled
system, as is the intervention. The possibility that some prodromes

**Box 10.5** Monitoring

This has four objectives:

1. To develop a baseline measure against which changes
   can be discerned and compared;

2. To reinforce the discrimination of the changed percep-
   tual, cognitive and affective processes through use of
   appropriate labels;

3. To educate individuals, their carers and professionals
   about the precise nature of the 'relapse signature';

4. To promote clients' engagement with services, and to
   share responsibility for prodrome detection between individuals, carers and professionals.

may spontaneously remit (due, for example, to personal coping responses) suggests a two-stage strategy, in which the first includes increased surveillance of the ' at risk' mental state.

Early intervention seeks to intervene as early as possible in the process of relapse on the basis of information that relapse is probable. Where a pharmacological intervention is indicated, a targeted and time-limited oral dose of neuroleptics may be chosen in advance in consultation with the client. Figure 10.4 provides three individual case examples, from the Birmingham Early Intervention Study (Birchwood *et al.*, 1991).

In the first case (Figure 10.4a), SH achieved a baseline score of 13 on the ESS scale including the presence of idiosyncratic signs: racing thoughts, inefficient and confused thinking, poor concentration and a 'giggly' effect. He self-administered a targeted dose of 20 mg of Stelazine which was increased by 50% if an improvement was not observed within one week. His record clearly shows a steady improvement over six weeks with no breakthrough of either hallucinations or delusions.

The second case, a 28-year-old female with a three year history of multiple relapses, achieved a baseline score of eleven and the decision rule was a 20 point increase in the ESS scores, in the context of the following relapse signature: irritability and social withdrawal, entertaining thoughts about telepathic contact with people she once knew and having difficulty distinguishing dreams from reality. She self-medicated with Stelazine, and after five weeks her signs subsided (Figure 10.4b).

In the third case, targeting began when TS experienced his relapse signature, including: poor concentration, inefficient thinking, social withdrawal and a loss of appetite for up to a week accompanied by a change of ESS scores of 20 points. Again, the impact of self-medication was readily apparent and shown in Figure 10.4c.

A sense of ownership over these data should be fostered with patients and their families so that responsibility for initiating early intervention is a shared one; for example in the author's work, regular updated copies of the graphs are available to participants, many of whom are taught to interact with a computer-based system. Educating patients and relatives about early signs of relapse, collaboration in monitoring, feeding back to them information from the early signs interview and any detected prodromes should significantly raise the likelihood of future early detection and therefore intervention.

*Support and counselling*   Once a prodrome has been declared, the individual and family need intensive support. The psychological reaction to a loss of well-being, and the possibility that this may herald a relapse, places a significant strain on both parties, which if unchecked, could accelerate the decompensation process. The availability of support,

**Figure 10.4** The impact of early pharmacological intervention. See text for details. —, self-report; – – –, observer

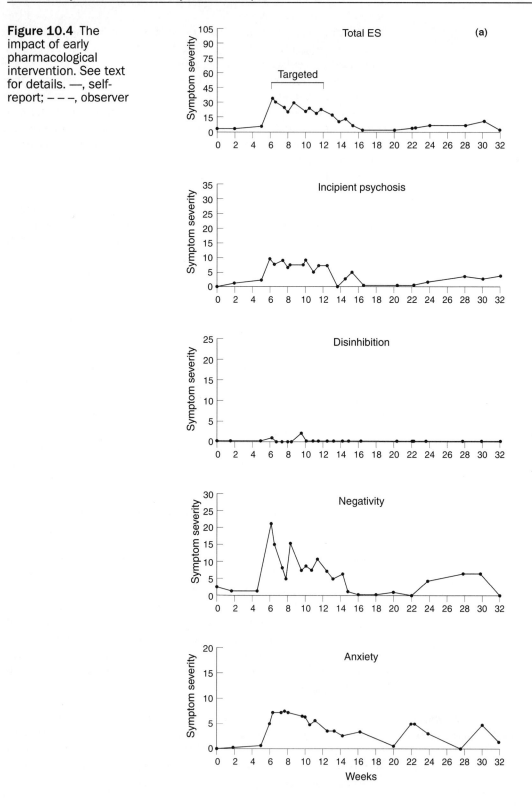

**Figure 10.4**
(*continued*)

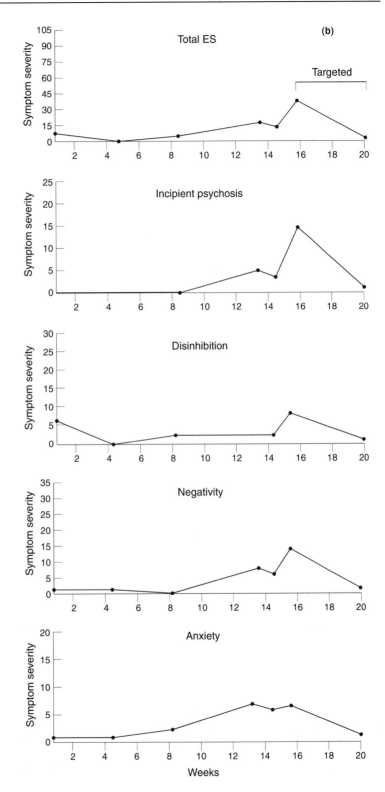

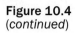

**Figure 10.4**
(*continued*)

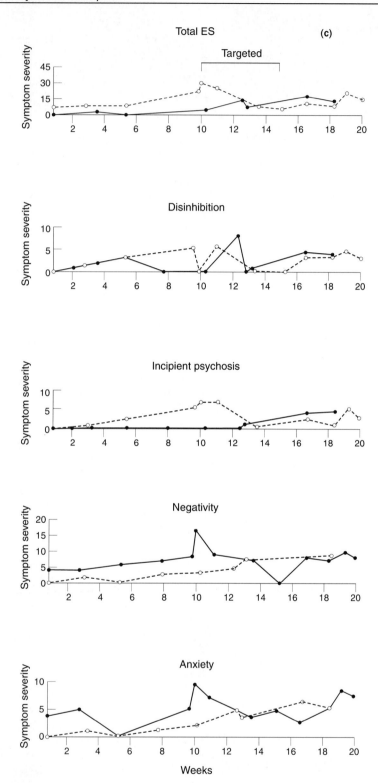

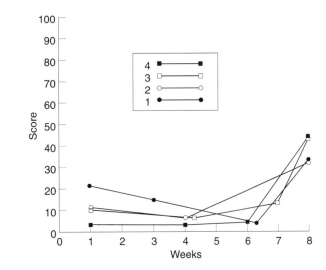

**Figure 10.5** Total E. W.S. : TF. EWS, early warning signs. 1, First relapse; 2, Second relapse; 3, Third relapse; 4, Fourth relapse

quick access to the team, the use of stress management and diversionary activities may help to mitigate these effects (Breier and Strauss, 1983).

Weekly, daily, or even inpatient contact can be offered, which serves to alleviate anxiety and emphasises the shared burden of responsibility. In routine clinical practice, most clinicians value the opportunity to utilise day care where admission is not deemed necessary but an element of decompensation is evident.

*Clarifying the relapse signature*    Impending or actual crises present an important opportunity to 'sharpen the image' of the signature for client, carer and professional; in this respect the crises can be reframed as an opportunity to acquire information that can facilitate control and prevention. Figure 10.5 illustrates a client who showed early relapse on more than one occasion. The prodromes of these episodes are juxtaposed in the figure. Considerable consistency in the nature and timing of the early symptoms is apparent, consistent with the signature concept. In the case of TF, the record clarifies that the time window is at least two weeks; the onset of 'psychotic thinking' coincides with increases in agitation and withdrawal. Two weeks before this, TF showed clear evidence of an improvement in these indices (agitation/withdrawal) followed by an abrupt deterioration. This, then, was incorporated into his signature, 'raising the question' of early relapse.

*COGNITIVE APPROACHES TO EARLY INTERVENTION*    The propensity of individuals to self-regulate their illness and the individual's search for meaning in disordered experience (Birchwood, 1995, 1996) offer options for a cognitive approach to the enhancement of self-care. Three components might be considered. The first step involves identifying the attributions that individuals make about their symptoms, which may include catastrophisation (e.g. 'I am relapsing and I can't control it'), the employment of an externalising attribution linked to the appraisal of changed mental life (e.g. 'something is happening *to* me') or social attribution (e.g. 'people are saying they're not interested in me').

Second, a modified form of cognitive therapy (CT) may be employed to facilitate reattribution that emphasises control: de-catastrophisation is a CT technique frequently employed in the management of panic attacks and involves the examination of supposed catastrophic consequences and emphasises those aspects that are within the client's control; verbal challenge, hypothetical contradiction and the search for alternatives (Chadwick and Lowe, 1990; Chadwick and Birchwood, 1994) are CT techniques that have found a therapeutic role in the management of delusional beliefs. Third is the use of stress management manoeuvres and the rehearsal of a coping repertoire, including the challenging of these various cognitions that disempower the individual. A small number of case studies have been conducted to develop these ideas, and a recent example is shown below (Birchwood, 1995, 1996).

*Case study: KF*    ***Assessment***
Six weeks into a training course at a local college, KF reported a diminution in her ability to sustain concentration on her studies and further disturbing symptoms including restlessness, anxiety, racing thoughts, low mood and loss of sleep. She also reported entertaining themes about a relationship with a famous actor and had begun to feel that people were talking about her on the bus, referring to her past sexual behaviour and fantasies and aspects of her family's feelings towards her. These referential ideas were often triggered while watching the television or travelling on her own. This constellation of symptoms conformed to her prodrome, and was confirmed to be an elevated score on the ESS scales from 8 to 28. Interview elicited three recurring cognitions associated with her distress:

1. 'I'm relapsing, it's my fault and I'm going right back to the beginning (of my recovery).'
2. 'I'm immature for having these sexual fantasies.'
3. 'Everyone knows about my past.'

***Intervention***
Within a collaborative atmosphere, the three cognitions were discriminated and addressed. The first two cognitions were generalised ones and appeared to be linked to periods of restlessness and agitation.

Regarding the first cognition, it was suggested that the tendency to relapse was a feature of the illness for which she bore no responsibility. She was invited to consider the case of her friends at the hostel where she lived who had shown signs of relapse following a stressful period and whether she would consider them responsible. She reasoned that to avoid training courses and the like was a sign of being defeated by her illness; at least she had tried. The factors within her control were reviewed. In order to decatastrophise her thinking about relapse, a short-term stress control measure was agreed involving a reduction in her attendance at college from four days a week to two, and similarly a reduction in the time she spent watching the television, as this was a trigger for her ideas of reference. To reinforce the stress attribution she was taught some anxiety management techniques including breathing control and muscular relaxation.

The cognition that she was immature was countered by asking her to consider whether this held true in the light of evidence of her past relapses. Even though her last relapse was a full one, she nevertheless managed to get to the point of returning to college: the fact that on this occasion she has caught her relapse early was offered as evidence for her learning greater control which would improve, and not adversely affect her recovery and well-being. Through a process of 'live' rehearsal she was encouraged to challenge these cognitions concurrently with employing the stress management techniques.

KF felt guilty and that 'someone of my age should not be having these (sexual) thoughts'. A distinction was made between her sexual fantasies and the re-emergence of the delusional theme about the famous actor. With regard to the former, therapy focused on normalising such fantasies and these were tested by encouraging her to discuss these in confidence with a trusted friend and her key worker. The thought about the famous actor was characterised as a 'fossilised' thought that had been laid down during the time of her life when her illness began (her teens) and which re-emerged on these occasions, and thus, it was suggested, had no meaning. As evidence of this she debated that this actor was no longer attractive to her and was simply a teenage idol. This reframing approach served to disengage her from the thought and enabled her to dismiss it.

The third, referential, cognition was examined by use of a verbal challenge centering on the motive and means by which others would try to achieve this. The fact that the referential ideas centred only on her guilty thoughts about her past was considered. She acknowledged that guilty thoughts do lead to 'paranoid vigilance' and day-to-day examples were identified to support this. This was tested by rehearsing some distraction techniques – it was predicted that the more she was able to distract her thoughts, the less she would experience referential thinking. This was made achievable through use of brief programmed bus journeys, which were the main setting conditions for her ideas of reference.

***Outcome***

KF was seen three times a week for two weeks. Her EWS score reverted to baseline as did her insight score. No pharmacological intervention was used and KF slowly increased her days at college.

***THE EFFICACY OF EARLY INTERVENTION***

In the opening section of this chapter it was argued that perceived loss of control over 'illness' (relapse, residual symptoms), the life goals this affects, as well as relapse itself can lead to deleterious outcomes for people with psychosis (depression/demoralisation, suicide, raised relapse risk). In addition to any further opportunities, early pharmacological and/or cognitive intervention which places the individual in the 'driving seat' may promote control and self-efficacy. The important evaluative questions then are as shown in Box 10.6.

**Box 10.6** Evaluative questions

1. Can pharmacological interventions initiated at the onset of apparent early symptoms slow down or arrest the relapse process?

2. Is cognitive early intervention effective and can it achieve similar or better outcome than pharmacological early intervention, and is their combination better than either alone?

3. Does the process of early intervention (education, collaborative monitoring etc.) improve clients' understanding and discrimination of prodromes and control of relapse and promote a 'collaborative' style of engagement with services?

***Pharmacological early intervention***

Many of the drug studies have involved withdrawing patients from maintenance regimes, monitoring clinical state and providing brief pharmacotherapy at the onset of a prodrome. This paradigm has been chosen with the goal of minimising drug exposure and therefore side-effects, without prejudicing prophylaxis, rather than as a means of controlling further relapse. This issue will be returned to at the conclusion of this section.

Three well-controlled studies have been reported using this paradigm (Box 10.7). Jolley *et al.* (1989, 1990) studied 54 stabilised, symptomatic and, thus, highly selected patients who were randomly assigned to active or placebo maintenance therapy conditions, with both receiving early drug interventions at the onset of a prodrome which involved the administration of 5–10 mg of haloperidol daily. Patients received a brief educational session about prodromes and early intervention on entry to the study, as reliance

**Box 10.7** Pharmacological early intervention studies

| | Maintenance and targeted | | Targeted only | |
| --- | --- | --- | --- | --- |
| | Jolley et al. (1990) | Carpenter et al. (1990) | Jolley et al (1990) | Carpenter et al. (1990) |
| Relapse – 1 year | 7% | | 30% | |
| Relapse – 2 year | 12% | 36% | 50% | 53% |
| Readmissions – 1 year | 7% | | 13% | |
| Prodromes | 27% | 1.6%/year | 76% | 3.18%/year |
| Side-effects | 55 | ? | 24 | ? |
| Drug-free period | 0% | 0% | ? | 48% |
| Non-adherence | | 19% | | 51% |

was placed on patients to recognise their early signs of relapse and to contact the clinical team. Outcome at one year revealed that significantly more patients experienced prodromal symptoms in the intermittent group (30% versus 7%), although there was good evidence that 'severe relapse' was not affected and was indeed low in both groups. Nevertheless, the large difference between the number of prodromes and number of relapses does suggest that prompt action can abort relapse in many instances. During the first year of the study, 73% of relapses were preceded by identified prodromal symptoms; during the second year this fell to 25%, as reliance was placed on patients and families to identify and seek assistance for prodromal symptoms. This suggests 'that the single teaching session at the start of the study does not provide patients and families with an adequate grasp of the intermittent paradigm ... ongoing psychoeducation should be an essential component of further studies' (Jolley *et al.*, 1990, p. 841).

Carpenter *et al.* (1990) report the outcome of a study of similar design to that by Jolley and colleagues with largely similar outcomes. However, in their study, not only was the intermittent regime less effective, it was also less popular: 50% refused to continue with the regime (versus 20% in continuous treatment), presumably due to the higher rate of prodromes and hospitalisations and perhaps also due to the fact that patients found the responsibility placed on them to recognise relapse an excessive one.

Gaebel *et al.* (1993) report a multicentre open German trial comparing maintenance and targeted medication, targeted medication alone ('early intervention') and no pharmacotherapy. Six 'prodromal' symptoms were measured by the participating psychiatrists using a four-point scale of severity on a regular basis; impending relapse was designed on the basis of a 'significant increase' in these symptoms, but was essentially determined by the psychiatrist. The study found that relapse under targeted pharmacotherapy alone (49%) was less than no pharmacotherapy

(63%) but was greater than maintenance and targeted pharmacotherapy combined (23%). This study suffered from a massive drop-out of over 56%, on a par with the Carpenter study, and no data are presented regarding selectivity of drop-outs by experimental condition. Unlike the other studies, the results do suggest that targeted medication alone is effective in controlling relapse compared to no treatment, but again the value and relative popularity of maintenance medication is clearly underlined.

The methodology used to identify relapse prodromes has relied heavily on patients' skill and their initiative to alert services. Jolley *et al.* (1990) have suggested that a brief educational session is insufficient for patients to sustain a grasp of the prodrome concept and early intervention; and the high drop-out rate noted by Carpenter *et al.* (1990) underlines its unpopularity. This experience suggests that this responsibility is viewed best as one that is very clearly shared between patient, carer and services.

Experimental designs ask specific questions and hitherto the early intervention studies have asked only limited questions, namely, whether a targeted regime alone yields comparable prophylaxis to one which combines maintenance and targeting yet minimises side-effects. The answer to this is clearly negative, although the Gaebel study does suggest that targeted treatment is not without benefit. For present purposes, therefore, our question then becomes: can a 'standard' dose maintenance medication combined with a targeting paradigm control relapse to an adequate degree?

The study by Jolley *et al.* found an unusually low rate of relapse over two years in the group receiving continuous and targeted regimes (12%), suggesting a possible additive effect. Marder *et al.* (1984, 1987) studied patients assigned to a low (5 mg) or standard (20 mg) dose maintenance regime of fluphenazine decanoate over two weeks and at the first sign of exacerbation the dose was doubled. If this failed, patients were considered to have relapsed; this occured in 22% taking the lower dose and 20% on the higher dose, with fewer side-effects in the former. Marder *et al.* found that lower doses carried a greater risk of relapse, but these were not 'serious' and were eliminated once the clinician was permitted to double the dose at the onset of a prodrome (the survival curves of the dosage groups were not different under targeted conditions). This was later followed up by a study of low-dose neuroleptic maintenance treatment in schizophrenia (Marder *et al.*, 1994) in which 36 patients were given 10 mg of fluphenazine hydrochloride under double-blind conditions following the appearance of operationally defined 'prodromes'. Prodromal symptoms were monitored weekly in each group using an individually tailored 'idiosyncratic prodromal scale' including the three most common symptoms arising from the baseline interviews with each patient and an informant, similar to the methodology outlined by Birchwood *et al.* (1989). Survival analysis beginning at the start of the second year demonstrated a significant reduction in relapse risk for those receiving active drug supplementation, and that they spent less time in psychosis during the second year and that patients and clinicians improved over time in their ability to detect 'true' prodromes. The study by Gaebel *et al.* (1993) found a similar rate of two-year relapse under maintenance and targeted conditions alone ($P < 0.001$). Overall these data suggest two conclusions: first, using pharmacotherapy alone, in maintenance and targeted forms, relapse can be reduced to 12–23% over two years; and second this can be achieved with a low dose regime. A cognitively oriented intervention would therefore have some further work to do to reduce relapse even further if it were to be combined with this 'ideal' form of pharmacotherapy.

Opportunities for cognitive early intervention do not rest on this consideration alone, however. There is first of all the problem of medication non-adherence (Hoge, 1990). Studies of clients' attitude to medication show that the prevailing view is ambivalent: a necessary evil (Pan and Tantam, 1989). This resistance is linked partly to the experience of dysphoria and other drug side-effects (Hogan *et al.* 1985) and to a perception that treatment is coercive and disempowering.

Non-adherence has been associated with youth, compulsory detention (Buchanan, 1992) and its excessive use among Black groups (Sashidharan, 1993). Cognitive and pharmacological early intervention approaches that are essentially client driven may find favour with those who are disaffected by prescriptive approaches. In the wider arena of psychological interventions, a titration of drug dose against family intervention has been reported (Falloon and Pederson, 1985; Hogarty *et al.*, 1988); the cognitive approach to early intervention, if successful, may similarly offer options that allow medication to be used more sparingly than at present, thus maximising its efficacy and attractiveness.

*Collaborative early intervention*

Collaborative early intervention as described here is an attempt to confer, in a practical sense, empowerment in relation to relapse by placing the individual in the 'driving seat' determining when and if and how intervention should take place. We are presently in the midst of a trial of this approach but we are able to present indirect evidence that the impact of collaborative early intervention is a positive one.

Box 10.8 shows a comparison of 35 patients taking part in our early intervention project two years pre- and post-trial entry (i.e. non-first episodes). This shows a sharp decline in rates of re-admission including compulsory admission and time spent in hospital. We believe the style of service provision is facilitating the engagement with services of a difficult client group who were selected as young, high relapse risk, and predominantly inner city residents. We are also collecting data on a group of clients who

**Box 10.8** Analysis of admissions and days in admission 2 years pre- and post-trial entry (Those entering the trial after a first admission are excluded)

| | Pre-trial entry | Post-trial entry |
|---|---|---|
| No. (%) of patients admitted | 26(74%) | 9(26%) |
| Total no. of admissions for group | 31 | 10 |
| No. of compulsory admissions | 13 | 1 |
| Days in hospital | 2781 | 729 |

*n* = 35 patients

have spent two years in the early intervention programme, and comparing them with a case-matched control group on their ability to discriminate and clarify their prodrome, their understanding of the significance of these symptoms and their attribution of these symptoms, and fear and control of relapse (Davis *et al.*, in press).

*Cognitive early intervention*

There are as yet no studies which have attempted to evaluate cognitive early interventions using single cases or group studies. As we have seen, there is little as yet in the way of theory guide to such an approach. Stress-vulnerability is a general theory which would offer stress management intervention linked to the cues or stresses and to the client's cognitive and emotional stress responses. If our model is correct, then once in prodrome, cognitive and attributional processes would come into play that might exacerbate stress (e.g. catastrophic thoughts about relapse) as well as driving delusional thought about externalising attribution process.

Since prodromes are neither regular not prolonged occurrences, developing these interventions will be fraught with difficulty (in contrast to cognitive therapy for psychotic symptoms or panic disorder). This will necessitate the use of considerable rehearsal as a prelude to *in vivo* management of the kind described for KF. There are immense opportunities here, particularly as it holds out the hope of engaging a client group who are traditionally resistant and for whom the approach outlined in this chapter will have face validity.

*CONCLUSION*

The clinical application of early signs monitoring offers considerable opportunity for improving care. However, if the encouraging results of the early intervention studies employing targeted medication are to be realised in clinical practice, careful thought must be given to the identification of individual 'relapse signatures', the design of monitoring methodology, the training of mental health professionals and the nature of the service response to secure these advances for the well-being of people with psychosis.

The relationship between early signs of decompensation and actual psychotic relapse remains unclear. There is unlikely to be a simplistic relationship and the evidence suggests that false positives and negatives will occur. We have discussed a number of means to improve the specificity of early signs information using additional information relating to idiosyncratic signs for a given individual.

Experienced staff, engaged in long-term clinics supporting patients often have years of regular contact with the client and can provide useful information concerning certain key changes which in themselves might go unnoticed but which, for a given individual, may be highly predictive of relapse. The fuller 'relapse signature' that is thus obtained can be incorporated into the early signs monitoring procedure and used as a hypothesis to predict specific idiosyncratic signs which will occur at a subsequent relapse of a given individual. Any additional early signs information observed at this relapse can be added to the signature, thereby increasing the accuracy of prediction with each relapse.

The strategy of close monitoring by highly trained personnel is impractical in routine care. On the other hand, the use of close monitoring staff for particular target groups with a high relapse risk is limited by the ability to reliably select high potential relapsers. The methodology adopted by Birchwood *et al.* (1989), harnessing the experiences of patients and their carers in a routine service setting, may be possible to apply clinically. This offers the potential for documenting information relating to early signs of relapse for a substantial group of patients, with relatively limited input of professional time. However, it is still possible that a substantial group of patients, who retain very little insight or lose interest very early in decompensation, may be unable or unwilling to entertain self-monitoring, and are also least likely to consent to observation by another. There are no easy solutions to these problems, although education about the illness may, in some cases, improve insight and permit key people in the individual's life to monitor and recognise specific early warning signs, and to initiate preventative strategies such as seeking professional help promptly if relapse is predicted.

Notwithstanding its potential therapeutic value, the notion of self-monitoring does raise a number of concerns about sensitising patients and carers to disability, promoting the observations as critical responses, burdening individuals and carers further with requests for repetitive information at frequent intervals, or increasing the risk of self-harm in an individual who becomes demoralised by an impending relapse. There is no real evidence that self-monitoring is likely to increase the risk of self-harm; indeed, florid and uncontrolled relapse may be more dangerous and more damaging. Engaging patients and carers more actively in the management of the illness may also promote a sense of purposeful activity and have therapeutic benefits *per se*. The repetitive nature of the procedure may be self-defeating in the long term and indeed wasteful in well-stabilised patients. Instituting monitoring at times of stress may be a reasonable alternative to continuous monitoring. Those individuals who develop expertise in monitoring through a number of relapses may develop and sharpen the signature in the minds of professionals and carers alike. Despite the many limitations, if early signs monitoring fulfils even part of its promise, it may for many patients with recurrent episodes, promote learning and lead to increased opportunity for combined efforts to control exacerbations due to stress.

*DISCUSSION*
*QUESTIONS*

♦ Is the concept of the prodrome a misnomer? Relapse may be a continuous process, not a staged one. The failure of a prodrome to predict relapse may be the result of the intervention of a treatment, particularly self-control strategies.

♦ Is the relapse signature best viewed as an 'at risk' mental state?

♦ Are the early symptoms of relapse indicative of a cognitively mediated stress response?

♦ Cognitive approaches to early intervention have clinical validity but they have yet to be subject to empirical validation.

*FURTHER READING*

♦ Birchwood, M.J., Smith, J., Macmillan, F. *et al.* (1989) Predicting relapse in schizophrenia: the development and implementation of an early signs monitoring system using patients and families as observers. *Psychological Medicine*, 19, 649–656.
This emphasises the individualised nature of early symptoms of relapse and the carer's role in their detections.

♦ Birchwood, M.J. (1995) Early intervention in psychotic relapse: cognitive approaches to detection and management. *Behaviour Change*, 12, 2–19.
A cognitive analysis of the individual's appraisal of the 'at risk' mental state.

♦ Herz, M.I. and Lamberti, J.S. (1995) Prodromal symptoms and relapse prevention in schizophrenia. *Schizoprenia Bulletin*, 21, 541–551.
A review of the status of prodromes arguing that the moderate sensitivity of prodromes to predict relapse must be interpreted within the stress-vulnerability perspective.

♦ Marder, S.R., Wirsching, W.C., Van Putten, J. *et al.* (1994) Fluphenazine vs. placebo supplementation for prodromal signs of relapse in schizophrenia. *Archives of General Psychiatry*, 51, 280–287.
A ground breaking study showing that targeting medication at the onset of a prodrome can help to reduce relapse after twelve months in people receiving low dose medication.

**REFERENCES**

American Psychiatric Association (1994), *Diagnostic and Statistical Manual*, 4th edn. Washington: APA.

Birchwood, M. (1995), Early intervention in psychotic relapse: Cognitive approaches to detection and management. *Behaviour Change*, 12, 2–19.

Birchwood, M. (1996), Cognitive assessment of voices. In: Chadwick, P., Birchwood, M. and Trower, P. (Eds) *Cognitive Therapy for Delusions, Voices and Paranoia*. Chichester: Wiley.

Birchwood, M., Smith, J. and Cochrane, R. (1992), Specific and non-specific effects of educational intervention for families living with schizophrenia: a comparison of three methods. *British Journal of Psychiatry*, 160, 806–814.

Birchwood, M., Mason, R., Macmillan, J.F. and Healy, J. (1993), Depression, demoralisation and control over psychotic illness: a comparison of depressed and non-depressed patients with a chronic psychosis. *Psychological Medicine*, 23, 387–395.

Birchwood, M., Smith, J., Macmillan, F. and McGovern, D. (1991), *Early intervention in psychotic relapse: a controlled trial*. London: Department of Health.

Birchwood, M., Cochrane, R., Macmillan, F., Copestake, S., Kucharska, J. and Cariss, M. (1992), The influence of ethnicity and family structure on first-episode schizophrenia: a comparison of Asian, Afro-Caribbean and White patients. *British Journal of Psychiatry*, 161, 783–790.

Birchwood, M., Smith, J., Macmillan, F. *et al.* (1989) Predicting relapse in schizophrenia: the development and implementation of an early signs monitoring system using patients and families as observers. *Psychological Medicine*, 19, 649–656.

Breier, A. and Strauss, J.S. (1983), Self control in psychiatric disorders. *Archives of General Psychiatry*, 40, 1141–1145.

Buchanan, A. (1992), A two-year prospective study of treatment compliance in patients with schizophrenia. *Psychological Medicine*, 22, 787–797.

Carpenter, W.T., Hanlon, T.E., Summerfelt, A.T., Kirkpatrick, B.M., Levine, J. and Buchanan, R.W. (1990), Continuous versus targeted medication in schizophrenic outpatients. *American Journal of Psychiatry*, 147, 1138–1148.

Chadwick, P. and Birchwood, M. (1994), The omnipotence of voices. A cognitive approach to auditory hallucinations. *British Journal of Psychiatry*, 164, 190–201.

Chadwick, P. and Lowe, C.F. (1990), The measurement and modification of delusional beliefs. *Journal of Consulting and Clinical Psychology*, 58, 225–232.

Davis, E., Birchwood, M., Smith, J., Macmillan, F. and McGovern, D. (submitted), Discriminating the early warning signs of relapse: the impact of a monitoring system. *British Journal of Clinical Psychology*.

Davis, J.M. and Casper, R. (1977), Anti-psychotic drugs: clinical pharmacology and therapeutic use. *Drugs*, 14, 260–282.

Derogatis, L., Lipman, R. and Covi, L. (1973), An outpatient psychiatric rating scale – preliminary report. *Disorders of the Nervous System*, 36, 323–330.

Falloon, I. and Pederson, J. (1985), Family management in the prevention of morbidity of schizophrenia: the adjustment of the family unit. *British Journal of Psychiatry*, 147, 156–163.

Gaebel, W., Frick, U., Kopcke, W. *et al.* (1993), Early neuroleptic intervention in schizophrenia: are prodromal symptoms valid predictors of relapse? *British Journal of Psychiatry*, 163, 8-12.

Heinrichs, D., Cohen, B. and Carpenter, W. (1985), Early insight and the management of schizophrenic decompensation. *Journal of Nervous and Mental Disease*, 173, 133-138.

Herz, M. and Melville, C. (1980), Relapse in schizophrenia. *American Journal of Psychiatry*, 137, 801-812.

Herz, M.I., Symanski, H.V. and Simon, J. (1982), Intermittent medication for stable schizophrenic outpatients. *American Journal of Psychiatry*, 139, 918-922.

Herz, M.I. and Lamberti, J.S. (1995), Prodromal symptoms and relapse prevention in schizophrenia. *Schizophrenia Bulletin*, 21, 541-551.

Hirsch, S.R. and Jolley, A.G. (1989), The dysphoric syndrome in schizophrenia and its implications for relapse. *British Journal of Psychiatry*, 156, 46-50.

Hogan, T.P., Awed, A.G. and Eastwood, M.R. (1985), Early subjective response and prediction of outcome to neuroleptic drug treatment in schizophrenia. *Canadian Journal of Psychiatry*, 30, 246-248.

Hoge, S.K. (1990), A prospective multicentre trial of patients refusal of antipsychotic medication. *Archives of General Psychiatry*, 47, 949-956.

Hogarty, G.E., McEvoy, J.P., Munetz, M.R. *et al.* (1988), Dose of Fluphenazine, familial expressed emotion, and outcome in schizophrenia. *Archives of General Psychiatry*, 45, 979-805.

Hogarty, G.E., Anderson, C.M., Reiss, D.J. *et al.* (1991), Family psychoeducation, social skills training and maintenance chemotherapy in the after care treatment of schizophrenia: II. Two year effect of a controlled study on relapse and adjustment. *Archives of General Psychiatry*, 48, 340-347.

Jolley, A.G., Hirsch, S.R., McRink, A. and Machanda, R. (1989), Trial of brief intermittent neuroleptic prophylaxis for selected schizophrenic outpatients: clinical outcome at one year. *British Medical Journal*, 298, 985-990.

Jolley, A.G., Hirsch, S.T., McRink, A. and Wilson, L. (1990), Trial of brief intermittent neuroleptic prophylaxis for selected schizophrenia outpatients: clinical and social outcome at two years. *British Medical Journal*, 301, 837-842.

Jorgenson, P. (in press), Early signs of psychotic relapse in schizophrenia. *British Journal of Psychiatry*.

Kumar, S., Thara, R. and Rajkumar, S. (1989), Coping with symptoms of relapse in schizophrenia. *European Archives of Psychiatric Neurological Science*, 239, 213-215.

Loebel, A., Lieberman, J.A., Alvir, J.M.J., Mayerhoff, D.I., Geisler, S.H. and Szymanski, S.R. (1992), Duration of illness and outcome in first-episode schizophrenia. *American Journal of Psychiatry*, 149, 1183-1188.

Malla, A.K. and Norman, R. (1994), Prodromal symptoms in schizophrenia. *British Journal of Psychiatry*, 164, 487-493.

Marder, S.R., Mintz, J., Van Putten, T., Levell, M., Wirsching, W. and Johnston-Cronk, K. (1991), Early prediction of relapse in schizophrenia: an application of receiver operating characteristic (ROC) methods. *Psychopharmacology Bulletin*, 27, 79-82.

Marder, S.R., Van Putten, T., Mintz, J., Levell, M., McKenzie, J. and Faltico,

G. (1984), Maintenance therapy in schizophrenia: new findings. In: Kane, J. (Ed) *Drug Maintenance Strategies in Schizophrenia*. Washington: American Psychiatric Association, pp. 31–49.

Marder, S.R., Van Putten, T., Mintz, T., Levell, M., McKenzie, J. and May, P.R.A. (1987), Low and conventional-dose maintenance therapy with fluphenazine decanoate. *Archives of General Psychiatry*, 44, 518–521.

Marder, S.R., Wirsching, W.C., Van Putten, J. *et al.* (1994), Fluphenazine vs. placebo supplementation for prodromal signs of relapse in schizophrenia. *Archives of General Psychiatry*, 51, 280–287.

McCandless-Glincher, L., McKnight, S., Hamera, E., Smith, B.L., Peterson, K. and Plumlee, A.A. (1986), Use of symptoms by schizophrenics to monitor and regulate their illness. *Hospital and Community Psychiatry*, 37, 929–933.

McGlashan, T.H. (1988), A selective review of North American long-term follow-up studies of schizophrenia. *Schizophrenia Bulletin*, 14, 515–542.

Mueser, K.T., Bellack, A. and Blanchard, J. (1992), Comorbidity of schizophrenia and substance abuse: implications for treatment. *JCCP*, 60, 845–855.

Norman, R.M.G. and Malla, A.K. (1995), Prodromal symptoms of relapse in schizophrenia: A review. *Schizophrenia Bulletin*, 21, 527–539.

Overall, J.E. and Gorham, D.R. (1962), The Brief Psychiatric Rating Scale. *Psychological Reports*, 10, 799–812.

Pan, R. and Tantam, D. (1989), Clinical characteristics, health beliefs, and compliance with maintenance treatment: A comparison between regular and irregular attenders at a depot clinic. *Acta Psychiatrica Scandanavica*, 7, 564–570.

Sashidharan, S.P. (1993), Afro-Caribbeans and schizophrenia: the ethnic vulnerability hypothesis re-examined. *International Review of Psychiatry*, 5, 129–144.

Shepherd, G. (1990), Case management. *Health Trends*, 22, 59–61.

Smith, A. and Birchwood, M. (1990), Relatives and patients as partners in the management of schizophrenia. *British Journal of Psychiatry*, 159(suppl.14), 57–61.

Subotnik, K.L. and Neuchterlein, K.H. (1988), Prodromal signs and symptoms of schizophrenic relapse. *Journal of Abnormal Psychology*, 97, 405–412.

Tarrier, N. Barrowclough, C. and Bamrah, J. (1991), Prodromal signs of relapse in schizophrenia. *Social Psychiatry and Psychiatric Epidemiology*, 26, 157–163.

Wing, J.K., Cooper, J. and Sartorius, N. (1974), *The Description and Classification of Psychiatric Symptomatology: An Instruction Manual for the PSE and CATEGO Systems*. London: Cambridge University Press.

Yung, A., McGorry, P., McFarlane, C.A., Jackson, H.J., Patton, G.C. and Rakkar, A. (1996), The prodromal phase of first episode psychosis: past and current conceptualisations. *Schizophrenia Bulletin*, 22, 283–303.

# CHAPTER 11

# The Administration and Monitoring of Neuroleptic Medication

## Peter Pratt

KEY ISSUES

- ◆ Terminology, differences between neuroleptics, dose equivalence and cost
- ◆ Benefits and hazards of drug treatment
- ◆ Balancing risks and benefits
- ◆ Involving patients in their own treatment
- ◆ Role of the pharmacist

INTRODUCTION    This chapter explains the role of neuroleptics in the treatment and management of psychoses. The rational basis of drug treatment is explained, but the reader is directed to specific texts such as the British National Formulary for prescribing details of individual drugs. The benefits and side-effects of treatments are explained in such a way that the information can readily be incorporated into explanations for patients and carers. To differentiate the real and apparent differences between the various neuroleptics, dose equivalents and the financial implications of neuroleptic treatment are also described. Emphasis is placed on the importance of optimising treatment through systematic assessment and treatment planning in collaboration with the patient and their carers, and access to a specialist pharmacist in the multidisciplinary team.

TERMINOLOGY    Before discussing medication used in the treatment or management of serious mental health problems, it is important to establish a clear understanding of the terminology used in relation to drugs and drug treatment and to dispel myths and misconceptions. Even the word 'drug' has connotations of illegality, addiction and overall unpleasantness. 'Medicine' may be a preferable term but many wrongly assume this to refer to the liquid form of the preparation. To avoid confusion, it is important to be clear about the context in which the words are used and to avoid any preconceived judgements about drugs or medicines being inherently 'good' or 'bad'. If the drugs are to be judged, then it should be the way in which they are prescribed, taken or otherwise used that should be judged good or bad, rather than the drugs themselves.

Clearly precision is needed when dealing with medication, but there are times when terminology is used loosely, to describe a concept, rather than an accurate description of the chemical structure or pharmacology of the drug. For instance a patient may be described as 'being treated with phenothiazines' when in fact they are taking haloperidol. Although haloperidol is not a phenothiazine, in this situation the word phenothiazine may have been loosely used to mean 'phenothiazine or other groups of drugs used in similar conditions'; other terms taken to have a similar meaning are 'neuroleptic', 'antipsychotic', 'tranquilliser' and 'major tranquilliser'. In addition to this, most drugs have brand names as well as an approved or generic name, which can cause more confusion.

Undoubtedly these drugs do have tranquillising properties; they may produce a feeling of indifference or tranquillity, and in some circumstances, often in low doses, they are used solely as a sedative or tranquilliser. However, the primary aim of treatment is usually to reduce or relieve the symptoms of psychoses, so perhaps the most appropriate term for these medicines is 'antipsychotic'. This should not be taken to indicate complete specificity of the action of the drugs and some people prefer to use the term neuroleptic, which was a term introduced in the 1950s to indicate compounds which reduce extrapyramidal function. There are now antipsychotics available which appear to have relatively little effect on extrapyramidal function, yet the terms 'antipsychotic' and 'neuroleptic' have become interchangeable and are mainly used in a general, rather than literal sense.

By convention, a systematic way of naming chemicals has been developed. For example a chemical made up of 17 carbon atoms, 19 hydrogen atoms, 1 chlorine atom, 2 nitrogen atoms and 1 sulphur atom would be written as $C_{17}H_{19}ClN_2S$. As the position of these atoms is important in determining the properties of the chemical, the convention tells us this chemical is called 2-chloro-10-(3-dimethylaminopropyl)phenothiazine. In everyday practice, the use of such chemical terminology for drugs would become unworkable, hence the development of a system giving these chemicals an 'approved' name. In this example the approved name of the chemical is chlorpromazine.

Clearly there can only be one chemical or approved name for a given substance, but in clinical practice people are not given the raw chemicals as their medicine, the chemical has to be presented in a way which makes it possible to administer. To manufacture the medication as a tablet, liquid or injection, a pharmaceutical company will compress a quantity of the chemical with other ingredients such as binding and bulking agents and give the end product a particular colour and shape depending on the mould and the type of dye or colorant used. The first company to make chlorpromazine called their medicine 'Largactil'. Therefore, products made by this company which contained the drug 'chlorpromazine' had the brand name 'Largactil'. Once the patent had expired, other drug companies started to make tablets containing chlorpromazine. They could also give brand names to their products, such as 'Chloractil' produced by DDSA pharmaceuticals, or leave their tablets with no brand name apart from the name of the active ingredient – chlorpromazine.

As one would expect, the major difference between any 'branded' product and an unbranded one is price. There may also be other minor differences such as colour or shape, but from a pharmacological perspective there is no difference between a product with a brand name Largactil and one with a brand name Chloractil: they both contain the same drug – chlorpromazine – and as long as the dose (number of milligrams) is the same, one would expect the same pharmacological effect from both products. Yet these apparently minor or cosmetic differences between brands could present a major concern for those prescribed the drugs. If the name, colour and shape of the tablet change they may be concerned that their medication has been changed or they may believe they have been given the wrong medication. Time spent explaining some of these practical issues around medication, such as brand names, will help reduce these concerns. It is also worth pointing out that mistakes with medication are very rare, but they do happen, and unexpected changes in the appearance or 'name' of medication should be checked.

***DIFFERENCES BETWEEN NEUROLEPTICS***

The British National Formulary states that the difference between the various antipsychotic drugs is less important than the variability in patient response to the individual drug. In practical terms this means that there does not appear to be a major difference between any of the available neuroleptics (with the exception of clozapine) in terms of efficacy. There are, however, major differences between the various agents in terms of potency, tolerability, side-effect profile and cost. Traditionally the neuroleptics are classified according to their chemical structure, which gives rise to the 'family' groups, shown in Box 11.1.

**Box 11.1** Families of neuroleptics

| Approved name | Brand name(s) |
|---|---|
| *The phenothiazines* | |
| Chlorpromazine | Largactil, Chloractil |
| Methotrimeprazine | Nozinan, Veractil |
| Promazine | Sparine |
| Pericyazine | Neulactil |
| Pipothiazine | Piportil |
| Thioridazine | Melleril |
| Fluphenazine | Moditen, Modecate |
| Perphenazine | Fentazin |
| Prochlorperazine | Stemetil |
| Thiopropazate | Dartalan |
| Trifluoperazine | Stelazine, Terrazine |
| | |
| *The butyrophenones* | |
| Haloperidol | Haldol, Fortunan, Serenace |
| Trifluoperidol | Triperidol |
| Benperidol | Anquil |
| Droperidol | Droleptan |
| | |
| *The thioxanthenes* | |
| Zuclopenthixol | Clopixol, Clopixol Acuphase |
| Flupenthixol | Depixol |

*Other neuroleptics from different chemical classes include*

| | |
|---|---|
| Sulpiride | Dolmatil, Sulparex, Sulpitil |
| Clozapine | Clozaril |
| Pimozide | Orap |
| Loxapine | Loxapac |
| Risperidone | Risperdal |

Other neuroleptics under development include: Sertindole, quetiapine, olanzapine, ziprasidone and amisulpiride.

Since the introduction of chlorpromazine more than 40 years ago, clozapine so far appears to be the only significant development in terms of efficacy. The majority of newer antipsychotics, such as sulpiride and risperidone, do, however, appear to have a reduced propensity for extrapyramidal side-effects, which may lead to improved tolerability and compliance. Other developments have been the production of different formulations of the antipsychotics, such as long-acting 'depots', or liquid preparations.

**EFFICACY** It appears that, with the possible exception of clozapine, all the currently available neuroleptics are equally effective in controlling psychotic symptoms (Kane and Marder, 1993). This is not surprising as all the neuroleptics share the effect of postsynaptic dopamine $D_2$ blockade. Although this is clearly an oversimplification, $D_2$ blockade is still commonly felt to be one of the most important factors in the antipsychotic effects of these drugs. As well as being effective against psychotic symptoms the neuroleptics also have a general tranquillising effect, which leads to their use in the control of acute behavioural disturbances. Other conditions where neuroleptics may be used include the control of emesis and intractable hiccups.

Schizophrenia is the only well-established indication for long-term use of neuroleptics. Even so, these drugs can by no means be described as curative; at best they can be described as having some beneficial effect in 70–80% of cases. In the first few days of treatment, neuroleptics will primarily affect behaviour. Delusions and hallucinations may take several weeks to respond. The so-called negative symptoms of social withdrawal, flat effect and poverty of speech may take months – if indeed they do respond at all to drug treatment (Breier *et al.* 1987).

**BENEFITS OF DRUG TREATMENT**

The benefits of neuroleptic medication have been clearly demonstrated in numerous studies (Kane, 1996). There can be no doubt that these agents are effective both in the treament of acute schizophrenic episodes and in preventing relapse. Although neuroleptics will control symptoms in up to 80% of cases, the nature of improvement can vary quite significantly between individuals. In some cases the benefit of symptom control is outweighed by the unpleasant and disabling side-effects of medication. In other circumstances the drugs may have little or no effect on the more disabling features of schizophrenia, such as loss of motivation and emotional blunting. Indeed some of the side-effects of conventional neuroleptics may mimic or exacerbate these symptoms. Overall there will be some 20–30% of people who will not respond to conventional antipsychotics (Anon, 1995).

Before embarking on treatment with neuroleptics it is essential that a full review is undertaken and a medical assessment must be made to exclude any organic causes of psychoses. Any physical abnormalities such as impaired cardiac function must be taken into account when establishing a treatment plan. For any individual, the purpose of drug treatment should be clear. This can best be achieved by evaluation of response in target symptoms. In the early stages of drug treatment these symptoms are most likely to be behavioural; in time, other symptoms will usually respond, but for some people response may be little more than a reduction of distress.

Traditionally the more sedative neuroleptics have been advocated in the acute management of psychoses, particularly where behavioural disturbance exists. In practice this has often led to high doses of neuroleptics being inappropriately used – primarily for their sedative side-effects (Peralta *et al.*, 1994). In view of the dangers of higher doses, and the tolerance that develops to sedative effects, it is advisable to use conventional doses of neuroleptics, with adjunct sedatives such as lorazepam to control behavioural disturbance. Although some practitioners have viewed this as inappropriate 'polypharmacy', in practice any negative aspect of 'polypharmacy' is outweighed by the ability to separate the sedative and antipsychotic elements of treatment, and thereby more accurately titrate the dose of the individual drug to the desired effect.

Once the initial symptoms have been controlled, people with schizophrenia are significantly more at risk of a relapse if they discontinue neuroleptic medication (Davis, 1975). In a naturalistic follow-up Johnson (1979) found improvement in both social functioning and reduced relapse rates, in patients who remained on drugs for 12 months. However, there are a small number of people who will remain symptom free without medication. Although the number of people who remain symptom free after the first episode is reported to be between 10% and 30% (Hogarty and Ulrich, 1977; Keks *et al.*, 1995), there continues to be a view that for the majority, outcome may be worse than this. Unfortunately, there is no sure way of distinguishing those patients who will relapse and those who will not. Therefore, it is generally accepted that medication should be continued for one to two years after the first episode, before treatment is gradually withdrawn (Kane, 1996).

In an attempt to reduce the frequency and severity of relapse in more chronically ill patients (i.e. those who have experienced two or more episodes of relapse) consideration should be given to continuing medication long term. Even with continued medication around 15–20% of patients may relapse within one year and up to 30% within two years. Only 20% will survive for up to five years without a relapse (Johnson, 1990). The protective effect of neuroleptics does not appear to be cumulative as an increase in relapse rates will be found if neuroleptic drugs are subsequently discontinued, even after several years of treatment.

Although this chapter deals with medication, successful pharmacotherapy can only occur against a background of intensive psychosocial support and the role of non-drug factors in preventing or exacerbating relapses must not be overlooked. Psychosocial interventions used in conjunction with medication can be effective in minimising relapse (Davies, 1994).

## DOSES OF NEUROLEPTICS

Paradoxically, the wide safety margin of neuroleptics may be considered responsible for some of the inappropriate ways in which they have been used in the past. Some psychiatrists have talked about there being 'no such thing as a maximum dose' in psychiatry, and 'the dose you need is the dose that works'. In some cases this has led to very large doses of neuroleptics being prescribed. Patient non-response has been simply explained by inadequate absorption, leading to higher doses being prescribed (Thompson, 1994).

There is now overwhelming evidence that there is no advantage in prescribing higher doses of neuroleptics, either in the acute situation or for longer-term maintenance. In a review of current issues around antipsychotic drugs in schizophrenia, Jain *et al.* (1988) remarked that rather than further research into the area of dosage, priority needs to be given to dissemination of knowledge to clinicians, many of whom take pride in their ability to remain comfortable when giving massive doses of neuroleptics.

In the UK, the Royal College of Psychiatrists has published a consensus statement on the use of high-dose antipsychotic medication (Thompson, 1994). This report resulted from the growing concern that neuroleptic drugs may be implicated in sudden unexplained deaths of psychiatric patients. In terms of the effects of dose, high doses of neuroleptics were defined as that which exceeds the advisory upper limit for general use in the British National Formulary (BNF), or product licence. For patients receiving medication under the Mental Health Act, the doses of neuroleptics should be within BNF limits, unless specifically recorded otherwise.

If someone is receiving more than one neuroleptic – a practice often referred to as polypharmacy – there is the additional danger that several neuroleptic drugs may be used, each within the so called BNF limit, but together producing a cumulative adverse effect. Individual prescribers occasionally advocate the advantages of combinations of neuroleptics, but there is still no conclusive evidence that using neuroleptic drugs in this way either increases the benefit or reduces the harm associated with the drugs.

Although the primary effects of neuroleptics are thought to be associated with their capacity to block dopamine $D_2$ receptors, drugs like clozapine have been found to have pharmacological effects on other neurotransmitter symptoms. The mixing of different types of neuroleptics could therefore be seen as some sort of pharmacological cocktail, designed to mimic the profile of drugs like clozapine, resulting in improved efficacy. Not only is there no evidence that this strategy is helpful, but in some cases patients end up receiving the equivalent of massive doses of neuroleptics, with clinicians believing their prescribing is safe as the amount of each drug is 'within BNF limits'. Despite the lack of established benefit and obvious hazards associated with combinations of neuroleptics, it is interesting to speculate that future research may establish the value of such therapy as we develop a greater understanding of how drugs work in schizophrenia.

**CHLORPROMAZINE EQUIVALENCE**

There are currently in excess of 20 different neuroleptics available in the UK. For each drug or preparation the relative harm/benefit ratio can be established for an individual, but this makes comparison between agents difficult. In a previous section it was stated that the difference in response between individuals was probably greater than the difference between the various drugs. In clinical practice there will often be a great reluctance to accept this. Patients may describe very unpleasant experiences from the side-effects of one type of drug as opposed to another. Unfortunately the relative difference in dose between the drugs is often overlooked when comparing the effects of one drug against another. Although some of the newer neuroleptics may differ, in many cases the variation in severity of side-effects experienced by people taking the drug can be explained by the fact that they are taking relatively more of one type of drug than another. In short, an understanding of the relative potencies of the different neuroleptics is important in explaining the different effects people may experience with the various neuroleptics.

Consider an individual patient who has been prescribed one 10 mg tablet of haloperidol which results in a very unpleasant and frightening side-effect such as an acute dystonic reaction. If that patient's drug treatment is then changed to one 100 mg chlorpromazine tablet, twice a day, the patient may perceive that they are being given more drugs as they are receiving more milligrams and double the number of tablets. If that patient does not then suffer the same side-effects with chlorpromazine, they will conclude that chlorpromazine is a better (or less hazardous) drug for them than haloperidol. Observation of these phenomena will also be taken into the 'clinical experience' of people caring for the patient. Events such as this lead to unhelpful impressions about the difference between drugs. In this example the patient is receiving around three times the amount of haloperidol, compared with chlorpromazine, therefore to draw a realistic comparison between the drugs the patient would have needed to have been prescribed five or six 100 mg chlorpromazine tablets, which would produce a markedly different response.

Despite the reservations of an oversimplification of the dopamine theories of schizophrenia, there is a reasonable correlation between the ability of a neuroleptic drug to block postsynaptic dopamine $D_2$ receptors and the number of milligrams required to produce an antipsychotic effect.

This leads to the concept of 'chlorpromazine equivalents'. That is, each antipsychotic drug can be expressed in terms of the number of milligrams required to produce an equivalent degree of dopamine $D_2$ blockage as 100 mg of chlorpromazine. This enables us to compare relative potencies of the different neuroleptics. Someone receiving a high potency neuroleptic such as haloperidol will require significantly fewer milligrams to produce the same antipsychotic effect as someone receiving a low potency drug like chlorpromazine or thioridazine. Once the concept of equivalence is grasped, it is important to remember that the premise upon which it is based is an oversimplification based on *in vitro* receptor binding studies, and the notion that antipsychotic effect is $D_2$ receptor blockade. It does not take account of interpatient variables in absorption, nor the other pharmacological effects contributing to antipsychotic effects.

Although numerous textbooks contain tables of antipsychotic equivalents concern has been expressed at the variation in equivalence quoted from various sources (Dewan and Koss, 1995; Foster, 1989). Major differences in equivalence appear in relation to the higher potency neuroleptics (Box 11.2).

**Box 11.2** Differences in equivalence

| | BNF equivalence (mg) | Reported range (mg) |
|---|---|---|
| Chlorpromazine | 100 | 100 |
| Fluphenazine | 2 | 2–5 |
| Haloperidol | 2–3 | 1–10 |
| Thioridazine | 100 | 50–120 |
| Trifluoperazine | 5 | 3.5–8 |

By using tables like that in Box 11.2, it is possible to compare the relative amounts of neuroleptics that different people may receive, or compare different treatments the same person has had over time. If the chlorpromazine equivalence is used to predict the maximum dose of neuroleptic, a somewhat inconsistent picture is found when comparing the maximum BNF advisory dose and the calculated maximum dose (Box 11.3).

**Box 11.3** Comparison of doses

| | BNF advisory maximum dose (mg) | Calculated equivalence (mg) |
|---|---|---|
| Chlorpromazine | 1000 | 1000 |
| Fluphenazine | 20 | 20 |
| Haloperidol | 100(200) | 20(40) |
| Trifluoperazine | None | 50 |

In practice the maximum dose of any drug is determined by clinical studies demonstrating subjects' ability to 'tolerate' high doses of drugs, not the relative chlorpromazine equivalence. Nevertheless this concept can be useful in both understanding and explaining the effects of different neuroleptics.

## HAZARDS OF DRUG TREATMENT

Despite the well-established benefits of neuroleptic medication in both symptom control and preventon or reduction of a relapse, there are significant risks associated with its use. The disabling nature of some of these side-effects may understandably result in patients discontinuing their medication. Rather than considering the benefits of drug treatment outweighing their symptoms, for some patients a more realistic appraisal of their treatment options is the balance of the catastrophic effects of the disorder and the unpleasant and disabling side-effects of medication. Once symptoms have subsided, it is sometimes difficult for some patients to accept the risks and consequences of a relapse if they discontinue their medication. When they are feeling well it is difficult to accept that a relapse may not only result in a return of distressing 'symptoms', but could also include family, social and occupational breakdown or self-harm.

When considering the hazards of treatment, it is not possible simply to look at treatment as either harmful or not. The question can only be considered in the context of the benefits of drug treatment. For an individual, it is the relative balance between benefit and harm from drug treatment that must be established.

## SIDE-EFFECTS OF NEUROLEPTICS

Standard texts such as the BNF provide a useful summary of the different side-effect profiles of the neuroleptics. One mistaken criticism about the BNF is that too little detail is given about individal neuroleptics, with side-effects often listed as 'see under chlorpromazine'. The simple reality is that most neuroleptics do produce a similar range of side-effects (Box 11.4) with certain drugs differing in the degree or severity of one type of side-effect over another.

Even if we knew the precise areas of the brain involved in schizophrenia, the neuroleptics are not 'smart drugs', they do not selectively and exclusively target areas of the brain. Once the drug is absorbed, the neuroleptic will act on various sites within the body. Blockade of dopamine $D_2$ receptors is felt to be important therapeutically within the mesolimbic area, whereas the blockage of these receptors within the nigrostriatal tract is responsible for many of the parkinsonian type movements induced by the drugs. It is possible to control some of these extrapyramidal side-effects by the administration of anticholinergic (antimuscarinic) agents (Box 11.5).

**Box 11.4** Side-effects
of neuroleptics

The more common, or serious side-effects associated with neuroleptics include:

*Antimuscarinic*: dry mouth, blurred vision, urinary retention, constipation

*Sedation*

*Cardiovascular*: postural hypotension, cardiac arrhythmias, tachycardia

*Extrapyramidal*: dystonia, parkinsonism, tardive dyskinesia, akathisia, temperature dysregulation, neuroleptic malignant syndrome

*Endocrine disturbances*: galactorrhoea, hyperprolactinaemia, amenorrhoea

*Sexual dysfunction*: impotence, delayed ejaculation

*Reduced seizure threshold*

*Haematological reactions*: agranulocytosis

**Box 11.5**
Anticholinergic drugs

| Approved name | Brand names | Formulations available |
|---|---|---|
| Benztropine | Cogentin | Tablets, Injection |
| Benzhexol | Artane, Broflex | Tablets, Liquid |
| Orphenadrine | Disipal, Biorphen | Tablets, Liquid |
| Arpicolin | Kemadrin | Tablets, Liquid, Injection |
| Biperiden | Akineton | Tablets, Injection |

These drugs do have a range of side-effects as well as the potential for abuse. If they are necessary to control extrapyramidal symptoms, their use should be reviewed and treatment gradually withdrawn after one month. If extrapyramidal symptoms return, and the dose of neuroleptic cannot be reduced, the drugs should be re-introduced and attempts made to reduce and withdraw the drugs every two or three months. There is no justification for the long-term regular prescribing of these drugs. Some patients take the drugs intermittently on a when required 'prn' basis which is fine, as long as the drugs continue to relieve extrapyramidal symptoms.

The neuroleptics may also cause a range of other side-effects related either to dopaminergic inhibition in other areas or as a consequence of interfering with non-dopaminergic systems. The antimuscarinic drugs have no useful effect on these side-effects, and in some circumstances may exacerbate the condition. If a person is using these agents to control the side-effects of neuroleptics, it is essential that they are fully aware of which side-effects the drugs will help and which they won't. There is a common misconception that antimuscarinic agents are general antidotes for all the side-effects of neuroleptics.

*Acute dystonic reactions*    Acute dystonic reaction occurs due to contraction of involuntary muscles, commonly involving those of the head and neck. This may be manifest as the tongue protruding (torticollis), the neck may arch backwards and sideways with the mouth open, the jaw may become locked (trismus) or the gaze may become fixed, followed by upwards rotation of the eyes (occulogyric crisis). Rarely the respiratory muscles may be involved, which could be life threatening and should be treated as a medical emergency, with the immediate parenteral administration of anticholinergic agents.

If these reactions occur, they usually do so soon after treatment is initiated or increased (days or weeks). The effect is dose related and therefore high potency drugs are often implicated. They may last for a few minutes or several hours. Young males less than 30 years of age appear to be more at risk. The patient remains aware of the events, which become distressing and frightening. Although the condition will remit as plasma levels of neuroleptics fall, the distressing nature of these side-effects warrants treatment with anticholinergic drugs.

The risk of developing an acute dystonic reaction will be reduced if careful attention is given to the dose and rate of dose increases of neuroleptic. Although routine co-administration of anticholinergic is not generally recommended, some clinicians advocate the practice when starting treatment in susceptible people. As these side-effects may be the first experience patients have of taking neuroleptics, their reluctance to continue taking the drugs, following such a reaction, is understandable.

*Akathisia*    Also referred to as 'restless legs syndrome', in which patients may describe a particularly unpleasant feeling of inner restlessness. One patient has described feeling like 'wanting to jump out of their skin'. They may continuously move in an attempt to satisfy this feeling. It can be mistaken for an increase in psychotic agitation, resulting in more, rather than less neuroleptic. The condition may manifest as constant pacing, tapping the feet or shifting the legs. Women may be more commonly affected than men.

Akathisia develops more slowly than the acute dystonic reactions and may become apparent after days or weeks of treatment. Unlike the dystonias, akathisia is not helped by antimuscarinic drugs. Beta-blocking agents (e.g. propranolol), or a benzodiazepine (e.g. diazepam) may be more useful. The most appropriate strategy is to reduce the dose of neuroleptic, although this may not always be feasible.

***Pseudo parkinsonism***   Neuroleptics do not cause Parkinson's disease, but they can induce the classical features of parkinsonism: muscle rigidity, tremor, generalised slowing of movements (bradykinesia), shuffling gait and excessive salivation. The effects may occur within days or weeks of starting neuroleptics and appear to be dose related. Patients may look 'drugged' as their facial expressions and voluntary movements are reduced or lost. These symptoms occur in around the same time frame as akathisia (days to weeks) and appear to affect women more commonly than men. The symptoms are controlled by anticholinergic agents, but as the effect is dose related, initial consideration should be given to reducing the neuroleptic.

At one time it was felt that the development of parkinsonian symptoms was a useful indication that the neuroleptic had been given in effective antipsychotic doses; this is an oversimplification. It is possible to use neuroleptic drugs effectively without using doses that cause the more overt symptoms of parkinsonism. Many of the newer neuroleptics (olanzapine, sertindole, clozapine, risperidone and sulpiride) appear to cause either no or fewer extrapyramidal side-effects than the traditional neuroleptics, even when used in equivalent doses.

***Tardive dyskinesia***   After neuroleptic agents have been taken long term (more than six months) involuntary movements, commonly of the mouth, lips and tongue, may develop. The tongue may roll round the mouth occasionally flicking out, lips may be repetitively pursed, the cheeks puffed and a constant chewing motion may be observed. Other movements may include ticks and facial grimacing, increased blinking and whole body rocking movements. These movements may be particularly stigmatising and isolating, as the patient looks 'odd'. The social interaction that commonly occurs between people is unlikely to happen with someone sticking their tongue out, constantly smacking their lips and rocking backwards and forwards.

Women may be more at risk than men, but the prevalence does increase with age (Bristow and Hirsch, 1993). Despite a range of studies examining the effects of various treatments, there is as yet no established effective treatment (Cavallaro and Smeraldi, 1995). Treatment with vitamin E or clozapine may prove to be beneficial, but for the moment this remains speculative. Anticholinergic drugs are not effective and may worsen the condition; the only strategy is to reduce or remove the neuroleptic. In the early stages of neuroleptic withdrawal, tardive dyskinesia may appear to worsen, but this is usually temporary and eventual remission is possible. Unfortunately there is a proportion of patients in whom the condition remains, despite withdrawal of the neuroleptic.

Although prevention is by far the best strategy, this may be difficult. The main risk factors for tardive dyskinesia appear to involve the patient, rather than the drug (Cavallaro and Smeraldi, 1995). Overall, age appears to be the most important risk factor with duration of treatment and dose of neuroleptic being the major pharmacological risk factors. In an attempt to prevent the occurrence of tardive dyskinesia patients should be assessed every 6–12 months for evidence of involuntary movements, particularly the tongue. Neuroleptic drugs should only be used, or continue to be used, where there is clear evidence of benefit.

*Neuroleptic malignant syndrome*

Neuroleptic malignant syndrome unfolds over one to three days and consists of raised body temperature (hyperthermia), muscle rigidity, fluctuating levels of consciousness, increased heart rate and labile blood pressure. Massively raised levels of creatinine phosphokinase are also found. Although rare (reports vary between 0.02% and 3.2%), it can be fatal if not recognised and promptly dealt with. The syndrome can develop at any time during the course of treatment with neuroleptics and appears to affect men more than women. Dehydration and concomitant treatment with lithium appear to be additional risk factors.

Anyone developing neuroleptic malignant syndrome should be treated as a medical emergency and neuroleptics should be immediately withdrawn. This may be difficult with patients receiving long-acting 'depot' neuroleptics. Treatment is aimed at reducing temperature and ensuring the maintenance of vital functioning. Anticholinergic drugs are not thought to be helpful and may interfere with the body's natural cooling mechanisms. Dantroline and bromocriptine have both been advocated as helpful. Once the syndrome has subsided there will be a dilemma over whether or not to reintroduce neuroleptics. The risk of recurrence is said to be about 50%. Whenever possible the decision to re-start neuroleptics must involve the patient. In practice this may be difficult, as the reason for re-introducing neuroleptics will normally be because the patient has relapsed. The risk of recurrence will be less if low potency drugs (e.g. sulpiride) are used and treatment delayed for up to two months.

*Hyper-prolactinaemia*

Due to their effects on the anterior pituitary dopaminergic receptors, neuroleptics cause a rise in prolactin and other hormones. This may lead to a variety of problems including: lack of, or irregular menstrual periods (amenorrhoea), reduced libido, breast enlargement and breast tenderness. Females and occasionally males may start producing milk (lactating). Although these effects are rare, if they do occur, their occurrence is often quoted as having little significance. However, for most patients it will not be helpful to dismiss effects like these as insignificant. Not least the suppression of menstruation may lead females to wrongly conclude they are no longer at risk of pregnancy and fail to take contraceptive precautions.

**Sexual dysfunctioning**

Neuroleptics affect sexual functioning in a variety of ways. Males may find it more difficult to obtain or maintain an erection, ejaculation may be delayed, or sometimes retrograde ejaculation occurs where the ejaculate passes 'backwards' into the bladder. The quality of orgasm can be affected and females may report an inability to reach orgasm. Due to the generalised tranquillising effects of the neuroleptics people may become indifferent to sex, which may further compromise their ability to maintain relationships. Although tolerance may develop to some of these effects, dose reduction or a change in type of neuroleptic are the main options for treatment. A simple explanation and reassurance that these effects are a predictable consequence of neuroleptic treatment often helps to allay anxiety about the cause of the problems. The side-effects are not permanent and any drug-related impairment of sexual functioning will resolve if the drug is withdrawn.

**Effects on the blood**

Neutropenia, agranulocytosis and aplastic anaemia occur rarely during treatment with neuroleptic drugs, with the exception of clozapine. Reports of agranulocytosis report an incidence of 1 in 10 000 and 1 in 500 000 people treated with traditional phenothiazines. Clozapine carries a significant risk of inducing neutropenia (around 3%) and agranulocytosis (around 0.7%). In normal circumstances the risk would not be considered acceptable, but as clozapine is the only treatment available that has been clearly shown to offer some possibility of response where other neuroleptics have failed, the risk may be acceptable. In the UK the availability of clozapine is restricted to psychiatrists and pharmacists registered with the clozapine monitoring scheme. This ensures patients do not receive clozapine unless both the psychiatrist and the pharmacist are aware that their patient has had a satisfactory blood test every week for the first 18 weeks of treatment, every two weeks up to one year and every month thereafter.

**Effects on the cardiovascular system**

Low potency neuroleptics commonly cause postural hypotension, causing patients to become dizzy on standing. In the elderly this may be particularly problematic. Thioridazine is a low potency neuroleptic often advocated as a drug causing less extrapyramidal disturbances. This has led to its common use in the elderly, where although it may cause fewer problems with parkinsonism it is more likely to induce postural hypotension. Neuroleptics also have a direct effect on cardiac functioning, altering conduction. Electrocardiogram (ECG) changes may occur, which can be serious in some patients or those taking other treatments affecting the heart. Higher doses of pimozide have been reported to be particularly risky and routine ECG is now recommended prior to using this drug.

*Antimuscarinic effects*    As well as blocking dopamine receptors many neuroleptics, particularly the low potency ones, will also affect acetylcholine. One positive effect of this may be the reduced propensity for causing extrapyramidal disturbances. The pharmacological effect from this type of neuroleptic can be considered similar to taking a combination of a dopamine blocking compound plus an anticholinergic agent. The antimuscarinic side-effects are commonly described as 'anticholinergic effects'. These will manifest as blurred vision, dry mouth, urinary retention and constipation. If a patient is given an anticholinergic such as procyclidine (Kemadrin) to control the parkinsonian side-effects of the neuroleptic, these anticholinergic side-effects will be exacerbated.

*Weight gain*    Many patients find the weight gain associated with neuroleptics unacceptable. Although this problem is associated with most neuroleptics, chlorpromazine and clozapine appear to be the most commonly implicated. Careful attention to diet may be helpful, but is an unrealistic option for some people. Assuming a neuroleptic continues to be indicated, weight gain may be reversed by changing to an alternative agent.

*Secondary negative symptoms*    In many ways this should be considered the most severe and disabling side-effect of the neuroleptics. The whole purpose of giving neuroleptics is to reduce, suppress or relieve the symptoms of illness, and to prevent these recurring. To some degree they are effective particularly against the so-called positive symptoms such as hallucination and delusions. The preceding section has demonstrated there is sometimes a price to pay for this, but in the majority of cases drug treatment can be managed in such a way that the benefits of treatment outweigh these problems or side-effects. To date, with the possible exception of clozapine, neuroleptics do not appear to provide substantial benefit in people suffering the so-called 'negative' features of schizophrenia. These include apathy, withdrawal, flat mood, slow speech and movement. These symptoms will result in demotivation, social isolation and lack of self-care leading to patients failing to achieve a meaningful existence and eventually losing contact with any supporting service. Interestingly, it is often the presence of 'positive symptoms' that may actually be keeping patients in contact with services. Once these positive symptoms are controlled, there could be a danger that patients will be lost.

Although there is no doubt that the emotional withdrawal, poverty of speech and diminished self-interest are features of schizophrenia, there continues to be debate over the question of how many of these negative symptoms are drug induced, or by how much neuroleptics exacerbate the pre-existing condition (Coffey, 1994). For example, general slowness of movement (bradykinesia) is a feature of drug-induced parkinsonism. This will present difficulties of interpretation. Has the patient become slow and less spontaneous as a consequence of treatment, or is this just another symptom of their illness? Being clear about 'target symptoms' before initiating drug treatment may help clarify the question, but these symptoms may exist before treatment, and may not become apparent until the more florid symptoms and behaviour have been controlled by drugs.

As the newer neuroleptics (such as sulpiride, clozapine, risperidone, olanzapine and sertindole) appear to have less propensity to cause parkinsonian symptoms, it may be postulated that they are less likely to induce the secondary symptoms associated with bradykinesia. This probably explains why many of the studies attempting to establish the value of these agents in the treatment of negative symptoms are inconclusive or 'suggest', rather than demonstrate, benefit (Cunningham Owens, 1996).

## BALANCING THE RISKS AND BENEFITS OF NEUROLEPTICS

All drug treatment, no matter what it is used for, should be on the basis of a balance between the beneficial effects and the problems associated with treatment. If the benefits outweigh the problems, drug treatment should be continued. If they do not, it should be stopped. If a proper balance between the benefits and harm from drug treatment is to be maintained in conditions like schizophrenia, drug treatment must be adjusted over time to match or take account of the variation in the nature, consequence and severity of the disorder for the individual and their circumstances. There may be some people for whom a relapse results in violence, harm or even death. In these cases few people in our society would argue against the importance of preventing a relapse almost regardless of the consequences of terms of side-effects for the individual. However, this represents the minority of patients. The question of 'benefit' or 'risk' is much less obvious for the majority of patients.

The preceding sections have listed both the benefits and hazards (or side-effects) of treatment. Some people may be tempted to concentrate on the hazards, to emphasise a view that drug treatment must not be used; others may concentrate on the benefits – the removal of symptoms and the prevention of a relapse. Clearly neither extreme is either helpful or true. Comprehensive lists of side-effects can be frightening and require detailed explanation of the likelihood of occurrence. It is uncommon to suffer the whole range of side-effects reported with all the neuroleptics. Many of the side-effects are proportional to the dose used. Therefore, dose adjustment is perhaps one of the most useful strategies in optimising treatment.

### Rating scales

The use of rating scales can help bring an objective assessment, both to the degree of improvement as a result of drug treatment and to the assessment of side-effects. In studies assessing neuroleptic drugs these rating scales are commonly used, but in routine clinical practice there is sometimes a reluctance to develop such systematic assessments. Examples of instruments measuring symptoms include the Brief Psychiatric Rating Scale (BPRS) (Overall and Gorham, 1962), the Manchester scale (KGV) (Krawiecka et al., 1977), the Positive and Negative Syndrome Scale (PANSS) (Kay et al., 1987) and the Scale for the Assessment of Negative Symptoms (SANS) (Anreasen, 1982) (see Chapter 6 for brief review of measures).

Measures of side-effects include the Liverpool University Neuroleptic Side Effect Rating Scale (LUNSERS) (Day et al., 1995) which enables people with schizophrenia to rate their own side-effects. It covers a comprehensive range of neuroleptic side-effects (51) as well as 10 red herring items such as hair loss and dark urine. As the scale takes between 5 and 20 minutes to complete, there is no reason why it cannot be widely used in practice. Simpson and Angus (1970) developed a scale around 30 years ago which measures extrapyramidal side-effects. It consists of 10 extrapyramidal symptoms, scored from 0 (absent) to 4 (severe). The Abnormal Involuntary Movements Scale (AIMS) (Guy, 1976) is a 12 item scale measuring primarily dyskinesias; as with the Simpson and Angus, movements are scored from 0 (absent) to 4 (severe).

*Cost of treatment*   When considering drug treatment the question of 'balance' should not be restricted to consideration of side-effects and benefit from treatment; consideration should also be given to the financial implications of drug treatment which is clearly an expenditure of health care resources which can usually be readily identified.

Health care demands continue to exceed the resources available, which effectively means that expenditure in one area denies the opportunity for that money to be spent elsewhere. This simple fact is often glossed over when claims are made that newer (and more expensive) drugs can 'save money' by enabling patients to be discharged from hospital. If we say the cost of keeping someone as an acute psychiatric inpatient is around £200 per day, then a drug costing £10 per day looks excellent value for money. By prescribing this drug a saving of up to £190 per day can be claimed! In practice this £190 is never realised; it cannot be if the bed and all the staff associated with it still exist. In most cases, where the use of a more expensive drug enables a patient to be discharged the bed (and staff) continue to exist. The actual financial implication of using the 'new' drug is therefore a total expenditure of £210.

From a purely pragmatic perspective it may appear better value for money to have a higher turnover of patients in hospital. The claims that more expensive drugs facilitate this need to be assessed on an individual basis. It is important to remember that discharging a patient does not save money, unless the bed is dismantled and the staff dismissed. This will focus the mind on ensuring the right balance is struck between older (cheaper) and newer (expensive) drugs.

There are two areas where cost is a major issue, the actual cost of the drug and who pays for the drug. The cost of the drug is a question of balancing health care resources, the question of who pays for the drug can sometimes have a bearing on treatment. Within the National Health Service, drugs may be charged to the hospital, or NHS Trust budgets or general practitioner budgets. Patients do not pay for their drugs; some people pay a tax for using the health service, in the form of a prescription charge. Unfortunately this method of tax collection is a significant disincentive for someone already reluctant to take medication. Some people may even have to pay a second prescription charge (tax) on the medication prescribed to counteract the extrapyramidal side-effects of the original medication.

## COMPLIANCE

'People who are ill take medication, people who are not don't.' 'Taking medication is a sign of weakness.' 'All drugs stop working after a time as your body gets used to them.' 'You don't need to keep taking medication once you are better.' 'You should be able to get better on your own, without the help of drugs.' 'You cannot cure mental illness with drugs.' 'Everyone thinks there is something wrong with you if you are on medication.' 'You cannot get a job, or drink alcohol when you are on medication.' 'I don't believe in drugs.'

These are just some of the views of many ordinary people, and even some care workers. Many people just do not like the idea of taking medication, so for someone with a mental illness where they may not even agree they are ill, it is not surprising that 'compliance' or doing what you are told with medication is sometimes a problem. Corrigan *et al.* (1990) report 'non-compliance' with medication to be as high as 80% in psychotic patients.

It was against this background of so-called non-compliance with medication that 'depot' neuroleptics were developed. These are injections of the neuroleptic ester, formulated in vegetable oils, such as coconut oil or sesame oil. The esterification of the neuroleptic does not change its effect. It just enables the drug to be released more slowly and therefore last longer. From some patients' point of view, assuming equivalent doses, there is no difference in effect or side-effect between neuroleptics given as tablets, liquid, injection or as a long-lasting depot injection (the decanoate). The only difference is how quickly the drug produces an effect and how long the drug remains in the body.

The administration of depot neuroleptics may reduce the incidence of covert non-compliance; but if a patient is determined not to take medication, the prescribing of neuroleptics in this way will do nothing more than confirm the fact that the patient is not receiving medication. For some people, regular injections of depot neuroleptics, together with the regular contact and review by community psychiatric nurses can be an important factor in successful treatment. Perhaps the biggest problem when using depot neuroleptics arises because some patients continue to receive medication, sometimes for many years, without consideration of the continued risks or benefits of treatment. With oral medication if a patient does 'nothing' they end up with no medication, whereas with depot medication a patient doing 'nothing' continues to receive medication – assuming that they continue to attend a 'depot clinic' or receive visits from a community mental health nurse.

Compliance aids have been another 'technical' development aimed at improving the compliance of patients with their medication. These devices comprise small plastic boxes, labelled for each day of the week, and separated into dosage times of breakfast, lunch, dinner and bedtime. One week's supply of medication can thus be laid out in advance so that the patient can easily see if they have forgotten a dose. These devices can be extremely helpful for people who want to take their medication, but just forget. They can also be useful in group homes where each person's medication can be checked at a glance, by carers. But, like depot medication, they will not address the most important factors in ensuring correct drug treatment – the motivation, attitude, and beliefs of the patient.

There are times, usually in the acute phase of the illness, when people refuse their medication. The Mental Health Act allows patients to be given medication against their will and so treatment is ensured. There is no such provision for the long-term enforceable administration of neuroleptics, even though they may benefit the majority of people with schizophrenia.

Patients must be involved in decisions about their treatment. It could be argued that even the term 'compliance' is wrong, when talking about medication. The use of this word suggests patients should 'comply', that is, do as they are 'told'. This assumes patients have no say in their own treatment. Instead the use of the word 'alliance' has been suggested as a means of reinforcing the concept of involving patients (and significant others) in the process of drug treatment. Whichever word is used, the important point is that patients must genuinely be involved in their own drug treatment.

*INVOLVING PATIENTS IN THEIR OWN TREATMENT* There are a number of ways in which a person can be involved in their own treatment, so that they have some choice and control over their prescribed medication. Without knowledge, a patient cannot be expected to make informed decisions about their treatment. They will have subjective experiences of the drugs and their illness, they may even have been given long lists of side-effects and benefits of medication, but unless time is spent ensuring that the patient understands the information and what it means for them, the exercise will be little more than tokenistic. Education alone does not necessarily improve compliance with medication (Macphearson *et al.*, 1996). For those who are not averse to taking medication, behavioural interventions focusing on drug taking and using visible cues and prompts does lead to better compliance (Macphearson *et al.*, 1996), however it is important to remember that the whole point of successful drug treatment is achieving the right balance between benefits and hazards of the illness and treatment.

One common misconception is that telling patients about the side-effects of medication will inevitably result in them stopping treatment and suffering relapse. Most of the support for this comes from professionals' experience of patients who have found out about side-effects from 'someone else' and then stopped their medication. The issue here is that the patient's trust in the professional is often lost, rather than the side-effect itself. The problem could be primarily a failure in the relationship between patient and professional. Patients may say 'they didn't tell me about that side-effect – what else haven't they told me?' By understanding the positive as well as the negative side to medication, patients are more likely to accept and participate in successful treatment, and most importantly develop a trusting relationship over drug treatment.

## ROLE OF THE PHARMACIST

A multidisciplinary team in psychiatry traditionally includes nurses, psychiatrists, occupational therapists and social workers. With a few notable exceptions, pharmacists are generally not included as part of the team. Given the fact that the whole of a pharmacist's training is around drugs and drug treatment and that specialist postgraduate training in psychiatric pharmacy can be undertaken by pharmacists specialising in the field, it is difficult to understand why they are not generally involved in all mental health teams, particularly when decisions around drug treatment are often so complex. Pharmacists have a key role in medication review and in providing information.

The only reliable indication for a patient to receive a particular neuroleptic is a previous response. Someone with a long history of mental health problems may have received many drugs over the years; a time consuming but systematic review of previous treatment, by a pharmacist, can help identify the most appropriate treatment for an individual. When drug treatment appears to have failed, a review by a pharmacist can often identify gaps in treatment or drugs that may have produced partial response.

Some hospitals or NHS Trusts encourage mental health teams to formulate treatment plans, which include the need for review and support by a specialist pharmacist, before treatment with some of the more expensive neuroleptics can be approved. The purpose of this is not to use pharmacists to curtail expenditure on new drugs *per se*, but to ensure the right balance is struck between the important factors that make up successful drug treatment.

In an ideal world patients and their important family, friends or carers would know everything they needed to know about their treatment. However, pressure on time, different priorities of mental health workers, and a lack of knowledge on their part, mean that patients do not always get their questions about drug treatment addressed. Referral to a specialist pharmacist who is part of the multidisciplinary team is one way of ensuring all patients have enough information to help them make informed decisions about their drug treatment. Specialist pharmacists can also run open forums, where patients and/or carers can discuss 'anything they like' to do with drug treatment.

One of the barriers to successful team work could be professional rivalry. Some psychiatrists may perceive a pharmacist as a threat, looking to take over their prescribing role. Viewing a pharmacist in this light misses the point that successful drug treatment in psychiatry is about finding the balance between numerous factors for the individual patient, rather than being about the power to prescribe.

*CASE STUDY*   Mr Jones is a 35-year-old gentleman. He has a 10-year history of schizophrenia and has been treated with neuroleptics. He lives in a flat with his dog, but gets very troubled by his neighbours who, he believes, spy on him. He also continuously feels the local newspaper sends people to break into his house to spy on him and interfere with him.

Three years ago, this situation led him to take an overdose which required treatment in intensive care and dialysis. Following the overdose he was admitted to a psychiatric hospital where he was given chlorpromazine 200 mg and 25 mg amitriptyline per day.

Mr Jones refused to take a higher dose of medication as he felt his body could not tolerate it following his overdose. After four weeks on the psychiatric ward he was still concerned about his neighbours and the local paper, but felt if he just got on with his own business in his flat they would not bother him. He was discharged to be followed-up by a community mental health nurse (CMHN) and his general practitioner.

Soon after his discharge Mr Jones stopped taking his chlorpromazine, and was re-admitted one month later in a very distressed condition as he believed the local paper had put up cameras to spy on his every movement. He initially refused medication, but eventually agreed to have 5 mg trifluoperazine (but no more). Over the next two weeks, he became much less distressed and was discharged back to his CMHN. Again he stopped his medication, but agreed to take 12.5 mg fluphenazine decanoate as a depot injection every two weeks.

Last year Mr Jones refused to have anything to do with his CMHN because he felt she was now working for the local paper. A few weeks later he was re-admitted to hospital. He had become very distressed as he felt people from the local newspaper were once again breaking into his flat to spy on him; he also believed they interfered with him in the night and gave him renal failure. Mr Jones was invited to meet the pharmacist to discuss his concerns about medication and renal failure. Following this, a medication review was completed. This revealed that for the past 10 years Mr Jones had never been completely free of psychotic symptoms, but his delusions and distress normally responded to neuroleptics within two to three weeks.

Some of the team felt that Mr Jones' history indicated that he was resistant to treatment and so should be offered clozapine. However, as he had never received any neuroleptic up to BNF maximum doses he could not be considered treatment resistant and clozapine was not pursued at the time.

Mr Jones was grateful for the opportunity to spend time talking about his fears of drug treatment. The team agreed that the 'target symptom' was the distress associated with delusions concerning the newspaper and neighbours. This was clearly documented and he agreed to take trifluoperazine, increasing at 5 mg per week until the target symptom was controlled.

After four weeks Mr Jones was much less distressed, and he expressed a strong desire to return to his flat. He still felt the newspaper people might be spying on him, but he did not feel this would prevent him from getting on with things.

This presented a dilemma; Mr Jones was less distressed from his psychosis, he had no side-effects from neuroleptics, but his past history and continued concerns about medication indicated that he would soon stop taking medication and relapse. However, for more than 10 years Mr Jones had never been free of his delusions and it was agreed that his treatment plan would be to continue to attempt to treat his delusions. This would involve changing to a second neuroleptic and then clozapine, unless side-effects compromised treatment. A great deal of time was spent explaining the rationale of treatment, particularly the reasons for regular blood testing with clozapine.

Over the next 2–3 months, Mr Jones received trifluoperazine up to 40 mg per day, with little change in his symptoms with medication; he then agreed to change to flupenthixol, initially as tablets, and then up to 100 mg every two weeks as a depot injection. During this time Mr Jones' delusions remained, and so clozapine was started. Initially Mr Jones accepted clozapine and blood tests, but after three months became quite concerned about continuing to have his blood tested. He had also started gaining weight, which concerned him greatly and he felt sleepy most of the time.

Mr Jones has now had the opportunity of benefit from drug treatment, but clearly higher doses or more complex treatment were offering no benefit in terms of the quality of his life over his previous treatment. The final part of Mr Jones' treatment plan was to revert to 5 mg trifluoperazine which was the dose he was happy to take, but which was only partially effective in controlling his psychotic symptoms. The only other factor that changed was that Mr Jones was less concerned about this drug affecting his 'renal failure'. He was happy to remain in contact with his CMHN who continued to monitor both his compliance, his symptoms and his concerns about medication.

This case should not be seen as one where drugs have failed; they have not. The important points here are that a clear plan – involving the patient – was established and drug treatment was discussed fully with the patient. When drug treatment failed to achieve the predetermined goals it was changed and finally the optimum dose and role of drug treatment for this individual were established.

*CONCLUSION*

For the majority of neuroleptics at an equivalent dose, the differences between the various agents are less important than the difference in response between individuals; although generalisations can be made about neuroleptic drugs as a group, patients should not be considered as a homogeneous group and individual characteristics in attitude towards medication and response to drugs must be recognised. It is clear that neuroleptic medication has an important role in the support of people with serious mental health problems; by controlling distress, controlling some symptoms of psychosis and preventing relapse, it can be crucial in enabling people to live independently. However, since side-effects and adverse effects are an inevitable consequence of taking neuroleptic medication, the aim of treatment must be to achieve a balance between the consequences of the illness and the consequences of treatment. In this regard, the patients are the experts: they experience the negative and positive effects of medication and, given adequate and accessible information, they can decide where the balance lies. Indeed, without sufficient information and understanding of their prescribed medication, patients will often decide to cease taking tablets but it is not the case that more information leads to greater fear and greater likelihood of 'non-compliance'. It is, therefore, essential to involve the patient in decisions about their treatment. Furthermore, given the importance of medication in the treatment of a great many people who have serious mental health problems, it is essential for all workers and patients to have access to accurate, contemporary information on medication, and for those with particular difficulties related to medication to have direct access to a pharmacist who is able to develop a specific treatment plan. For this reason, all mental health teams should include specialist pharmacists.

*DISCUSSION QUESTIONS*

◆ What should be included in a patient educational package about drug treatment in schizophrenia?

◆ How do you establish the balance between the benefits and hazards from treatment in your clinical practice?

◆ If the government reduced the availability of neuroleptics to three, which three would you insist on being available?

*FURTHER READING*

◆ Tyrer, P.J. (Ed) (1982) *Drugs in Psychiatric Practice*. London: Butterworth.
Although almost fifteen years old, this book still provides an excellent basis for learning about drug treatment in psychiatry. Despite the obvious limitations around 'new' drugs this book should be considered a standard text for anyone involved with psychotropic drugs.

◆ Healy, D. (1993) *Psychiatric Drugs Explained*. London: Mosby Year Book Europe Ltd.
A non-technical book, giving perhaps more of an insight into what people think and feel about psychotropic drugs, rather than an academic account of drug treatment. The book should be used as a means of broadening one's view of medication.

◆ British Medical Association and The Royal Pharmaceutical Society of GB (1996) *British National Formulary*.
Published every six months, the BNF details the indications, side-effects and price range of prescribable medication in the UK. Each chapter contains an introduction to each type of drug outlining the relative place of the drugs within the group.

◆ ABPI (1996) *Compendium of Data Sheets and Summaries of Product Characteristics*. Datapharm publications.
An annual publication containing comprehensive details of licensed medication. Anyone involved in the prescribing of medication should be aware of all the information contained in the product data sheet or summary of product characteristic.

◆ Cooper, J.R., Bloom, F.E. and Roth, R.H. (1991) *The Biochemical Basis of Neuropharmacology*. Oxford: Oxford University Press.
This book provides an in-depth account of the pharmacology of psychotropic medication and the biochemistry of central functioning.

**REFERENCES**    Anon (1995), The drug treatment of patients with schizophrenia. *Drug and Therapeutics Bulletin*, 33, 81–86.

Anreasen, N.C. (1982), Negative symptoms in schizophrenia. *Archives of General Psychiatry*, 39, 784–788.

Breier, A., Wolkowitz, O., Doran, A. *et al.* (1987), Neuroleptic responsivity of negative and positive symptoms in schizophrenia. *American Journal of Psychiatry*, 144, 1549–1555.

Bristow, M.F. and Hirsch, S.R. (1993), Pitfalls and problems of the long term use of neuroleptic drugs in schizophrenia. *Drug Safety*, 82, 136–148.

Cavallaro, R. and Smeraldi, E. (1995), Antipsychotic-induced tardive dyskinesia recognition, prevention and management. *CNS Drugs*, 4, 278–293.

Coffey, I. (1994), Options for the treatment of negative symptoms of schizophrenia. *CNS Drugs*, 1, 107–118.

Corrigan, P.W., Liberman, R.P. and Engel, I.D. (1990), From non-compliance to collaboration in the treatment of schizophrenia. *Hospital and Community Psychiatry*, 41, 1203–1211.

Cunningham Owens, D.G. (1996), Adverse effects of antipsychotic agents: do newer agents offer advantages? *Drugs*, 6, 896–930.

Davies, T. (1994), Psychosocial factors and relapse in schizophrenia. *British Medical Journal*, 309, 353–354.

Davis, J.M. (1975), Overview maintenance therapy in psychiatry, I: schizophrenia. *American Journal of Psychiatry*, 132, 1237–1245.

Day, J.C., Wood, G., Dewey, M. and Bentall, P.A. (1995), Self-rating scale for measuring neuroleptic side effects validated in a group of schizophrenic patients. *British Journal of Psychiatry*, 166, 650–653.

Dewan, M.J. and Koss, M. (1995), The clinical impact of reported variance in potency of antipsychotic agents. *Acta Psychiatrica Scandinavica*, 91, 229–232.

Foster, P. (1989), Neuroleptic equivalence. *Pharmaceutical Journal*, 243, 431–432.

Guy, W. (1976), ECEDU *Assessment Manual for Psychopharmacology, revised version*. Bethesda, Maryland: US Department of Health, Education and Welfare.

Hogarty, G.E. and Ulrich, R.F. (1977), Temporal aspects of drug and placebo in delaying relapse in schizophrenic outpatients. *Archives of General Psychiatry*, 34, 297–301.

Jain, A.K., Kelwala, S. and Gurshon, S. (1988), Antipsychotic drugs in schizophrenia: current issues. *International Clinical Psychopharmacology*, 3, 1–30.

Johnson, D.A.W. (1979), Further observations on the duration of depot neuroleptic maintenance therapy in schizophrenia. *British Journal of Psychiatry*, 135, 524–530.

Johnson, D.A.W. (1990), Pharmacological treatment of patients with schizophrenia. Past and present problems and potential future therapy. *Drugs*, 39, 481a–488a.

Kane, J.M. (1996), Schizophrenia. *New England Journal of Medicine*, 334, 34–41.

Kane, J.M. and Marder, S.R. (1993), Pharmacologic treatment of schizophrenia. *Schizophrenia Bulletin*, 19, 287–302.

Kay, S.R., Fiszebein, A. and Opler, L.A. (1987), The positive and negative syndrome scale (PANSS) for schizophrenia. *Schizophrenia Bulletin*, 13, 261–276.

Keks, N.A., Copolov, D.L. and Burrows, G.D. (1995), Discontinuing antipsychotic therapy: A practical guide. *CNS Drugs*, 4, 351–356.

Krawiecka, M., Goldberg, D. and Vaughan, M. (1977), A standardised psychiatric assessment scale for rating chronic psychotic patients. *Acta Psychiatrica Scandinavica*, 55, 299–308.

Macphearson, R., Jerrom, B. and Hughes, A. (1996), A controlled study of education about drug treatment in schizophrenia. *British Journal of Psychiatry*, 168, 709–717.

Overall, J.E. and Gorham, D.R. (1962), The brief psychiatric rating scale. *Psychological Reports*, 10, 799–812.

Peralta, V., Cuesta, M.J., Caro, F. and Marinez-Larrea, A. (1994), Neuroleptic dose and schizophrenic symptoms. A survey of prescribing practices. *Acta Psychiatrica Scandinavica*, 90, 354–357.

Simpson, G.M. and Angus, J.W.S. (1970), A rating scale for extrapyramidal side effects. *Acta Psychiatrica Scandinavica* (suppl 212), 45, 11–19.

Thompson, C. (1994), The use of high dose antipsychotic medication. *British Journal of Psychiatry*, 164, 448–458.

# CHAPTER 12

# The Assessment and Management of Risk

## Steve Morgan

*KEY ISSUES*

♦ Identifying categories of 'risk'

♦ Linking the procedures developed in secure and inpatient environments to dispersed community practice

♦ Case materials to illustrate the complexity of the assessment and management issues

♦ The need for a coordinated clinical and management strategy, recognising the individual context of risk

♦ The application of intensive case management principles in developing a collaborative approach to work with high risk clients

*INTRODUCTION*  The concept of risk is closely interwoven with the general perceptions of severe mental illness held by public and professionals alike. Historically, institutional care has upheld the notion that the risks to the public can be eliminated by its confinement within the institution, and minimised for professionals through its containment within restrictive schedules for daily functioning (Goffman, 1961; Lloyd, 1995). Though the last decade has seen a proliferation of published material on psychiatric inpatient violence, it is arguable whether this is representative of a worsening level of risk within the institutions or reflects an increased interest in the subject (Crichton, 1995a; Sayce, 1995). The policy shift to community care has been accompanied by a growing concern that levels of risk will inevitably increase within the public domain. Indeed, Shepherd (1995) reminds us that although 'care' is theoretically possible in the community, the practical and legal freedom enjoyed by the service user makes 'control' impossible, in all but the most extreme circumstances.

Media attention has only served to intensify public concern and fear, focusing attention on the stereotypical 'religious fanatic' or 'mad axeman' (Philo *et al.*, 1993). We should not minimise the tragedy and impact of the fatalities that have resulted from the actions of some individuals experiencing severe mental illness (Ritchie *et al.*, 1994). However, Sayce (1995) draws our attention to just how unbalanced this whole debate becomes when it is spearheaded by media attention and government response. She reminds us that the vast majority of people with serious mental health problems are not violent individuals, yet they have to live with a stigmatised 'presumed guilty' label, which they are often unable, or not given the opportunity, to disprove. Diagnosis is not a reliable predictor of violence; incidents are more likely to be linked to a situational response or an intoxicated state independent of mental state. Indeed, public and professional debates largely neglect the fact that people with mental health problems are most likely to experience violence as victims (Sayce, 1995; MIND, 1994; Prins, 1993; Department of Health, 1993), in a variety of ways (Box 12.1).

**Box 12.1** Users of services as victims

People with mental health problems are most likely to experience violence through:

◆ childhood sexual and physical abuse;

◆ adulthood domestic violence;

◆ discriminating attacks in the neighbourhood and community;

◆ inpatient abuse and assault from patients and staff;

◆ deaths through the use of neuroleptic medications;

◆ suicide.

Although the prediction of risk is an imprecise art, the literature reflects a recent growth of interest in the area, and increasing certainty about the factors that may underpin good practice. Crichton (1995b) suggests that there is a '...shift of current good practice away from a position where there can be a one-off decision about a patient's dangerousness, towards a continuing process of risk management' (p. 3). Thus, the emphasis is moving from the legal concept of dangerousness towards a decision-making concept of risk founded on careful on-going assessment rather than hunches or gut reactions. This is not to deny the value of gut reaction in prompting full re-assessment of risks. However,

**Box 12.2** An
empowering approach

> In the context of risk, an empowering approach should
> include a combination of:
>
> ♦ understanding the service user's expression of their real
>   and perceived experiences of risk;
>
> ♦ open discussion and enquiry into past, current and future
>   potentials for risk behaviour;
>
> ♦ encouraging and supporting service users to exercise
>   their rights to choices and opportunities to learn from
>   positive 'risk-taking'.

the challenge is not only to develop a response that limits the potentially negative aspects of client risk, but to achieve this through a broadly collaborative and empowering approach so that the service user and service provider reach an understanding and, as far as possible, an agreement.

The ultimate beneficiaries of an effective risk management strategy should be the service users, the public and the service providers alike.

## THE MEANING OF RISK

Before examining the assessment and management of levels of risk it is useful to explore the different interpretations of the term in its daily use. Dictionary definitions broadly point in two directions: a positive outlook, through upholding the notion of a challenge, a gamble, the weighing of pros and cons, the chance of a new experience, an opportunity to be gained or achieved; and a negative concept of danger, loss or the chance of damage or injury, largely linked to fear of detrimental outcomes.

Risk is what you are left to carefully consider when you have discounted all the certain variables. Yet in the consideration of experiences associated with mental health, very little can be attributed the tag of certainty: the service user experiencing severe and enduring mental health problems is exposed to a wide range of uncertain variables and risk factors. In the NHS Executive (1994) introduction to supervision registers, three broad categories of risk are delineated: aggression and violence, suicide and self-harm, and severe self neglect. These broad categories are developed in greater detail through this chapter. However, although these may represent a service or governmental view of risk, it is essential not to lose sight of the service user's more practical daily experiences of risk. These may include some or all of those listed in Box 12.3.

Whatever aspect of risk is being considered, its assessment will essentially comprise an examination of past experience, observed

**Box 12.3** Daily
experiences of risk

◆ Social isolation through loss of family and friends.

◆ Loss of social and economic status through the stigma associated with mental health problems.

◆ Threatened or real loss of home.

◆ Loss or deprivation of basic freedoms and human rights.

◆ Distressing contact with the criminal justice system.

◆ Relapse of illness and hospital admission, loss of community tenure.

◆ Victimisation in an unsympathetic and fearful community.

◆ Intentional or unintentional exploitation by community support workers.

in relation to the present circumstances, with a view to predicting potential future outcomes. However the assessment of risk is approached, it will inevitably impact on service users, their carers, and professional workers alike. If the assessment and management of risk is to be comprehensive, effective and owned by all, it must be a collaborative venture.

*SAFE INSTITUTION AND RISKY COMMUNITY?*

In relation to aggression, violence, suicide and self-harm, institutional settings of medium to high security are assumed to possess an advantage regarding the assessment of and response to risk. Although the pressure cooker effect of high security institutional living may predispose itself to higher incidences of risk behaviours, the frequency of contact and well-rehearsed routines of intervention and containment enable a more continuous assessment of and response to potential and actual situations (Lloyd, 1995). Even the lower security open psychiatric wards are expected to implement a teamwork approach to the assessment and management of risk, with an expectation of quick response back-up from other hospital staff and security in exceptional circumstances.

The situation outside the institution presents a very different set of circumstances. Vaughan and Badger (1995) remind us that, 'By contrast, workers in the community are far more exposed to risk with considerably less support. Their clients are much more likely to be unknown quantities in terms of risk potential. Opportunities to get close to the client in order to pick up early signs of difficulties are often limited to brief contacts ... once or twice a week.... Furthermore, many are notoriously difficult to keep track of....' (p. 79). In addition, despite the need to work in pairs or in neutral/ safer locations where there is known to be a high risk (or where the level of risk is unknown), community workers frequently work alone – a major contributing factor to low staff morale and/or stress (Carson, 1994).

The question should not reasonably be one of an either/or situation regarding the institution or the community. Although the notion of institutional care is progressively changing, there will always remain a need for open and secure inpatient facilities. Some people experiencing severe mental health problems will have an ongoing but intermittent need for asylum in order to relieve themselves of the pressures of daily living. Similarly, there will be a need for secure provisions for those who are deemed to pose too great a risk for release into the community at any given time (Department of Health/Home Office, 1992). The reality of changing patterns of acute bed use in recent years, has been an overall reduction in bed numbers leading to: a raised threshold for admission and consequently higher occupation of beds by higher risk patients; and increased throughput leading to some people being discharged sooner than ideally would be liked, or sent on extended leave into the community whilst still under legal restriction (Ritchie *et al.*, 1994; Grounds, 1995).

At a political level, the question surrounding the management of high levels of risk is one of how the predicted need for secure beds can be achieved in the areas where they are most needed. The practical question is how can the good practices of risk assessment, developed in specialist institutions, be promoted in the more varied and dispersed conditions of the community.

*HIGHLIGHTING SERVICE FAILINGS*  The report of inquiry into the care and treatment of Christopher Clunis (Ritchie Report, 1994) represents an authoritative call for the careful coordination of a clinical and management strategy for assessing and managing risk. The details of the tragedy that resulted in the need for the inquiry have been widely publicised: Jonathan Zito was fatally stabbed by Christopher Clunis on an underground station platform in December 1992, while Clunis was in an acute state of relapse of paranoid schizophrenia. The personal and psychiatric history of Christopher Clunis is thoroughly documented in the report, so will not be repeated here. However, it is important to recall a number of the critical findings and recommendations that inform us of the failings that result when detailed individual assessment and careful coordination of services are lacking.

As a result of 10 reported assaults (four of a serious nature), frequently involving knives, the Police and Criminal Justice System were regularly involved (including two prisons). Rather than specifically condemning any one individual, service or agency, the Ritchie Report (1994) documents a cumulative pattern of failure and missed opportunities. The over-riding failure is that of inade-

**Box 12.4** Clunis' involvement with services

Lambeth, Southwark and Lewisham Health Commission (1994) summarise Christopher Clunis' involvement with services between 1986 and 1992 as follows:

 8 Hospitals
13 Consultant Psychiatrists
 5 GPs
 5 Community Psychiatric Nurses
 4 Social Workers
 5 Housing departments
 4 Hostels
 1 Occupational therapist
 4 Bed and Breakfast facilities

quate communication, liaison and transfer of information between the numerous agencies involved:

♦ poor liaison between individuals from different agencies;
♦ a lack of managed coordination between health and social services;
♦ Section 117 after-care procedures not closely implemented;
♦ poor liaison across geographical boundaries as well as service sectors;
♦ a failure to adopt assertive outreach, or to address early warning signs of relapse;
♦ a failure to obtain a full, accurate and verified history;
♦ a failure to involve the original GP.

At an individual practitioner level several deficiencies appear to have been repeated, with the alarming conclusion that the whole training of professionals may be inadequate in the area of work with high risk clients:

♦ failure to verify an accurate history, compounded by an over-reliance on Christopher Clunis' own deluded accounts;
♦ a lack of awareness of the location and contacts of family members;
♦ repeated treatments of Christopher Clunis as an itinerant homeless person;
♦ a failure to chart the relationship of offending behaviours to mental disorder, resulting in a failure to acknowledge the rule of best predictor of future behaviour being past behaviour.

If you do not assess the risk, you cannot adequately manage the risk; public and professionals alike will be exposed to the risk. The Ritchie Report (1994) stated, '... there are examples in the story of Christopher Clunis where poorly considered and sometimes misleading predictions led to false reassurance about his potential for dangerous behaviour' (p. 119).

*AGGRESSION AND VIOLENCE: ASSESSING THE EVIDENCE*

Much of the available work on risk associated with aggression and violence concentrates on the experience of forensic services; generally inpatient services, specifically secure facilities. The incidence of risk in community settings has received far less attention (Vaughan and Badger, 1995). The clinical assessment of dangerousness and the provision of regional secure units became closely linked through the Butler Report (Home Office/Department of Health and Social Security, 1975). At this time dangerousness was defined as relating to the cause of 'serious physical injury or lasting psychological harm'. Yet a major difficulty in assessing dangerousness and measuring factors related to aggression and violence has been the inconsistency of definitions across studies (Wykes *et al.*, 1994). Some fail to give a clear definition, whereas others vary in their inclusion of physical injury to staff and/or others, psychological harm, threats and verbal abuse, or destruction of property. Furthermore, research in this area has examined different aspects of dangerousness, for example behavioural factors, aspects of personality, contextual factors and triggers (Wykes *et al.*, 1994). However, the importance of personal and psychiatric/forensic history is emphasised throughout the literature (Whittington and Wykes, 1994; McClelland, 1995). The assumption that the best predictor of future behaviour is past behaviour is, however, somewhat problematic; it leads to an individual with a history of violent behaviour being permanently labelled as a high risk. This begs the question: Can the management of an assessed high risk effectively reduce the level of risk?

Although a person's history must be considered in the assessment of risk, this must not lead to a general discounting of other factors, particularly the context in which violence occurs for an individual. If past behaviours are accepted as the baseline factor of assessment, much further research is needed into the relative weightings of the myriad of other factors which will overlay past history. However, relative weightings of factors also hold the danger of misguiding some practitioners towards prioritising certain elements of assessment, with the potential to play down other factors which may be particularly significant in individual cases. This dilemma is due to statistical evidence leading all individual instances of clinical practice, when most humans do not fit the statistical norm so precisely.

Wykes *et al.* (1994) question why, given the length of time and volume of published material on the assessment of risk, the psychiatric professions still find it difficult to achieve a consensus view on what constitutes violence, and what are the defined protocols for its prediction. Their study of assessment tools currently available leads them to conclude that the choice of assessment instrument will vary depending on the particular question being addressed. It would appear that there are still more questions than clear answers. Despite the difficulties involved in the accurate prediction of risk of violence, some commentators suggest that evidence is weighted against violent incidents being out-of-the-blue or spontaneous. Rather, violence or aggression usually arise out of the interaction of observable factors (McDonnell *et al.*, 1994). Prins (1986) argues that it is unhelpful to view an offence in isolation from its situational context; it is more productive to consider an individual in relation to dangerous situations than simply to see him as a dangerous individual. In any given case, it is therefore more effective to place the emphasis of risk assessment on the interaction of multiple factors.

The prediction of the likelihood of violence is an assessment that clinicians are expected to make on a daily basis. Yet the only clear conclusion from the evidence to date is the need for more research into the categories, subcategories and weighting of factors in any given situation so that decisions can be based on reliable clinical tools for risk assessment. In the meantime however, risk assessment factors must refer to: the individual client, the individual worker(s), the immediate environment (home, office, centre) and the community. Risk management factors must include: clear operational procedures, clear individualised plans and common sense. The case study of Michael (Boxes 12.5 and 12.6) demonstrates the implementation of risk management strategies based on a structured assessment.

## SUICIDE AND SELF-HARM: ASSESSING THE EVIDENCE

The *Health of the Nation* targets, which currently guide the prioritisation of suicide prevention services, aim to reduce the suicide rate in the general population by 15%, and the psychiatric population by 33% by the year 2000 (Department of Health, 1993). These targets may prove to be somewhat ambitious when the innumerable causes and methods for attempting suicide, and the difficulties encountered in its effective prediction and prevention are considered. Suicide prevention cannot solely focus on individual care and interventions. The *Health of the Nation* guidance manual on suicide prevention (NHS Health Advisory Service, 1994) emphasises the role of service providers, purchasers and Regional Offices in the development of sensitive and effective services and interventions through:

♦ strategic considerations by purchasers to improve the quality of services, for example: establishment of multidisciplinary audit meetings on suicide; local prison suicide prevention groups and/or a locality based suicide prevention group;

♦ strategic measures by purchasers to promote prevention and early intervention services, for example: commission a specialist

**Box 12.5** Case study of Michael: background/history

Aged 30, white, English, youngest of three siblings, all male, Michael describes an unhappy childhood. Neglected by parents who invested expectations in their eldest two sons, and bullied at school for being an apparent misfit and a loner. Homosexual development only incurred disappointment and disgust from the family, and Michael describes the harbouring of early fantasies of violent revenge. Isolated and quick tempered, Michael suffers frequent feelings of low self-esteem, intimidation from authority figures, and occasionally seeks solace in alcohol and drugs. Long periods of unemployment have only been interrupted by a spell working in a turf accountant's office, and as a male prostitute.

Michael was diagnosed with schizophrenia five years ago, and has a history of seven admissions to psychiatric hospital wards during this time. Variable compliance with medication has resulted from ambivalence towards his diagnosis and experience of severe dystonic reactions to depot medications. Psychotic symptoms have not always been evident causes for admissions to hospital; Michael can present as very agitated, anxious and distressed with suicidal ideas, and more recently with homicidal plans. He can become obsessional in behaviour patterns, and particularly anxious at times of discharge. He is generally guarded in his interpersonal interactions with professionals, but will engage with specific individuals while remaining distant and aloof from most. Physical health is characterised by obesity and ataxic gait caused by low back pain and sciatica. Infrequent pseudo-epileptic experiences have been assessed as a manifestation of hospital discharge anxiety.

Michael's forensic history is a recent development which he closely identifies as being a reaction to his perceived exploitation by individuals of the 'gay' community. Initially plunging a hunting knife into the wall of his community support worker's office, Michael was extremely distressed by a specific sexual relationship. On being discharged from inpatient care on the grounds that he was not experiencing psychotic phenomena, Michael became further enmeshed in relationships which he found unsatisfactory, and finally stabbed a man in the neck whom he perceived had encouraged then rejected him. Michael attempted to hang himself while in police custody, was remanded in prison, and finally received a two year suspended sentence.

Michael expressed no remorse while on remand, and on release expressed more elaborate homicidal fantasies to his community support workers. On interview he felt rejected by mental health and criminal justice systems, expressed feelings of hopelessness and aimless drifting, and concern that his actions shocked him to the point of not being able to predict what he may be capable of doing in the future. He also felt he was experiencing strong suicidal urges in the face of release rather than hospital transfer, on the basis that he had no future, and would in future be seen as 'the offence rather than as a person'.

**Box 12.6** Case study of Michael: assessment and management of risk

| Area of concern | Risk assessment factors | Risk management |
|---|---|---|
| 1. PAST BEHAVIOUR | Childhood traumas<br>Violent fantasies of revenge<br>Forensic history with use of weapons | Assess and document all sources of information<br>Supervision Register (to prioritise Michael in service) |
| 2. MENTAL HEALTH | Psychotic symptoms<br>Reactive distress levels<br>Hopelessness and rejection<br>Low self-esteem | As 1 above<br>Formal assessment of Homicidal/suicidal thoughts<br>Informed assessment by keyworker<br>Balance negative risk with positive risk-taking to generate hope |
| 3. SOCIAL FUNCTIONING | Poor quality interpersonal relationships<br>Exploitative relationships<br>Social/psychological impact of occupational choices | Supportive counselling<br>Consider personal interests for alternative activities<br>Discuss perceptions of past occupations |
| 4. PERSONALITY FACTORS | Poor stress coping mechanisms<br>Impulsive actions<br>Experience and attitude to aggression and violence | Psychology assessments<br>Anger management and stress coping strategies |
| 5. MEDICATION | Variable compliance with prescribed medication<br>Perceived rejection by medical services<br>Abusing illegal drugs | Regular reviews involving Michael and CMHT staff<br>Close liaison between consultant psychiatrist and GP practice<br>Discuss impact of abusing substances on mental state with Michael |
| 6. PHYSICAL HEALTH | Impact of back pain and sciatica on mental state | Monitoring by keyworker<br>Liaison with GP |
| 7. WARNING SIGNS | Increasing levels of distress<br>Avoidance of direct questions<br>Perceived rejection by partners and service providers<br>Preoccupation with weapons<br>Planned intent of homicide/suicide | Regular monitoring with Michael and keyworker<br>Supervision register with all relevant workers aware of identified early warning signs |

(continued)

**Box 12.6** (*continued*)

| Area of concern | Risk assessment factors | Risk management |
|---|---|---|
| 8. STAFF FACTORS | Frequency of contacts<br>Experience of keyworker<br>Cover arrangements<br>Serious incident inquiry | Weekly contact, clear dates and times, with flexibility for additional responses in times of distress<br>Allocating two senior workers with experience working with high risk<br>Clear plans to cover leave, communicated to Michael and all workers<br>Guidance to staff from Inquiry report |
| 9. ENVIRON-MENTAL FACTORS | Location of meetings<br>Worker punctuality<br>Potential weapons at location<br>Availability of back-up support | Home visits by TWO workers with a mobile phone<br>Identify circumstances which contraindicate home visits<br>Worker punctuality for clearly dated and timed meetings<br>Service location contacts with ONE worker, but needing prior precautionary checks of back-up support |
| 10. COMMUNITY FACTORS | Distressing memories related to flat<br>Negative attitudes towards local area<br>Communication between several agencies | Application and supportive letters for housing transfer<br>Keyworker coordinating lines of communication and accurate information exchange |

after-care service for people who deliberately harm themselves; produce specialist information for vulnerable groups; prioritise training for all staff working with people who are at high risk of suicide;

♦ comprehensive planning at a local level to ensure that a balanced range of interventions and services is available; that adequate numbers of staff are available and that staff receive appropriate training and ongoing clinical supervision; that role and needs of relatives are considered in the assessment and management of risk, and in the provision of support to those suffering bereavement;

♦ recognition of the importance of interagency collaboration, so that services are developed on a basis of shared values and principles and communication is clear and comprehensive.

The assessment of risk is, however, not confined solely to attempted suicides, but to a range of harming activities that may impact on health, fatally or otherwise. Suicide attempts may have a planned intent, or may be a call for help. Cutting and self-mutilating behaviour, and the abuse of addictive and/or harming agents (e.g. alcohol, drugs, solvents) may have a further role in the call for help.

There appears to be no truth in the myth that people who talk about their suicide plans will not enact them. A number of studies into completed suicides have identified high percentages of people who have discussed their ideas with psychiatric professionals and/ or GPs shortly before they enacted them (Lewisham and Guy's Audit Committee, 1995). Similarly, there appears little evidence to support the notion that open discussion of suicidal plans brings about an increased likelihood of them being enacted. Empathic understanding of the underlying distress can reduce the enactment by enabling the person to experience a perception of care and understanding (Vaughan and Badger, 1995). This complex evidence poses particular problems for the practitioner who has the responsibility of assessing the likelihood of self-harm or suicide. Hawton (1994) summarises a number of reasons why prediction can be so difficult:

♦ suicide is rare, and the predictors are crude;
♦ research is mainly into completed suicides, so has limited use in more generalised prediction;
♦ short-term risk and long-term risk are different;
♦ most risk factors, with the exception of gender, fluctuate in magnitude;
♦ most studies report group characteristics, in practice every individual differs.

The different nature of suicidal factors serves to complicate the whole picture of prediction. Several attempts have been made to categorise risk factors (Charlton *et al.*, 1993; Vaughan, 1995), with an agreement on some of the major contributors to risk, e.g. previous psychotic history, past incidences of self-harm, and social circumstances. Vaughan (1995) has attempted to draw these factors into a more clearly defined hierarchy of risk, with successive steps from self-harming through to completed suicide. However, he reminds us to use any such categorisation with caution, because of the complexity of individual circumstances and situational context.

*Risk assessment factors* (Box 12.7)   Hawton (1994) suggests that assessment of suicide risk in an individual requires attention to an additional range of less tangible factors, such as: emotional ties to family members; trust in the clinician; likely impact of treatments, and awareness of potentially misleading clinical outcomes.

**Box 12.7** Suicide: Risk assessment factors

♦ Previous history of suicide attempts and self-harming.

♦ Psychiatric history; with particular reference to depressive conditions characterised by feelings of hopelessness and helplessness. It is estimated that the incidence of depression increases suicide risk by some 500%, with a 15% overall suicide rate associated with the affective disorders. Schizophrenia carries an estimated 10% suicide rate, most specifically linked to persecutory experiences of a delusional or hallucinatory nature.

♦ The incidence of substance abuse (alcohol and drugs) is second only to depressive illness as a contributory factor in relation to suicidal behaviour. The significant characteristics are the depressing effect on the central nervous system, and the disinhibiting release of destructive behaviours.

♦ Age-related component: over 50s have an increased risk, largely linked to aspects of loss and social isolation. Recent evidence has highlighted males in late teenage years and early-20s as a significant peak in suicidal statistics though the analysis is conflicting in its attribution to long-term unemployment as the cause of.

♦ Gender: more women attempt suicide, but more men succeed. This statistic is reflected in the preferred modes of suicide behaviour, women favouring overdoses, and men preferring carbon monoxide poisoning or more violent but certain methods.

♦ Relationship factors: more single, widowed and divorced people attempt suicide than married people.

♦ Definite statements of planned intent, particularly with the absence of others in the stated plan, and an increasing degree of irreversibility of the plan. These factors greatly increase the level or risk.

♦ Groupings of negative life events close together, leading to a depressive condition, significantly increases the level of risk.

***Risk management factors***    Vaughan (1995) outlines stages of suicide risk from possible/slight up to completed suicide, and suggests the types of interventions that may be relevant at the different stages, as follows:

♦ ventilation of suicidal feelings;
♦ tackling social and interpersonal difficulties;

- increased frequency of contact and supervision;
- formal psychiatric assessment;
- removing potential dangers e.g. drugs, weapons;
- voluntary and compulsory admission to hospital;
- first aid, or admission to hospital casualty units;
- comfort and support to significant others, in the event of a completed suicide.

Communication with the client should be clear and open. A potentially suicidal person is more likely to benefit from an honest acknowledgement of their situation, and a focused and decisive approach. Since the details of the situation can often confuse assessment of the seriousness of the potential outcomes, a problem-solving approach may help. By isolating small, manageable portions of the overall problem, this approach can help the worker to understand and manage the situation, and it can help the client to achieve a sense of hope through the identification of small, specific and realistic goals. It is essential that the client and worker collaborate in a supportive relationship within which they may construct their own resolutions to the life-threatening situations they experience. Ultimately, it is important for workers to be aware that guarantees of prevention are not possible. The worker, agency and remaining family and/or informal supports must all have access to support in the event of a completed suicide. The case study of Valerie (see Boxes 12.8 and 12.9) demonstrates the way in which careful assessment can highlight specific factors known to be associated with suicide and inform the subsequent management of that risk.

*SEVERE SELF-*
*NEGLECT:*
*ASSESSING THE*
*EVIDENCE*

People experiencing serious and long-term mental health problems are likely to be at risk of severe self-neglect. This is widely assumed to be a consequence of the common 'negative symptoms' of schizophrenia (Bouricius, 1989; Barnes, 1994), but is also a common feature of the extreme experiences of most other psychiatric diagnoses. Yet, despite its widespread occurrence, as a category of risk it appears to receive little or no attention in the literature. Perhaps this is a result of expectations that it will be dealt with more as a symptom requiring practical intervention, and less as a serious risk to the individual which also impinges on the sensitivities of the general public. Indeed, severe neglect does seem to be something more confined behind closed doors or easily ignored in the street if a dishevelled individual passes by. It is more likely to be passed off by the lay-person as an unfortunate adjunct to the social problem of homelessness, to be dealt with by the nameless agencies who run soup-kitchens and night shelters, or even simply seen as further evidence of an uncaring government.

**Box 12.8** Case study of Valerie: background/ history

Late-30s, mixed race, English, the youngest of three siblings, Valerie describes an unhappy childhood, constantly trying to please family members but denied affection or attention in return. She is the victim of physical and psychological abuse by her parents and elder brother. Valerie felt all blame was attached to her for any family difficulties and the eventual parental divorce. Frequently locked in a dark cellar-like room as punishment by her mother, and the constant criticism and verbal abuse from her father served to severely undermine her confidence. Attempts to seek attention at school included challenging older children, resulting in severe beatings. Valerie interpreted this situation as giving her attention, and describes herself as being 'numb to the pain'.

Married with two children, Valerie is determined not to repeat her own parents' mistakes in her responses to her own children, but is also acutely aware of the negative effect on them of her suicidal behaviours and psychological disturbance. She married a dominant partner, initially perceiving that she would have a role through serving his needs, but also struggles with her own desires for more independence.

A ten-year psychiatric history is characterised by periods of severe depression, three hospital admissions, and several serious suicide attempts, including overdosing, attempted hanging and cutting. Psychotherapeutic approaches have triggered her fragility over early life experiences, resulting in further self-harming behaviours, suicidal plans and threats to staff while intoxicated. Poor self-image has resulted in periods of eating disorders, abuse of laxatives and Epsom salts; ambivalence about her own sexuality has caused marital and other interpersonal relationship difficulties. Distrust of medical treatments has occasioned Valerie to abuse drugs and alcohol in response to her experiences of depression.

Valerie's most recent suicidal plan involved detailed questioning of her community workers about the likelihood of killing herself if she dropped electrical equipment into the bath with her. The initial question developed into further inquiries about the dangers to her children returning home and rushing into the bathroom – would they be electrocuted also, or would there be a fire?

Valerie planned to lock the front door with the key remaining in the lock to prevent easy access by family members. She also planned to drink sufficient alcohol in advance to numb the pain.

**Box 12.9**  Case study of Valerie: assessment and management of risk

| Area of concern | Risk assessment factors | Risk management |
|---|---|---|
| 1. CHILDHOOD TRAUMAS | Sexual abuse<br>Physical abuse<br>Emotional abuse | Encourage discussion of distressing material at her own pace, through trusted working relationships<br>Negotiate home and telephone contacts with Valerie<br>Valerie to take responsibility for initiating these discussions |
| 2. MENTAL HEALTH | History of depression<br>Alcohol abuse on a daily basis<br>History of drug abuse<br>Poor self-image and low self-esteem<br>Eating disorder | Regular assessment of mental state by keyworker<br>Discouragement of early morning alcohol use with early termination of meeting when she is intoxicated (leaving an encouraging written note with a time for next meeting)<br>Help Valerie link image and esteem difficulties to multiple abuse experiences |
| 3. PHYSICAL HEALTH | Abuse of laxatives and Epsom salts | Encourage a planned reduction |
| 4. RELATION-SHIPS | Fluctuating quality of marital relationship<br>Intense despair linked to contact with parent or siblings<br>Poor adjustment to mother's death<br>Dependency issues on individual workers (after a long period of building trust) | Ventilating conflicting views of her marriage<br>6 monthly meetings with husband (with Valerie's permission) to encourage his expression of concern<br>Encourage expression of feelings about her family within the supportive one-to-one relationship<br>Discuss her difficulties with change and workers reasons for changing jobs (not linked to negative views of Valerie)<br>Emphasise the team approach (several workers not one)<br>*(continued)* |

**Box 12.9** *(continued)*

| Area of concern | Risk assessment factors | Risk management |
|---|---|---|
| 5. SUICIDE AND SELF-HARMING HISTORY | Serious suicide attempts<br>Daily self-harming through arm cutting and cleansing in very hot water<br>Elaboration of planned intent in discussions with keyworker | Plan agreed with Valerie to avoid hospital admissions (reflecting her ownership of personal responsibility)<br>Alternative constructive methods of tension release<br>Monitor development from ideas to planned intent (early warning sign) |
| 6. STAFF FACTORS | Frequency and type of contacts<br>Gender considerations for material in discussion | CMHT keyworker home visiting on 7–10 day basis<br>GP staff contact by telephone twice weekly<br>Support reception/secretarial staff to maintain boundaries when Valerie engages them in distressing details on the telephone<br>Engagement with male worker over a 12-month period has given Valerie a first opportunity to discuss her history with a male in this manner |
| 7. COMMUNITY/ AGENCY FACTORS | Potential splitting and conflict CMHT and GP staff | Regular review meetings between teams with Valerie's knowledge (invitation to attend always refused to date) |

The subcategories of self-neglect to be considered in the assessment of risk are:

◆ the development of serious physical disability or illness, as a result of neglect;

◆ a relapse into a serious mental state that would endanger general health and well-being, clearly identified as caused by neglect of self and/or treatment;

◆ the development of a serious environmental health problem that may endanger the individual, carers or other visitors.

***Risk assessment factors (general)*** Despite the lack of evidence in the literature, there are clearly a number of factors which are unequivocally associated with self-neglect and which might alert the mental health worker to increased risk and the need for specific support (Box 12.10).

**Box 12.10** Self-neglect: risk assessment factors

♦ A previous history of severe mental illness resulting in episodes of severe self-neglect, including environmental health problems through deteriorating condition of accommodation.

♦ Progressively deteriorating physical condition.

♦ Repeated non-compliance with treatment and/or support consistent with evidence of self-neglect.

♦ A progressive neglect of personal appearance, hygiene and daily living skills.

♦ The hoarding of rubbish and persistent neglect of rotting food.

♦ A denial of danger from malfunctioning appliances, e.g. cooker or fire.

♦ The disconnection of essential services, e.g. water, gas, electricity, as a direct consequence of neglect and denial.

♦ Leaving home with doors unlocked and open.

It would be dangerous to assume that any one of these factors alone is sufficient to declare severe self-neglect to be present at a high level of risk. It is much more clear if a combination of a number of these factors exists, and is supported by evidence that they arise out of denial or avoidance of expected 'normal' social controls and limits on personal behaviour. Furthermore, this should not be seen as an exhaustive list, but as an indicator of the directions severe self-neglect may more commonly take.

*Risk management factors*   In assessing and managing risk of severe self-neglect and its consequences, mental health workers need carefully to evaluate their own threshold of what constitutes problematic neglect. Moral and ethical issues around freedom of choice should enable individuals to adopt standards below the accepted social norm, without penalty. It is often necessary for workers to revise their expectations and focus on maintenance and survival rather than endeavouring to meet higher level needs associated with progression and growth.

The focus of management should be on engaging in a working relationship with the client. Where direct contact is avoided by the client, it may occasionally be necessary to monitor the individual's well-being through indirect contact, letting them know that support is available if and when they want to avail themselves of it. Close liaison with the formal and informal networks of support will enable close monitoring, even when the keyworker is in indirect contact only. It may also enable support to informal carers who frequently feel neglected. Education, information and dialogue on concerns around neglect are essential. This should include giving the client clear guidance on what and when actions may need to be taken without their specific consent. Again, it may be necessary to negotiate specific functions with the client through indirect contact (telephone messages and letters). Ultimately a decision may need to be made by an individual worker to involve the treatment and support team in order to invoke mental health or public health legislation. The individual client may not be sectionable under mental health law, but may still be liable as a citizen under public health law.

The assessment and management of severe self-neglect is made all the more difficult by the absence of formalised tools, and the influence of personal moral and ethical standpoints in relation to civil liberties and freedom of choice to live as you wish. The relative absence of violence to others makes this a less contentious public issue. Nonetheless, its discovery brings severe condemnation of uncaring services, with little or no respect for potential existence of 'eccentric' personal service user wishes. The case study of Nancy (Boxes 12.11 and 12.12) illustrates how the risk of severe self-neglect is most frequently associated with a combination of many aspects of neglect, not simply one or two predominant factors.

*COORDINATED CLINICAL AND MANAGEMENT STRATEGIES*

The case studies of Michael, Valerie and Nancy serve to illustrate the complexity of decision-making related to risk. The frequently wide network of supportive individuals and agencies may contribute significantly to the assessment and management, but as repeated inquiries have shown, they may greatly hinder the process through poor lines of communication and conflicting plans. The need for a clearly coordinated strategy towards the whole conceptualisation of risk is developed by Carson (1990, 1994) and tragically illustrated by the Ritchie Report (1994).

The guidance on the introduction of supervision registers (NHS Executive, 1994) is intended to be a method of administering a coordinated management strategy for targeting existing resources on the clients who represent the highest levels of need. Tyrer and Kennedy (1995) suggest that the hitherto widespread disinterest in standardised planning procedures for identifying service needs, gaps and risks, has only served to weaken the argument around the poor resourcing of community care. They support the validity of supervision registers for negotiating properly targeted investment, and for distributing risks and responsibilities across senior management rather than simply scape-goating individual clinicians.

This positive outlook on the guidance for introducing supervision registers is far from universal; indeed, it is more widely

**Box 12.11** Case study of Nancy: background and history

Late 40s, British, white, the eldest of two siblings, Nancy describes a normal and reasonably happy childhood, with good academic achievements and a place at an Oxbridge college. Both parents have died of cancer in recent years. Her younger sister is married with three children, but Nancy has lived a relatively isolated life having few close friends at school, one sexual relationship whilst at college, but no close friendships since that time. Her sister visits occasionally, but has experienced periods of depression herself, and finds the intensity of Nancy's disabilities too much to cope with at times. Nancy was initially given a diagnosis of schizophrenia at the age of 19, while pursuing academic studies. Attention has been drawn to her increasingly suspicious and preoccupied behaviours, with a rapid deterioration of concentration and quality of work. Eight hospital admissions have occurred in the intervening period, six of them as compulsory admissions under the Mental Health Act legislation, all characterised by patterns of suspicion, isolation and extreme self-neglect, non-compliance with treatment or support, and a pre-occupation with 'the curse' that dictates her thoughts and actions.

viewed with scepticism. McCarthy *et al.* (1995), while attempting to grapple with the true practicalities of implementing a version of the guidance in a deprived inner city location, nevertheless suggest '... we are aware that there is no evidence that placing a patient on the register will have any impact on the likelihood of the patient committing further offences' (p. 198). In addition to the challenges against their costs and effectiveness, the registers have been further questioned on the grounds of their basic legality (Harrison, 1994), and on the issues of confidentiality as service users become even more suspicious of service providers' intentions (Crepaz-Keay, 1994).

The further development of 'supervised discharge' (Department of Health, 1995) fares little better in terms of critical acclaim. The central tenet, that service practitioners will now have the powers to take a client to a place of treatment and support as a part of the implementation of the coordinated care plan, is viewed with scepticism and dismay. Fulop (1995) suggests that this is a fudged compromise that meets the needs of no-one in particular, and yet remains glaringly under-resourced through a physical lack of places for people to be taken. Harrison (1995) further highlights the opposition to so-called powers that have no clearly identified purpose; that will ultimately only serve to damage fragile relationships and drive those in need of, but mistrusting services, further away from the support that they require.

**Box 12.12** Case study of Nancy: assessment and management of risk

| Area of concern | Risk assessment factors | Risk management |
|---|---|---|
| 1. MENTAL HEALTH | The 'curse' giving Nancy instructions to deny access to community workers<br>Stating her health is managed by a neighbouring Health Trust<br>Purchasing large quantities of unnecessary goods from a local street market (on unspecific instruction) | Switch the balance of direct and indirect contact (with more use of encouraging and supportive written notes)<br>Increase indirect contacts by liaison with informal carers, e.g. sister (who represents less of an 'authority' figure)<br>Formal assessments of mental state when indicated |
| 2. PHYSICAL HEALTH | Neglect of personal appearance and hygiene<br>Preventing access to district nurse changing dressings on a fractured leg | Using volunteer staff from a non-statutory agency to offer intensive support for daily living skills<br>Education on potential physical disabilities (using verbal and written information) |
| 3. ENVIRON-MENTAL | Growing collection of rotting food and rubbish inside the flat<br>Reduced space for walking on stairs and between rooms in the flat<br>Increased fire risk | Offering practical help to clear rubbish from flat<br>Support to neighbours fearful of infestation (and presenting threats to Nancy)<br>Local Authority Environmental Health Officers using public health law and threats to her tenancy (if she persists with the hoarding of rubbish in this manner) |

Carson (1990) reminds us that philosophies of risk should involve the whole organisation, not simply be left to isolated individual practitioners. Moreover, to be effective, strategies to manage risk need to respect the service user through incorporating principles of dignity, choice, independence and decision-making, not simply focusing on detention, treatment and coercive powers. Accurate prediction remains extremely difficult, but at least an integrated management strategy that prioritises and supports individuals to conduct flexible yet systematic assessments and responses, may encourage more collaborative decision-making with service users, without necessarily damaging the trusting relationship. How information is presented, and for what purposes, can be as influential as what is being presented. Information-sharing is the basis of relationships which maximise the choices, and subsequently the power, of users.

### INTENSIVE OUTREACH AND SUPPORT

Crepaz-Keay (1994) gives a critical account of the service users' perspective of supervision registers, but reminds us that the key element of support is the provision of a range of good quality services and the promotion of trusting working relationships between service users and service providers. This is supported further by the independent user evaluation of the Sainsbury Centre for Mental Health case management project (Beeforth *et al.*, 1994).

In relation to high-risk client groups with complex needs, case management has provided the basis for many of the recent clinical and legislative service developments, particularly the implementation of a care programme approach and care management (Bleach and Ryan, 1995). Morgan (1993) outlines the key elements of an intensive outreach and support service, where the focus is primarily on engaging clients in an effective working relationship, developing a comprehensive on-going assessment, and the coordination of resources across health and social care needs. The outreach element of the service has proved to offer the basis of a more user-empowering response to individual client needs (Morgan, 1996).

At a superficial level, the assessment and management of risk would appear to be contradictory to a user-empowering approach to service provision. However, if a progressive deterioration into high levels of risk generally results in serious dangers, loss of freedoms through compulsory hospital admissions, and a compounding stigma associated with mental health problems, addressing risk in a preventative manner would appear to be a significant and relevant focus of intervention. Clear communication of risk potentials is essential in order to confront them at an early stage of detection; whereas ignoring risk only serves to permit the development of its worst outcomes. It should be acknowledged that the subject matter of risk generally represents quite sensitive and disturbing personal material, and thus requires sensitively developed trusting relationships in which it may be effectively explored. For these reasons, it would appear that case management approaches of outreach, engagement and response to individual client needs, on their terms, based on accessible information, represent a useful framework for the development of clinical services for high risk client groups.

### CONCLUSION

Much of the current research and literature identifies the more common factors generalised to client groups, but not necessarily to the individual context of risk. Although recent reports of inquiry have rightly highlighted failures of communication and professional training, the vitally important call for an integrated clinical and management strategy needs to be flexible in its acknowledgement of the personal experiences and responses to risk factors. Issues of assessment and management need to be inextricably linked if they are to be effective in the developing practices of community teams. The value of the intensive outreach case management approach is the focus on engaging in a trusting working relationship on an individual level. This comprehensive approach to support needs should incorporate systematic evaluation of risk factors with the client, in a collaborative manner that values principles of service user empowerment.

*DISCUSSION QUESTIONS*

1. How can effective strategies for the management of risk be promoted within the principles of user empowerment?
2. How can the clinical assessment and practical management of risk be closely integrated in dispersed community settings?
3. How can well-researched weightings for the various factors identified in the assessment of risk be developed?
4. How can the negative stigmatising media image associated with the reporting of severe mental illness be addressed?

*FURTHER READING*

♦ Alberg, C., Hatfield, B. and Huxley, P. (Eds) (1996) *Learning Materials on Mental Health Risk Assessment*. Manchester: University of Manchester and Department of Health.

Since risk assessment and risk management are such complex tasks and require the training and experience that is acquired through professional practice, these materials have been developed as a multidisciplinary training resource. Each professional group brings to mental health risk assessment their own knowledge and expertise, all of which contribute to the understanding of each individual case. The materials are organised into modules, covering risk factors, interventions, legislation, special needs groups, ethics and exercise.

♦ Bibby, P. (1995) *Personal Safety for Health Care Workers*. Aldershot: Arena.

The growing evidence of violence against health care workers in primary and secondary health care settings requires a policy response from employers. This text offers guidance on developing a workplace personal safety policy, covering a wide range of environments in which health care workers are required to function. The aim is to recognise that services should be offered in a way that is sensitive to user needs, while establishing protection for all people involved.

♦ Bjorkly, S. (1995) Prediction of aggression in psychiatric patients: a review of prospective prediction studies. *Clinical Psychology Review*, 15, 475–502.

Five aspects of prospective studies are analysed: sample characteristics, setting and time perspective, predictor variables, criterion variables, and outcome. The review reveals predictive studies to be scarce, and overall predictive validity to be low. Attempts are made to offer suggestions for improving this situation.

♦ Kemshall, H. and Pritchard, J. (Eds) (1996) *Good Practice in Risk Assessment and Risk Management*. London: Jessica Kingsley.
This text brings together the key issues of risk assessment and management within the context of a wide range of social care settings. It aims to address questions of defining risk within particular work settings, accuracy of risk prediction, and the balance of managing risk with the rights of individuals. Extensive case study material is used throughout the text.

♦ Maltsberger, J.T. (1994) Calculated risks in the treatment of intractably suicidal patients. *Psychiatry*, 57, 199–212.
The intractably suicidal patient requires much time and energy from those involved in their direct support and care. It is recognised that keeping a clinical balance is difficult, that some services seek to exclude this type of person, and management decisions are fraught with concerns for tragic outcomes and potential litigation. The purpose of this paper is to review the clinical principles necessary for management and treatment, and the support and supervision required by staff involved in challenging working relationships.

*REFERENCES* Barnes, T.R.E. (1994), The assessment of negative symptoms. In: Barnes, T.R.E. and Nelson, H.E. (Eds) *The Assessment of Psychosis: A Practical Handbook*. London: Chapman & Hall, pp. 51–70.

Beeforth, M., Conlan, E. and Graley, R. (1994), *Have We Got Views for You: User Evaluation of Case Management*. London: Sainsbury Centre for Mental Health.

Bleach, A. and Ryan, P. (1995), *Community Support for Mental Health: A Handbook for the Care Programme Approach and Care Management*. London: Sainsbury Centre for Mental Health; Brighton: Pavilion Publishing.

Bouricius, J.K. (1989), Negative symptoms and emotions in schizophrenia. *Schizophrenia Bulletin*, 15, 201–207.

Carson, D. (Ed) (1990), *Risk-taking in Mental Disorder: Analyses, Policies and Practical Strategies*. Chichester: S.L.E. Publications.

Carson, D. (1994), Risk-taking and Risk-assessment in Mental Disorder Services. Report of study day 13.4.94. London: Lewisham and Guy's Mental Health NHS Trust.

Charlton, J., Kelly, S., Dunnell, K., Evans, B. and Jenkins, R. (1993), Suicide deaths in England and Wales: trends in factors associated with suicide deaths. *Population Trends*, 71, 34–42.

Crepaz-Keay, D. (1994), 'I wish to register a complaint...' *Open Mind*, 71, 5.

Crichton, J. (Ed) (1995a), *Psychiatric Patient Violence: Risk and Response*. London: Duckworth.

Crichton, J. (1995b), A review of psychiatric inpatient violence. In:

Crichton, J. (Ed) *Psychiatric Patient Violence: Risk and Response*. London: Duckworth, pp. 9–23.

Department of Health (1993), *The Health of the Nation, Key Area Handbook: Mental Illness*. London: HMSO.

Department of Health (1995), *Mental Health (Patients in the Community) Act 1995*. London: HMSO.

Department of Health/Home Office (1992), *Review of Health and Social Services for Mentally Disordered Offenders and Others Requiring Similar Services, Final Summary Report*, Cmnd 2088. London: HMSO.

Fulop, N. (1995), Cash in the community. *Guardian, Society supplement*, 8 March.

Goffman, E. (1961), *Asylums*. New York: Doubleday.

Grounds, A. (1995), Risk assessment and management in clinical context. In: Crichton, J. (Ed) *Psychiatric Patient Violence: Risk and Response*. London: Duckworth, pp. 43–59.

Harrison, K. (1994), Supervision registers: unethical, illegal and unenforceable. *Mental Health Nursing*, 14(5), 6–8.

Harrison, K. (1995), Growing opposition to an uncontroversial bill. *Open Mind*, 74, 5.

Hawton, K. (1994), The assessment of suicidal risk. In: Barnes, T.R.E. and Nelson, H.E. (Eds) *The Assessment of Psychoses: A Practical Handbook*. London: Chapman & Hall, pp. 125–134.

Home Office/Department of Health and Social Security (1975), *Report of the Committee on Mentally Abnormal Offenders*, Cmnd 6244 (The Butler Report). London: HMSO.

Lambeth, Southwark and Lewisham Health Commission (1994), Local responses to the Ritchie Report of three borough-based conferences held July/August 1994.

Lewisham and Guy's Audit Committee (1995), *Audit of Suicide Seminar* (6.9.95). London: Lewisham and Guy's Mental Health NHS Trust.

Lloyd, C. (1995), *Forensic Psychiatry for Health Professionals*. London: Chapman & Hall.

McCarthy, A., Roy, D., Holloway, F., Atakan, Z. and Goss, T. (1995), Supervision registers and the care programme approach: a practical solution. *Psychiatric Bulletin*, 19, 195–199.

McClelland, N. (1995), The assessment of dangerousness: a procedure for predicting potentially dangerous behaviour. *Psychiatric Care*, 2, 17–19.

McDonnell, A., McEvoy, J. and Dearden, R.L. (1994), Coping with violent situations in the caring environment. In: Wykes, T. (Ed) *Violence and Health Care Professionals*. London: Chapman & Hall, pp. 189–206.

MIND (1994), *Report on Deaths Caused by Neuroleptic Drugs*. London: MIND.

Morgan, S. (1993), *Community Mental Health: Practical Approaches to Long-term Problems*. London: Chapman & Hall.

Morgan, S. (1996), *Helping Relationships in Mental Health*. London: Chapman & Hall.

NHS Executive (1994), Introduction of Supervision Registers for Mentally Ill People from 1 April 1994. HSG (94)5. London: Department of Health.

NHS Health Advisory Service (1994), *Suicide Prevention: The Challenge Confronted*. London: HMSO.

Philo, G., Henderson, L. and McLaughlin, G. (1993), Mass Media Representation of Mental Health/Illness: Report for Health Education Board of Scotland. Glasgow: Glasgow University Media Group.

Prins, H. (1986), *Dangerous Behaviour, the Law and Mental Disorder*. London: Tavistock.

Prins, H. (Chairman) (1993), Report of the Committee of Inquiry into the Death in Broadmoor Hospital of Orville Blackwood. 'Big, Black and Dangerous?' London: S.H.S.A.

Ritchie, J.H., Dick, D. and Lingham, R. (1994), *The Report of the Inquiry into the Care and Treatment of Christopher Clunis*. London: HMSO.

Sayce, L. (1995), Response to violence: a framework for fair treatment. In: Crichton, J. (Ed) *Psychiatric Patient Violence: Risk and Response*. London: Duckworth, pp. 127–150.

Shepherd, G. (1995), Care and control in the community. In: Crichton, J. (Ed) *Psychiatric Patient Violence: Risk and Response*. London: Duckworth, pp. 111–126.

Tyrer, P. and Kennedy, P. (1995), Supervision registers: a necessary component of good psychiatric practice. *Psychiatric Bulletin*, 19, 193–194.

Vaughan, P.J. (1984), Steps Towards Suicide. *Community Care*, 26 July, 14–16.

Vaughan, P.J. (1995), *Suicide Prevention*, 2nd edn. Birmingham: Pepar Publications.

Vaughan, P.J. and Badger, D. (1995), *Working with the Mentally Disordered Offender in the Community*. London: Chapman & Hall.

Whittington, R. and Wykes, T. (1994), The prediction of violence in a health care setting. In: Wykes, T. (Ed) *Violence and Health Care Professionals*. London: Chapman & Hall, pp. 155–173.

Wykes, T., Whittington, R. and Sharrock, R. (1994), The assessment of aggression and potential for violence. In: Barnes, T.R.E. and Nelson, H.E. (Eds) *The Assessment of Psychoses: A Practical Handbook*. London: Chapman & Hall, pp. 211–227.

# CHAPTER 13

# Training for the Workforce

## Kevin Gournay and Tom Sandford

**KEY ISSUES**

*Factors underpinning current training initiatives*

♦ Results of national and local enquiries (e.g. Clinical Standards Advisory Group, the care and treatment of Christopher Clunis)

♦ Policy changes and the development of community mental health teams

♦ Research findings and clinical effectiveness

♦ Influence of non-statutory organisations (e.g. the Sainsbury Centre for Mental Health, Dementia Relief Trust, National Schizophrenia Fellowship)

♦ New arrangements for commissioning education and training in the NHS

*Current training initiatives*

♦ Evolution of programmes

♦ Content of current courses

♦ Training outcomes

♦ Adequacy of preregistration programmes

♦ Case study – the West Midlands Regional Health Authority

**INTRODUCTION**

1997 has seen the publication of the Sainsbury Centre Review of roles and training for the mental health workforce. The report highlights some of the tremendous difficulties faced by the professions in attempting to deal with the rapidly changing arena of mental health care. The last 30 years have seen not only massive de-institutionalisation and changes in service provision, but the range of interventions/treatments available for serious mental illness has expanded considerably. At the same time training and education programmes for each of the mental health professions have been slow to develop. This chapter focuses on the training of the workforce and will conclude that training holds the key to delivering effective services and hence ultimately improvement in quality of life for those with serious mental health problems.

This chapter examines factors behind current training agendas including policy changes, the growth in community mental health teams and the recognition of the importance of applying the results of research to service settings. In addition we have been forced to examine the relevance and quality of our training programmes as a result of what we have learned from various national audit and standard setting initiatives and local enquiries into various tragedies involving mentally ill people. The chapter also examines the changes in the nature of education commissioning which are still occurring. Additionally, the influence of non-statutory bodies is considered and the benefits of such input are defined.

The description of the various training programmes available will be placed within the context of current research evidence and will highlight the need for courses to be designed in such a way as to be able to respond to emerging knowledge. The lack of proper evaluation of training programmes in mental health care is undoubtedly an issue which needs attention and an increasing recognition of this shortcoming leads one to question the adequacy of the basic qualification programmes in nursing, social work, psychology and psychiatry. Prior to the conclusion and summary, a recent example of good practice in education commissioning will be explored.

## FACTORS UNDERPINNING CURRENT INITIATIVES

De-institutionalisation programmes for the mentally ill have now been in progress for over 40 years and in the UK the process has continued to the point that in many areas hospital services are in a state of crisis with bed occupancy levels in some of our inner cities frequently rising to over 130% (Johnson *et al.*, 1997). Unfortunately the UK, as with most other countries, has been ill-prepared for relocating services in the community.

One of the central features of community-based services is the community mental health teams (CMHTs). Ideally these teams are multiprofessional, link with various agencies and provide a comprehensive service to those with serious and long-term mental health problems. However, a recent study of the country's CMHTs showed that these service units were organised in very different ways and there was wide variation in the nature and quality of interventions delivered (Onyett et al., 1995). The findings perhaps indicate that CMHTs need time to evolve and unfortunately the UK and other governments have not allowed for this need for evolution within a reasonable transition period. Onyett et al.'s report highlighted the need for CMHTs to focus on targeted populations with a specific battery of interventions which covered the spectrum of social, psychological and medical needs of the patient population. In its own way the research reflected the problem identified by Muijen et al. (1994) in their study of community psychiatric nurse teams in Lewisham. This work showed that merely re-configuring teams into new case management arrangements had no impact on client outcomes and the results of the study strongly suggested that CMHTs need appropriate training in order to achieve positive clinical and social change. There is vast anecdotal evidence that many of the staff of CMHTs have been relocated to these services from inpatient settings or from traditional community roles without proper preparation. The aforementioned studies were very influential in the establishment of the review of roles and training for the mental health work force, which was funded by the Sainsbury Centre for Mental Health and which published its report in June 1997 (Duggan, 1997). This review was chaired by Rabbi Julia Neuberger and comprised a number of individuals from various professional and user and carer backgrounds. The committee was supported by a large advisory group chaired by Sir Louis Blom Cooper. The group commissioned a number of projects through the Sainsbury Centre which examined the perspectives of users, carers, the professionals in the workforce and the various professional bodies. The report of the review team concluded that in order to deliver relevant and effective services there needed to be radical changes in the way that training and education for the workforce was organised and delivered. The report emphasised the need for much more joint training between various professions, rather than some of the rather tokenistic contributions made by some universities. At the same time the review made strong recommendations concerning the acquisition of core skills for all professions involved in work with those with serious and enduring mental health problems. Controversially, the report suggested that a mechanism be established for licensing, or at least regulating practitioners and that this mechanism is used across all professional groups.

There have been a number of very high profile tragedies involving people with mental illnesses and most of these have highlighted the need for specific training initiatives (Ritchie et al., 1994; Crawford et al., 1997). One failing which has been identified across virtually all inquiries is poor coordination of care. Most of these cases have been characterised by little or no communication between various people involved in the care of the patient. These deficits are due in part to structural problems in mental health services and in particular the way that health, social services and other agencies function separately as both commissioners and providers. Hopefully the Green Paper (Department of Health, 1997), which sets out four options for commissioners and providers working closer together, will lead to definitive changes in the way that mental health services are configured. Another aspect of the problem of care coordination however, is simply that mental health workers have traditionally confined their activities within their own agency and if care coordination is to be improved, mental health workers will need to work across agency boundaries to a greater extent. In order to do this specific training is required and an ability to communicate with a range of other individuals employed in different settings if of course central to the principles of assertive community treatment. In services where interagency working is established (for example in Sydney, Australia and in various parts of the USA), training events within services may often include workers from a variety of agencies. Joint training may be further facilitated by workers being seconded for various periods of time to other agencies so as to acquaint them with the problems and issues of that setting.

Various public enquiries have also highlighted the failure of mental health workers to undertake adequate risk assessments. In some cases (e.g. Raymond Sinclair, West Kent Health Authority, 1996) a reasonable risk assessment may have been made, but the results of that assessment were not communicated to other individuals involved in the patient's care. In the largest government-led initiative to conduct a systematic assessment of mental health services in the UK, the Clinical Standards Advisory Group Schizophrenia Committee carried out visits to a sample of eleven services across the United Kingdom during 1994 (Department of Health, 1995). The picture that emerged was of mental health services in a state of transition but, at the same time, displaying widely varying standards. The report certainly emphasised the need for training and education initiatives which should be responsive to the needs of a workforce operating in a rapidly changing environment. In many ways the report of this committee was pessimistic. For example, it showed that interventions such as family management and cognitive and behavioural therapy for psychotic symptoms were rarely seen in clinical practice. One of the central conclusions of this report, therefore, was that there was poor investment in training across the whole country, and a firm recommendation was made that we need to invest in proper education of the workforce.

In the last decade non-statutory charitable organisations have become increasingly important in the provision of education. In the late 1980s a unit called Research and Development in Psychiatry was set up by various charitable funds from the Sainsbury Family and eventually became established as the Sainsbury

Centre for Mental Health in South East London. From the outset, this organisation has recognised the need to develop innovations in training for the workforce. Its rapidly expanding training division has provided short, focused courses for a range of mental health professionals, non-professionals and users and carers across the country and has teaching input from a wide array of individuals from various professional, user and carer backgrounds. Recently the Sainsbury Centre has entered into partnerships with other voluntary organisations, for example the National Schizophrenia Fellowship, and more orthodox educational bodies such as the Institute of Psychiatry. The purpose of these partnerships has been to develop programmes which can be widely applied and which can be tested within research frameworks. Thus, for example, the Sainsbury Centre and the Institute of Psychiatry are beginning a multidisciplinary training programme in working with people with dual diagnosis commencing in September 1997. This same partnership is also working on the development of training videos across a range of issues in serious mental illness. These videos will also highlight good practice from various parts of the world.

In dementia care, the Dementia Relief Trust has set about training nurses in family care under the aegis of the Admiral Nurse Programme. There are now 10 Admiral Nurse posts located in North London and there are plans to disseminate the training more widely across the country. An evaluation of this programme, funded by the North Thames Regional Office of the Department of Health, is currently under way. The National Schizophrenia Fellowship (NSF) is rapidly developing a network of training programmes for carers delivered in a variety of ways. The NSF is being assisted in the planning and delivery of these programmes by the Sainsbury Centre for Mental Health. Encouragingly the NSF reports that local representatives of the organisation are now being invited to join Education Steering Committees in the various University Nursing Departments. However, such representation needs to be much more widespread and considerable thought needs to be given to the balance and choice of user and carer representatives on such bodies.

Perhaps the most important development to be funded by the voluntary sector has been the Thorn Initiative. The Sir Jules Thorn Trust donated £600 000 to develop two training courses for nurses at the Institute of Psychiatry and the University of Manchester. The central aim of this project was to develop a nurse practitioner analogous to the Macmillan Nurse in cancer care. A core principle of the course is the delivery of training in evidence-based interventions.

By the end of 1996, 85 nurses had graduated from the Thorn Programme in London and Manchester and a further 40 nurses were being trained during the academic year 1996–1997. By

October of 1997 these two Thorn Programmes will have been joined by new Thorn Programmes in Nottingham, at St Bartholomew's Hospital/City and Hackney Trust and the Royal College of Nursing Institute, London. In addition to these programmes, several others are at various stages of planning across the UK, including a new programme at Queen's University Belfast. The specifics of Thorn training and other programmes are discussed below in more detail.

*RESEARCH FINDINGS AND CLINICAL EFFECTIVENESS*

The need to apply research findings into clinical practice is of course paramount. However, although we are beginning to see which interventions should be applied, we do not, as yet, have a definitive picture of effectiveness of all mental health interventions. Lewis *et al.* (1997) have pointed out, for example, that the complete effectiveness literature on obstetrics and gynaecology has been reviewed and is being continually updated; the task for the mental health profession is truly Herculean. Lewis *et al.* have identified the need to review the literature systematically and conclude that there is a great deal more to do in order to provide a definitive picture of those mental health interventions that are effective. A recent example of how difficult it is to define an effective mental health intervention is found in the recent review of family interventions by Mari *et al.* (1996) which was carried out for the Cochrane Collaboration. This review stated rather guardedly that family interventions in schizophrenia were an effective, albeit comparatively expensive, treatment modality. However, the review covered only 12 randomised controlled trials and in this small group there were at least four differing versions of family intervention. Furthermore, each study used its own particular design and method. It is therefore tempting to say that the results of such a review still remain speculative rather than definitive, and that a great deal more research needs to be carried out on this important subject.

Although a great deal of prominence has been given to cognitive interventions, such as coping strategy enhancement (Tarrier, 1994), there are of course other psychological methods which have been shown to be effective. For example, Smith *et al.* (1996) reviewed nine studies of social skills training, conducted between 1983 and 1995 and argued that the efficacy of this approach was at least as good as family management. These authors suggested that more attention should be given to social skills approaches and the examination of how they may be used in combination with medication. The authors pointed out that when this is applied to populations with schizophrenia, the therapist needs to pay considerable attention to the cognitive deficits which are often associated with this illness. From the point of view of training, social skills approaches are labour intensive, as the method needs to use a considerable amount of workshop time, augmented by video feedback. This training process allows trainees to acquire skills in role-play, giving patients feedback, modelling and the other components of skill training such as monitored homework and graduated target setting. Such an approach needs the level of trainer input which has generally been beyond the reach of most traditional programmes and this expense needs to be recognised so that programmes may be costed accordingly.

Although medication remains the mainstay of treatment for schizophrenia, there is ample evidence (Bennett *et al.*, 1995; Sandford, 1996) that training in the management and monitoring of medication needs considerable attention. One study particularly showed that the CPNs in their sample had very poorly developed skills in the use and monitoring of medication, this perhaps reflecting the low level of skills training given on many of the CPN courses of the last two decades (Bennett *et al.*, 1996). More positively, research is now demonstrating that medication management skills can be simply defined and currently a team at the Institute of Psychiatry is testing a training package using community nurses and patients with a history of non-compliance. This study was prompted by the work of Kemp *et al.* (1996) at the Institute of Psychiatry who used a cognitive behavioural approach (CBT) with patients with a history of non-compliance, and in a randomised controlled trial showed that this approach led to improved clinical and social outcomes. The CBT treatment package relied on the use of motivational interviewing which is essentially an approach to help deal with treatment resistance and which has been used for some time in the substance abuse area (Rollnick and Miller, 1996). The core components of education and training in medication management which have been received by all nurses are shown in Box 13.1.

Those responsible for education and training need to be vigilant for interventions which show promise and which therefore have consequences for future education and training. For example, 'Personal Therapy' has been described by Hogarty *et al.* (1995) and although there is, as yet, no randomised controlled trial evidence to support its use, the work is showing some promise. The approach is essentially a long-term intervention with people with schizophrenia and emphasises a period of engagement which takes into account the considerable cognitive deficits which are often present in this illness. This initial process is followed by a programme of cognitive behavioural interventions which focus on social interactions and social perceptions. With regard to training, the difficulty with such an intervention is that it requires considerable knowledge of psychological theory and specific interventions and it is difficult to see how such interventions might be easily disseminated to large groups of mental health professionals.

**Box 13.1** Components
of training in
medication
management

♦ A basic knowledge of all types of medication and their
modes of action.

♦ A knowledge of side-effects of medications and skills in
detecting these side-effects and where possible the use
of valid and reliable measures (e.g. the Barnes Akasthisia
Scale, Barnes, 1989).

♦ The use of various educational strategies for use with
patients, their families and carers including the use of different media such as video information, leaflets and
group formats.

♦ Skills in recognising and managing non-compliance,
including the use of psychological strategies (e.g. motivational interviewing).

♦ Skills in using measures of clinical symptoms (e.g. the
KGV Scale, Krawiecka et al., 1977) and need (the Camberwell Assessment of Need, Phelan et al., 1995).

**COMMISSIONING
OF EDUCATION
AND TRAINING IN
THE NHS**

There have been several recent changes to the way that education
and training is commissioned in the NHS, and these should provide
for a more productive and efficient use of resources. Perhaps the
most noticeable change is that from now on, local consortia will be
responsible for buying places on various courses. These consortia
will comprise representatives of local trusts and, within each
region, varying numbers of consortia have been formed. Local
groups of trusts will, therefore, be able to consider the specific
needs of their geographical area and decide on an equitable basis
how the training and education budget should be spent. These
consortia will of course be advised by Regional NHS Executive
Officers and the Department of Health in turn, but decision-making
by these consortia will devolve a great deal more power to local
clinicians and managers. In addition to these changes in the
commissioning process there has been some rationalisation of the
fairly complex funding arrangements for the education of the
different professions. Now all non-medical education funds
(NMETS) are being placed within the same budget. This should
facilitate truly multidisciplinary courses where students and teachers can come from a variety of backgrounds and therefore
courses can be 'owned' jointly by several different professional
groups. The other important issue which will shape future initiatives is the location of all professional education and training within
university departments. Nurse education is now fully integrated
with the higher education sector in England, Scotland and Wales

and in Northern Ireland all colleges of health are now being assimilated into Queen's University Belfast. In the other mental health professions, education is now entirely based in universities and it seems likely that shortly after the turn of the century, all professional preparation in nursing, social work and occupational therapy will be at degree level. At the same time the clinical psychology profession is gradually shifting towards a doctoral qualification at the end of basic training and all training pro-grammes now have a greater emphasis on the acquisition of research skills. With universities becoming the sole provider of education the importance of current statutory bodies such as the national nursing boards will diminish because academic validation and regulation by universities will ensure that high standards are maintained. This issue is of course important for social work, occupational therapy and psychology, but in nursing the changes are likely to have considerable influence on the long-term survival of the National Boards, many of whose functions are now arguably largely redundant.

## CURRENT TRAINING INITIATIVES

### Evolution of training

The Sainsbury Centre Review of roles and training in mental health has highlighted that there are difficulties with the way that current training initiatives for all groups of mental health workers attempt to meet the demands of contemporary mental health services. For example, the review report makes the point that although education and training for psychiatrists is both lengthy and academically demanding, the process does very little to prepare psychiatrists for work in community settings. Similarly, it could be argued that clinical psychology training, like psychiatry, is of the highest academic standard and may train psychologists to become expert psychotherapists (of one persuasion or another), but current training programmes do little to help the psychologist meet the needs of the seriously mentally ill within the context of the community mental health team. Social work training has many obvious problems: for example the Mental Health Nursing Review (Department of Health, 1994) pointed to the difficulties which have arisen since social work training became generic. The problems of the profession are also compounded by the continuing split between health and social services provision which have led in many areas of the country to mental health social workers being no more than the office-bound brokers of services. Arguably, nursing has led the way in developing sound skills-based training programmes which hopefully could become a model for training for all mental health workers, regardless of their professional origin. Indeed, it is pleasing to note that the Thorn Programme (mentioned above and described below in more detail) has now opened its doors to workers of other professional and indeed non-professional backgrounds.

Nursing was the first profession to offer a systematic training in research-based interventions in the form of the nurse behaviour therapy programme (Marks *et al.*, 1977; Marks, 1985), which began some 25 years ago at the Institute of Psychiatry. This programme has been the subject of very careful evaluation, including the collection of outcome data from literally thousands of patients, as well as being subject to randomised controlled trial and economic analysis (Ginsberg *et al.*, 1985). The course has demonstrated that nurses can be trained in the same core skills as their psychiatrist and psychologist colleagues and can be at least as effective as colleagues from those professions. This experience adds weight to the argument set out in the Sainsbury Review recommendations, that all professions should be subject to training in core competencies.

As noted above, one of the most important developments in training was prompted by the donation by the Sir Jules Thorn Trust of a sum of money to develop training courses for nurses in research-based interventions in schizophrenia. In turn, seminal influences for this training came from those involved in training programmes for family work for schizophrenia (Barrowclough and Tarrier, 1992; Brooker *et al.*, 1994). Basic elements of this programme are shown in Box 13.2.

**Box 13.2** Basic elements of training programme

- ◆ Focus on psychosis.

- ◆ The adoption of a stress-vulnerability model.

- ◆ The introduction of trainees to a cognitive behavioural model.

- ◆ Direct linkage of clinical practice to training.

- ◆ An introduction of trainees to various therapeutic interventions aimed at improving outcomes for patient, family and carers.

- ◆ The training emphasises patient contact with structured clinical supervision.

- ◆ Outcomes from the course are evaluated by both the trainee and, where possible, an external evaluator.

Thus the Thorn programme has three equally weighted modules:

- ◆ Clinical case management including the use of valid and reliable assessment of mental state, the use of medication management strategies, brokering and networking and a range of other clinical skills.

♦ Behavioural and cognitive behavioural interventions for symptoms, including social skills training, cognitive strategies for managing hallucinations and delusions.
♦ Family work, including family education, family stress management and goal setting.

Training on this programme involves students attending one day a week for an academic year and acquiring skills and knowledge through a wide range of teaching methods. Skills training is reinforced by students taking newly acquired skills into the clinical arena and practising them and then feeding back to their trainers using written reports and tape recordings of patient contacts etc. At the same time as the Thorn Programme commenced in London and Manchester, the University of Woolongong in New South Wales began a very similar programme for nurses. One interesting modification of the Australian programme was the use of video conferencing and detailed high quality distance learning materials to reach students employed in inaccessible rural settings. Nevertheless, such students still attend the University Training Centre for skills based work and some students routinely make regular 800 mile round trips to attend for a one day workshop. Shortly after the Thorn programme commenced, Middlesex University began a Masters Degree in Mental Health Interventions, focusing on the same areas as Thorn, but requiring students to take an additional training in research methods and to produce a dissertation based on an empirical piece of research. Middlesex was the first programme to accept workers from backgrounds other than nursing, and students have included occupational therapists, social workers and graduates with social sciences degrees, but no professional training.

Shortly after the establishment of the Middlesex programme, the University of Sheffield launched a variety of training programmes up to and including Masters degree level which covered the same core topics as described above. However, the Sheffield programme has rightly paid considerable attention to working very closely with local service providers and their efforts at integrating education and service perspectives have been exemplary. The Sheffield programme is perhaps the most multidisciplinary skills-based course currently offered and has trained nurses, psychiatrists, psychologists, social workers and occupational therapists. The course is being rigorously evaluated with the emphasis of the research being placed on the factors that inhibit/enable the implementation of clinical skills in an organic service setting.

The Sainsbury Centre for Mental Health has also developed a number of training initiatives which range from academic partnerships with the postgraduate medical school at the Institute of Psychiatry to basic training for complete mental health teams. The total team-training initiatives involve all professions and the Sainsbury Centre trainers likewise include trainers from all professional backgrounds and users and carer representatives as well.

There are now a number of courses focusing on serious mental illness, using research-based interventions as the focus, being set up in various parts of the United Kingdom. Some of these programmes are new Thorn Centres (for example in Belfast, Nottingham and at the Royal College of Nursing Institute in London), while some are more akin to the Middlesex and Sheffield models (see below for the description of the programme in Birmingham).

It is pleasing to note that most of the above programmes have considerable advisory input from various user and carer representatives. Furthermore, both the Sainsbury Centre and the Institute of Psychiatry are now involved in the evolution of training programmes for users as case managers. Of course such ideas are not new and the Colorado programme for training users as case manager aides (Sherman and Porter, 1991) has been in existence for 12 years and versions of this training are now operating in more than 30 of the states of the USA. There is no doubt that users should be more fully involved in service provision and the Colorado experience demonstrates that users can be very effective in providing education about mental illness to other users and also helping with the process of engagement of people who tend to drop out of services or do not comply with their treatment.

*Training outcomes*  The Nurse Behaviour Therapy Programme stands out as an exception to the norm in that the outcome of this training has been carefully demonstrated with respect to outcomes on patients' clinical and social status. Furthermore, trainees from this programme have been carefully followed-up (Brooker and Brown, 1986; Newell and Gournay, 1994) and these follow-ups show that trainees report that they are still using the interventions they were trained in and still largely focus on the populations for which these interventions were intended. Nevertheless, even this very well-researched programme has very little data on the acquisition of skills *per se* and we can only speculate about which particular clinical skills are more, or less, important in determining patient outcomes. In the area of serious mental illness, there is little well-controlled evidence regarding training outcomes. Brooker *et al.* (1994) showed that CPNs can be trained to deliver family interventions in schizophrenia and that such training significantly improved clinical outcome and social functioning for clients and reduced minor psychiatric morbidity for carers. However, even if it is possible to demonstrate that family intervention training is effective, one of the problems is that trainees may not continue to use the approach after their training course is complete. Indeed this was the finding of a study by Kavanagh *et al.* (1993) who followed-up a cohort of mental health professionals who had received family intervention training in New South Wales. They found that some 18 months later, course graduates were either not using the training at all, or using it in an attenuated fashion.

There has been some attempt made to evaluate the outcomes of the Thorn Initiative. Trainees from the first three years of the programme identified four patients on their caseload and these patients have been evaluated by independent raters at the beginning of the students' training and then 12 months later. Data are still being analysed, but early results of the analysis show that patients seem to be benefiting from the trainee interventions. Although there are several dozen trainees and several hundred patients involved in this evaluative exercise, the data are uncontrolled and therefore interpretation needs to be cautious. What is essential in future is that new training programmes are subject to a proper randomisation procedure wherein suitable trainees are randomly allocated either to training or to a wait list control and patients on their respective caseloads are followed-up. Such a task is daunting as to achieve sufficient statistical power it is likely that the evaluation would need to encompass at least 200 trainees and 400 patients.

*Adequacy of pre-registration programmes*

Project 2000 represents the most significant change to nurse education since the training for Nursing State Registration was set up. Many of the aims of Project 2000 are laudable, although it is not clear how achievable all of them are. For example, although nursing is now a university-based discipline and is technically comparable with other undergraduate courses, the results of the recent research assessment exercise, wherein nursing achieved the lowest rating of all subjects, need to be taken into account. Leaving aside some of the general issues connected with nurse training, a central question to be addressed is whether pre-registration programmes, as they stand, equip nurses with the basic skills necessary to enter into contemporary mental health care as competent practitioners (the same question also applies, to a greater or lesser extent, to social work, occupational therapy and psychology). Given the current configuration of pre-registration programmes which was the subject of considerable criticism from the Mental Health Nursing Review (Department of Health, 1994), it is difficult to see how the curricula adequately address the challenges for providing the skills necessary for work within community mental health teams and acute inpatient settings. Key skills such as clinical case management (including the use of structured, valid and reliable methods of assessment, medication side-effects ratings and risk assessment), cognitive behavioural techniques and family interventions all require considerable skills-based training. Obviously such training needs to be provided at a postgraduate level, with some basics taught during undergraduate training. It is difficult to see how current courses which emphasise a considerable amount of psychological, sociological and nursing theory can equip students adequately with the necessary preparation.

*Case study*   A recent initiative which has been developed and steered by the West Midlands Regional Health Authority provides a model for the rest of the United Kingdom in how educational programmes in serious mental illness should be developed. The West Midlands Regional Health Authority covers a wide geographical area containing about 8 million people and includes the City of Birmingham, a number of smaller towns and cities as well as a variety of rural and suburban communities. The socioeconomic spread of the area is wide and Birmingham, of course, contains both ethnic and cultural diversity. Mental Health specialists in the NHS Regional office recognised that, like the rest of the UK, a large number of educational establishments provided a very wide range of courses in mental health care for a number of different professional groups. Examination of these programmes revealed that there was little evidence that the workforce was being provided with education and training which matched the twin demands of contemporary services and the available research evidence. The Regional Health Authority commenced their initiative by systematically seeking evidence about what training was available in the UK, what specific needs existed in the West Midlands Region and what training models could be developed within local education facilities. This process involved seeking views from both professionals and users and also taking a variety of expert advice (from within and outside the Region) concerning effective interventions and particular training models for the workforce. The steering group for the project therefore consisted of academics, clinicians and user and carer representatives. After various consultation exercises, the group agreed a specification of education and training which focused on approaches and interventions which were shown to be effective. The specification also included a requirement to use these approaches and interventions within the context of the specific characteristics of the West Midlands population, for example to reflect the diversity of ethnic and social groups and the changing nature of provision of mental health services. This specification was then sent to every educational establishment within the Region with an invitation to submit a fully costed proposal for a programme. Thus an open tendering exercise took place over several months. The process was facilitated by setting up a steering group comprising a range of people with different backgrounds and interests, from both within and outside the region. This group considered each application and eventually interviewed a short list of candidates. By the end of this process the Regional Health Authority decided to allocate resources to a programme at Birmingham University which had a principal aim of delivering training in research-based interventions in serious mental illness at various levels up to Masters Degree. The programme which commenced in October 1997 is aimed at all mental health professions and also students who do not have a specific professional background. The funding from the Regional Health Authority will allow for the appointment of teaching staff and pump-prime the project during its early development. Eventually the course will become self-funding in the sense that the places on the programme will be bought by local consortia which will pay the costs of the course. Students graduating from the course will have different levels of skills, but essentially these will cover methods of working within an assertive community treatment framework, with expertise in various psychological, social and family interventions. Perhaps the most important lesson from this particular case study is that one sometimes needs to start afresh rather than simply continuing to gradually develop programmes which may have been in existence for many years and for which there may not be any research evidence.

*CONCLUSION*    After many years of de-institutionalisation and a lengthy consideration of the issues concerning how community care and treatment can be best delivered, the mental health community has come to realise that research evidence needs to be the main driving force behind practice. Nonetheless it has to be recognised that research findings in mental health care are often ambiguous. Furthermore we are, unfortunately, a long way from finding a cure for any of the serious mental health problems, so that even the best of research-based practice may lead to only modest gains in the patient's clinical and social function. Nevertheless the realisation of the true importance of clinical effectiveness has demanded that we examine ways of ensuring that these interventions are used as widely as possible. The problem at the moment is that although we know what interventions we need to train professionals to undertake (and this is progress in itself) we do not necessarily know how we train, and, in the longer term, how we maintain skills.

Set alongside the huge education and training budget of the NHS properly controlled evaluations are essential. For many years we have assumed that some mental health interventions must be good because patients ask for them and staff like carrying them out. A classic example of this is found in counselling for adjustment disorders, and research findings from this area (Gournay and Brooking, 1994, 1995) can make sober reading. Such examples serve to emphasise that alongside all new training initiatives there must be attempts to evaluate how we train and educate. Government must realise that such evaluations will be expensive. The only method that will truly determine the effectiveness of training programmes is the randomised controlled trial, with due attention being given to a measurement of outcomes on both students and the patients that they apply their skills to. Ideally, such studies should also have an economic arm with the cost implications being explored in some detail. Evaluations which use the traditional educational research methods which are largely qualitative will be of little use on their own. To emphasise the size of the research task in this area, it is worth noting that any robust training evaluation will probably need to use a minimum of 200 trainees in order to achieve the required statistical power and that smaller samples would be beset by problems of individual variation of trainees and the heterogeneity of the patients they treat and care for. In summary therefore, training in relevant skills is the key to providing improved and appropriate care and treatment for the mentally ill; however, credible evaluation of what is being delivered is essential.

*DISCUSSION*
*QUESTIONS*

1. What factors have prompted the interest of policy makers in multidisciplinary training in mental health?
2. What changes are taking place in the commissioning of education/training in the NHS?
3. What skills should community-based clinicians be taught for their work with people who have serious mental health problems?

*FURTHER READING*

♦ Department of Health (1997) *Developing Partnerships in Mental Health*. Green paper. London: HMSO.
This Green paper published in the dying days of the last government sets out four detailed options for new structures in mental health services. It is worth reading in so far as it highlights the fact that there is probably no one ideal solution which will cover all mental health services in the UK. From the training perspective it highlights the need for multidisciplinarity and for readers of this chapter who are in managerial positions this paper is essential reading as it contains a great deal of food for thought and indicates areas where interagency tensions may arise.

♦ Marks, I., Connolly, J., Hallam, R. and Phillpott, R. (1977) *Nursing in Behavioural Psychotherapy*. London: Royal College of Nursing Publications.
Now 20 years old this book is still relevant today as the nurse therapy programme described covers the same basic problem areas and surprisingly, despite the current advances in treatment for neurotic disorders, many of the treatment techniques and measures remain as robust today as they were then. The detailed case material still makes for valuable reading as it highlights a range of issues connected with skill acquisition and supervision of therapists.

♦ Brooker, C., Falloon, I., Butterworth, A. *et al.* (1994) The outcome of training community psychiatric nurses to deliver psycho-social intervention. *British Journal of Psychiatry* 165, 222–230.

This paper makes for particularly valuable reading as it describes the study which examines the training of nurses in family interventions. The paper describes the process of measurement in some detail and the measures used in this study are now being increasingly applied by nurses using psychosocial interventions. There is particular emphasis on the effect of the illness on carers and this paper should be read in conjunction with the systematic review of family interventions by Mari *et al.* (1996) described below.

♦ Mari, J., Adams, C. and Streiner, D. (1996) *Family Intervention for Those with Schizophrenia*. The Cochrane Library, BMJ Publications (most recent amendment 23rd February 1996).

This systematic review of twelve studies of family interventions in schizophrenia is a very useful summary of the randomised controlled trials so far carried out and is probably the most definitive account of efficacy so far. Having said that, the review has a number of serious limitations including the fact that a number of studies involving different interventions have been drawn together and the total sample size of patients involved does not allow one to make other than the most tentative judgements about this mode of working. Indeed, the review highlights the arguably meagre results of considerable investment of time by the professionals involved.

♦ Sherman, P. and Porter, R. (1991) Mental health consumers as case manager aides. *Hospital and Community Psychiatry*, 42, 494–498.

This paper describes the outcome of the training programme for user case manager aides in Colorado. Although the data are now several years old, the results of this study have considerable impact on contemporary services in the UK. Detailed reading of the paper reveals just how much thought went in to plan this programme and how much preparation of the work place is necessary to ensure success. British readers who are interested in setting up such schemes should be aware that if they are to be successful a great deal of effort and, indeed, financial investment is required. Sherman and Porter's programme is not tokenistic and the paper is clear evidence that UK services have a long way to go before they even begin to address this important domain.

♦ Newell, R. and Gournay, K. (1994) British nurses in behavioural psychotherapy: a twenty year follow up. *Journal of Advanced Nursing*, 20, 53–60.

This study which followed-up a significant proportion of nurse therapists trained over a 20 year period provides detailed information about the practice of nurse therapists, highlighting the application of research based interventions but, at the same time, demonstrating that the different training centres are working with the same curriculum to produce different practitioners. Required reading for anyone involved in training or supervising nurse therapists.

**_REFERENCES_**    Barnes, T. (1989), A rating scale for drug-induced akasithisia. _British Journal of Psychiatry_, 154, 672–676.

Barrowclough, C. and Tarrier, N. (1992), _Families of Schizophrenic Patients: Cognitive Behavioural Intervention_. London: Chapman & Hall.

Bennett, J., Done, J. and Harrison-Reed, P. (1995), The community psychiatric nurse and neuroleptic medication. In: Brooker, C. and White, E. (Eds) _Community Psychiatric Nursing Research_, Volume III. London: Chapman & Hall.

Brooker, C. and Brown, M. (1986), Nurse behaviour therapy follow up. In: Brooking, J. (Ed) _Readings in Psychiatric Nursing Research_. London: John Wiley.

Brooker, C., Falloon, I., Butterworth, A. _et al._ (1994), The outcome of training community psychiatric nurses to deliver psychosocial intervention. _British Journal of Psychiatry_, 165, 222–230.

Crawford, L., Devaux, M., Ferris, R. and Hayward, P. (1997), _The Report into the Care and Treatment of Martin Mursell_. London: Camden and Islington Community Health Services NHS Trust.

Department of Health (1994), _Working in Partnership: A Review of Mental Health Nursing_. London: HMSO.

Department of Health (1995), _Clinical Standards Advisory Group: Schizophrenia_. London: HMSO.

Department of Health (1997), _Developing Partnerships in Mental Health_. Green paper. London: HMSO.

Duggan, M. (1997), _Pulling Together_. London: Sainsbury Centre for Mental Health.

Ginsberg, G., Marks, I. and Waters, H. (1985), A controlled cost benefit analysis. In: Marks, I. (Ed) _Psychiatric Nurse Therapists in Primary Care_. London: Royal College of Nursing.

Gournay, K. and Brooking, J. (1994), Community psychiatric nurses in primary health care. _British Journal of Psychiatry_, 165, 231–238.

Gournay, K. and Brooking, J. (1995), The community psychiatric nurse in primary care: an economic analysis. _Journal of Advanced Nursing_, 22, 769–778.

Hogarty, G., Cornblith, S., Greenwald, D. _et al._ (1995), Personal therapy: a disorder relevant psychotherapy for schizophrenia. _Schizophrenia Bulletin_, 21, 379–393.

Johnson, S., Ramsay, R., Thornicroft, G. _et al._ (1997), _London's Mental Health: a report to the King's Fund London Commission_. London: King's Fund Publishing.

Kavanagh, D., Clark, D., Piatkowska, O. _et al._ (1993), Application of cognitive behavioural family interventions for schizophrenia: what can the matter be? _Australian Psychologists_, 28, 1–8.

Kemp, R., Hayward, P. and Applewhaite, G. (1996), Compliance therapy and psychotic patients: a randomised controlled trial. _British Medical Journal_, 312, 345–349.

Krawiecka, M., Goldberg, D. and Vaughan, M. (1977), A standardised psychiatric assessment for chronic psychotic patients. _Acta Psychiatrica Scandinavica_, 55, 299–308.

Lewis, G., Churchill, R. and Hotopf, M. (1997), Editorial: systematic reviews and meta-analysis. _Psychological Medicine_, 27, 3–7.

Mari, J., Adams, C. and Streiner, D. (1996), _Family intervention for those_ *with schizophrenia*. The Cochrane Library, BMJ Publications (most recent amendment 23rd February 1996).

Marks, I. (1985), *Nurse Therapists in Primary Care*. London: RCN Publications.

Marks, I., Connolly, J., Hallam, R. and Phillpott, R. (1977), *Nursing in Behavioural Psychotherapy*. London: RCN Publications.

Muijen, N., Cooney, N., Strathdee, G., Bell, R. and Hudson, A. (1994), Community psychiatric nurse teams: intensive versus generic care. *British Journal of Psychiatry*, 165, 211-217.

Newell, R. and Gournay, K. (1994), British nurses in behavioural psychotherapy: a twenty year follow up. *Journal of Advanced Nursing*, 20, 53-60.

Onyett, S., Pillinger, T. and Muijen, M. (1995), *Making Community Mental Health Teams Work*. London: Sainsbury Centre Publications.

Phelan, M., Slade, M., Thornicroft, G. *et al.* (1995), The Camberwell assessment of need. *British Journal of Psychiatry*, 167, 589-595.

Ritchie, J., Dick, D. and Lingham, R. (1994), *The Report of the Inquiry into the Care and Treatment of Christopher Clunis*. London: HMSO.

Rollnick, S. and Miller, N. (1995), What is motivational interviewing? *Behavioural and Cognitive Psychotherapy*, 23, 325-334.

Sandford, T. (1996), Involving users in depot phenothiazine services. In: Sandford, T. and Gournay, K. (Eds) *Perspectives in Mental Health Nursing*. London: Bailliere Tindall.

Sherman, P. and Porter, R. (1991), Mental health consumers as case manager aides. *Hospital and Community Psychiatry*, 42, 494-498.

Smith, T., Bellack, A. and Liberman, R. (1996), Social skills training for schizophrenia: review and future directions. *Clinical Psychology Review*, 16, 599-617.

Tarrier, N. (1994), Management and modification of residual positive psychotic symptoms. In: Birchwood, M. and Tarrier, N. (Eds) *Psychological Management of Schizophrenia*. London: John Wiley.

West Kent Health Authority and Kent County Council Social Services (1996), *Report of the Inquiry into the Treatment and Care of Raymond Sinclair*. West Kent Health Authority.

***INFORMATION ABOUT EDUCATIONAL PROGRAMMES IN RESEARCH-BASED SKILLS (FOR WORK IN SERIOUS MENTAL ILLNESS)***

***Masters programmes***

MSc in Psychosocial Interventions, Sheffield University (offered as postgraduate certificate/diploma and Masters)

*Contact*: Mike Dudley, Course Tutor, Centre for Psychotherapeutic Studies, 15 Northumberland Road, Sheffield S10 2TT. Tel: 0114 222 2978

MSc Mental Health Interventions, Middlesex University (also Diploma Course)

*Contact*: Peter Ryan, Director of Training, Mental Health, Middlesex University, Queensway, Enfield, Middlesex EN3 4SF. Tel: 0181 362 5000

Thorn Programme, Institute of Psychiatry

*Contact*: Euan Hails, Programme Leader, Institute of Psychiatry, De Crespigny Park, London SE5 8AF. Tel: 0171 703 6333 Ext. 2583

Thorn Programme, Manchester University

*Contact*: Ian Baguley, Programme Leader, Coupland III Building, Coupland Street, Manchester University, Manchester M13 3PL. Tel: 0161 275 6267

## CHAPTER 14

# Serious Mental Health Problems in the Community

## Future Directions for Policy, Research and Practice

## Charlie Brooker and Julie Repper

*INTRODUCTION*

It is clear from the foregoing chapters that there is compelling evidence from research and practice to inform the development of flexible, continuous and effective services for people with serious mental health problems. There are also positive policy requirements to prioritise this client group and implement systems for monitoring and reviewing their needs and the support offered. Nevertheless, this evidence and guidance has been slow to permeate local services. This is not surprising when the scale of the task is considered. It appears that efforts to implement one particular service initiative or intervention are not sufficient: a range of adequately resourced community services are necessary to provide for multiple and fluctuating needs, and a complete change in philosophy and skills is required. For example, the introduction of case management does not lead to improved client outcome (Ford *et al.*, 1995) unless workers are using psychosocial interventions and have access to the necessary community facilities and services; efforts to train individual workers in family interventions have very limited impact when other members of the multidisciplinary team do not share a common approach and provide support (see Chapter 8); and the most sophisticated specific interventions cannot compensate for lack of housing and employment (Perkins *et al.*, 1998).

The development of acceptable, appropriate, accessible, efficient and effective services requires the support and collaboration of a number of key stakeholders. These include policy-makers, purchasers, multi-agency providers, practitioners, the general public and most importantly users and their carers, each of whom have a different role and a different perspective on the manner in which services should be delivered. Ultimately the treatment and care received by individuals and their families is the result of a complex interplay between these stakeholders in the three key areas of policy, research and local practice. This final chapter examines the intricate nature of this relationship further, drawing on the evidence and suggestions provided by contributors to the book, and concludes, finally, with a consideration of areas for further work – at the levels of policy, practice and training.

## DIFFERENT PERSPECTIVES ON THE DEFINITION OF 'SERIOUS MENTAL HEALTH PROBLEMS'

Perhaps nowhere is the potential conflict in the agendas of key stakeholders more manifest than in the question of how to define 'serious mental health problems'. Although the Department of Health has outlined the key elements that any such definition should comprise (safety, informal and formal care, diagnosis, duration and disability: SIDDD (Department of Health, 1995)), it has consistently left precise definition to local resolution. Indeed, in *Building Bridges* (Department of Health, 1995), the intention to arrive at a definition of serious mental illness based on standardised data from the operational definitions developed by local services is explicit (p. 11).

Although local services are beginning to define the client group they intend to focus upon, they are adapting the SIDDD criteria in different ways resulting in a wide range of definitions for serious mental illness and inevitably different numbers and characteristics in the prioritised client group. It is rarely clear how these definitions have been agreed: whether by estimating the numbers that are likely to meet criteria and matching this with resources; or by agreeing upon the type of work the service should be doing and generating a list of clients who would be included; by modifying examples of criteria for defining severe mental illness published elsewhere (e.g. Department of Health, 1991); or, as suggested by Peck in Chapter 2, through stakeholder groups to discuss and agree the core business of mental health services with representatives of all the different interest groups.

Whatever the mechanism for arriving at a definition of serious mental health problems, there is unlikely to be universal agreement. The severity of a mental health problem is uniquely experienced by users of services and their carers and it is hard to reconcile local pragmatic definitions with the perceived needs of every individual. Indeed, even if primary emphasis is placed on the demands of clients themselves for help, this does not solve the difficulties as some clients are clearly in a better position to make their demands heard than others. Moreover, there are societal concerns to be addressed: whether the problem is 'madness' or 'badness' and thus whether it should be seen as the preserve of health, or criminal justice services; and whether the problem is of a health or social nature (for example resulting from unemployment or poverty) and thus whether it should be met through health and/or social services.

For those who are deemed to have serious mental health problems, there are questions over which service should most appropriately be involved. Although people with problems such as pre-senile dementia, Huntington's chorea and alcohol-related brain damage might clearly fit locally defined criteria for prioritisation, there are frequently disputes over which service can best meet their needs. But perhaps the most difficult issue for local services – at a purchasing level as well as for individual practitioners – are the different views about appropriate prioritisation of primary and secondary care services. General Practitioners may, for example, demand priority for those clients who are placing most demands upon them (often those with acute, anxiety-based, traumatic or depressive problems), whereas health and social services purchasers, the police and local communities may demand priority for those most disturbed and disruptive clients who are causing difficulties elsewhere. This dilemma has proved particularly difficult to resolve for community mental health nurses (CMHNs) – the largest community mental health team resource. Results from the most recent national quinquennial census of CMHNs show that GP referrals continue to rise inexorably, from 24% in 1990 to 46% in 1996, and at the same time there have been large increases in the number of people with serious mental health problems on CMHN caseloads (Brooker and White, 1997).

Although various authors in this book have touched on the problem of defining the client group, it remains largely unresolved: there simply is no absolutely right answer, and strict adherence to fixed criteria will inevitably leave gaps through which people can fall. Services need to be clear about their 'core' business, but they need to be explicit in their consideration of who is best placed to serve whom, and committed to negotiation with other services and agencies to ensure that everyone receives the help that they need. Such principles of clarity, good communication, collaboration and flexibility are the basis of effective services for people who have serious mental health problems – however this group is defined – and these principles are reflected in many of the chapters in this book. Rather than prescribe rigid rules for decision making and practice, the authors frequently fall back on the principles underlying good practice, which are introduced in Chapter 1. These most notably emphasise the need for services to maximise the opportunities for individuals to take up valued roles within the community through support, education and information and by changing the demands, supports and expectations of that community. Perkins and Repper (Chapter 2) go further than this, however, to provide an integrative framework which has implications for all stake-holders, including those difficult and demanding clients who might fit local criteria for prioritisation but frequently do not fit into the services on offer. They stress the importance of providing services which are acceptable and accessible to all those who need them by listening to clients' wishes and finding ways of tailoring services to meet their requirements rather than expecting them to fit into rigid service rules, and by providing them with information so that they can make choices about their treatment, support and ultimately their lives.

*POLICY*   As illustrated by Box 1.1 (p. 6), the 1990s have witnessed a raft of both broad and with specific policy initiatives with implications for mental health services and with specific reference to people with serious mental health problems. These requirements and recommendations are driven by numerous interest groups with disparate agendas including the need to contain costs, to meet the expectations and demands of the general public, to implement research, to heed the voices of users and carers and their campaigning bodies, and to bow to the influence of professional bodies such as the Royal Colleges of Nursing and Psychiatrists. Not surprisingly, however, there are no easy ways of reconciling these different – even contradictory – views, consequently all policy brings with it particular difficulties in its implementation and implications.

Although politicians perpetuate the myth that the NHS continues to treat all comers whatever their problem, the potential demand for health services is infinite; more so as health services research becomes ever more ambitious and new treatments ever more costly. In the mental health arena, life events, political problems and everyday miseries are increasingly viewed as problems which require therapeutic solutions – as demonstrated by the suggestion that everyone should take Prozac to make them feel better than normal. Such demands have impossible resource implications: in the real world, rationing, targeting and prioritisation are inevitable and it falls on policy makers to make decisions about how available resources can be used most effectively and efficiently.

However, it is practitioners who must enact this policy. They are faced with ever greater and often conflicting demands; they have the difficult daily task of making political, ethical and clinical judgements about relative need, and they must reconcile themselves to either denying services to people who patently have some level of need, or managing a growing workload with inevitable consequences to the quality of the service they are able to provide. Such demands take their toll on the most important resource that the NHS possesses: the workforce. Indeed the findings of recent national research in this field by the Institute of Work Psychology at the University of Sheffield make worrying reading. Borrill *et al.* (1996) found that the mental health of those working in NHS Trusts is significantly worse than that of employees in the general population. Added to this, they report that within the NHS workforce, the mental health of managers, doctors and nurses is worse than that of other major occupational groups. Ongoing work in this study will report on the effectiveness of different interventions in improving mental health. In the meantime, there is a strong case for monitoring the levels of stress among mental health workers. In the Rehabilitation and Continuing Care Team in Tameside and Glossop NHS Trust in the north-west regional office area, Carson's measure of stress in community mental health workers is used alongside patient outcome and service use measures in an ongoing audit of the service (Brooker *et al.*, 1997). This allows changes in overall levels of stress to be observed and indicates key factors in accounting for stress levels. As year on year data are accrued, this information will also allow the efficacy of stress-reducing measures to be assessed.

The importance of good staff morale in services for people who have serious mental health problems is starkly illustrated in the Clinical Standards for Schizophrenia Report (Royal College of Psychiatrists, 1995), where this was stated to be the 'most important single feature distinguishing good (services) from poor' (p. 3). Among the interventions which might ameliorate stress and raise morale is clinical supervision. It is reassuring then that certainly the vast majority of CMHNs report that they receive clinical supervision although a worrying minority do not and, in addition, an important subgroup state that, although they receive clinical supervision, they gain no positive benefit from it (Brooker and White, 1997). It is clear that further research into differing models of clinical supervision, and the outcomes associated with these, are imperative if the morale of the workforce is to be sustained.

In Chapter 3, Peck has discussed the impact of *Working for Patients* (Department of Health, 1989a) and *Caring for People* (Department of Health, 1989b) on services for people with serious mental health problems and it is clear that the reforms were designed largely with the acute sector in mind. Nonetheless the heady rhetoric of the NHS reforms has helped to conjure up a scenario in which it is assumed that services are built on the local assessment of need and that subsequent allocation of resources is shaped by local discussion and partnership with purchasers, providers, carers and users. In reality, and as the Clinical Standards Advisory Group Report on Schizophrenia pointed out (Royal College of Psychiatrists, 1995), local contracting is still a sterile and unimaginative process whereby 'much of the same' continues to be replicated. Indeed, in this assessment of the standards of clinical care provided for people with schizophrenia, only one of the 11 districts examined had produced a plan to guide purchasing and contract arrangements. Other districts did not have a specific document to describe and define this strategy.

In considering the care of people with serious mental health problems who live in the community there are other special factors that affect the decisions taken by policy makers. One such factor is the political pressure that will always exist to reassure the general public that they are safe (hence the policy initiative to develop a continuous survey of public attitudes to mental illness). This, of course, may result in anti-libertarian measures, as some have suggested is the case with supervised discharge. As discussed by Steve Morgan in Chapter 12, this is frequently directly at odds with the needs of people with serious mental health problems themselves. A second factor relates more pragmatically to notions of public tolerance. Although, in theory, public attitudes reflect more tolerance and understanding of mental health problems, in practice 'Not In My Backyard' (NIMBY) campaigns are cruelly misinformed and vitriolic in some areas (Repper and Brooker, 1996). Such local opposition to mental health facilities leads to difficulty in siting facilities, and even to the closure of existing resources. The importance of public attitudes and behaviour toward people with mental health problems has been recognised by MIND who are currently running a major campaign to challenge stigmatisation and NIMBYism. However, this must compete with the distorted images of 'madness' presented in the media in a culture striving for perfection, dominated by a need for 'normality'. Indeed, the self-interested motives of the 'Me-decade' have seen a general rise in demonstrations and protests against developments that – although recognised as necessary – impinge on the lives of individuals and their families in the immediate locality.

Although accorded a much lower profile in the popular press, important steps are being made to acknowledge the value of people with mental health problems. One NHS Trust is currently working towards positively employing people with mental health problems and setting a short-term goal for 10% of its staff to have such difficulties. Indeed, in the US, some ex-patients' groups have excluded people from working in their services unless they have a history of, or current, mental health problems. Although such radical steps are yet to be seen in the UK, the role of service users has become increasingly recognised in the planning, provision and evaluation of services.

In short, it is all too clear that although people with serious mental health problems have been broadly prioritised in recent policy, the nature of specific policy requirements is both driven by, and has implications for, stakeholders with various agendas and contradictory interests. This appears to confirm Bulmer's (1986) observation that 'one of the principal characteristics of the policy-making process in industrial countries is that it is a process of adjustment between competing pressures exercised through the political process'.

**RESEARCH**  It would be reassuring to assume that policy is based on research about (unmet) needs, effective interventions and sound organisational models, but this is clearly not the case. Perhaps the clearest illustration of the limited place of research in the development of policy lies in the development of de-institutionalisation and community care – the cornerstone of mental health policy over the past three decades. When de-institutionalisation was initiated there was some evidence of the harmful nature of institutions but no research evidence of the benefits of community care – this has accrued in the last 20 years. Rather than emerging as a result of evidence of its benefits, the community care movement was based on a utopian ideal associated with the term 'community'; an association between 'community' and increased liberty for people with mental illness and a notion that community care might reduce the costs of care for people with mental illness, particularly in view of the restoration and upkeep costs of maintaining old institutions. Furthermore, therapeutic optimism was increasing as people with mental health problems appeared to be able to improve in novel post-war treatment regimes and the belief that community care would be possible was supported by the apparent effectiveness of psychotropic drugs coupled with increased optimism. This would appear to support Bulmer's suggestion that policy-making is more concerned with agreement between groups than it is with the quest for an objective rational truth (Bulmer, 1986).

A number of different models have been invoked to describe the relationship between research and policy-making and the assumptions that underpin these models. These are summarised in Box 14.1. Weiss (1986) has suggested that each of these 'ideal types' has advantages and disadvantages when applied to the real world and that no one archetype provides a satisfactory explanation of the policy-making process. It is perhaps naive to assume that the 'knowledge-driven' model exists, whereby policy is based on a synthesis of research evidence which also informs the purchasing of services and ultimately leads to improvements (or 'health gain') in the lives of people with serious mental health problems. There is, however, evidence of a 'problem-solving' model in operation. The national research and development programme has now commissioned two mental health programmes as shown in Box 14.2. Clearly there is symbiosis between the stated policy priority – people with serious mental health problems – and the topics that were commissioned.

What must be recognised however, is that research evidence is in itself limited; it cannot inform those interpersonal aspects of the caring process which are unique to relationships between particu-

**Box 14.1** Features of models that seek to explain the relationship between research and policy (adapted from Weiss, 1986)

| Name of model | Features of model |
|---|---|
| Knowledge-driven | Research process follows linear sequence: basic research, applied research, research development and finally widespread application. The notion that the very existence of knowledge 'pushes' development and use. |
| Problem-solving | Same linear sequence as for knowledge-driven model but information is lacking and so new research must be commissioned. The process in this model is: pending policy decision, identify missing knowledge, commission research, interpret findings, make policy decision. |
| Interactive model | Researchers are used by policy-makers as part of a larger group to discuss a solution to a policy problem in which 'expert knowledge' may be but one feature. Other skills that will be brought to bear include: political insight, opinion, and experience. |
| Political model | Research findings are used to bolster a case for a policy decision that has been taken on other grounds. Research as ammunition or 'grist to the mill'. |
| Tactical model | Commissioned research as 'proof' that policy-makers are serious about a problem. In this model research may be used as a delaying tactic ('we are waiting until the study has been completed and then it must be peer-reviewed'). |
| Enlightenment model | The permeation of concepts and perspectives from research over a period of time. The diffusion of findings through a wide range of channels including: journals, mass media and conversations between colleagues. Research in this model may challenge accepted truths (and overturn them). |

lar individuals. Furthermore, although evidence of effectiveness might exist, replication of the findings is not guaranteed; the application and implementation of findings of studies conducted on different populations, in different environments and at different times is not straightforward. Added to this, there are fundamental gaps in the body of knowledge available to inform policy and practice in relation to people who have serious mental health problems. First, existing research focuses mainly on people with schizophrenia rather than on the whole population with serious mental health problems. There is, as yet, little understanding of the

**Box 14.2**
Commissioned topics for national research and development programme for mental illness

National R & D Programme for Mental Health

1st Call for Proposals (1993)

◆ Community care of the severely mentally ill

◆ Methodology to establish the mental health needs of a particular population

◆ Mental Health of the NHS workforce

◆ Training packages for use in Primary Care and the Community

2nd Call for Proposals (1994)

◆ Training packages for use in primary and community settings

◆ Prevention

◆ Minority ethnic group

◆ Quality of life in residential care for the elderly mentally ill

Centrally commissioned Programme for research in mental health

Call for Proposals (1995)

◆ Facilitation of work at the interface between local authority social services departments, health services and other agencies having significant contact with people with severe mental illness

◆ Facilitation of work involving the interface between primary and secondary mental health care services

◆ The staffing and training implications of successful community mental health care

◆ Reducing the burden carried by informal carers of severely mentally ill people

◆ Reducing public fear and anxiety associated with mental illness

◆ The management in the community of challenging behaviour by people with severe mental illness or with learning disability

◆ The development of detection and treatment protocols in primary care.

application of the findings of studies (with carefully selected client groups) in routine practice (with clients who have a range of diagnoses and more complex needs). Where studies attempt to generalise to the whole population who have serious mental health problems, the attribution of findings to any particular intervention is problematic owing to the heterogeneous nature and needs of the client group and the range of interventions and services which might be used to meet these needs (Repper and Brooker, 1997). Clearly, for studies with such a potentially large number of variables, randomised controlled trials are not only limited in what they can tell us about the process of care, but also require very large numbers and are therefore practically difficult to organise and costly to run. Yet, syntheses of research evidence often rely solely on the results of randomised controlled trials so these reviews again have limited application to the population who have serious mental health problems in local services.

Second, added to the problems of defining the population, there are particular difficulties with the interpretation and application of research in local settings. Although many large research projects report the findings of 'model programmes', these results have to be tailored to local services with distinct characteristics, problems and resources. For example in one borough of London, the siting of community facilities for people with mental health problems is constantly thwarted or delayed by strong oppositional residents' groups (Repper *et al.*, 1997).

Third, there are aspects of service delivery in relation to people who have serious mental health problems which have been subject to very little research to date. For example, Brooker *et al.* (1996) have shown that evidence for the effectiveness of CMHNs is extremely limited even though they are widely regarded as the professional group that will actually provide the bulk of 'hands-on' care. In addition, community mental health teams are generally advocated as the most appropriate vehicle for the delivery and/or coordination of comprehensive community services, but as Steve Onyett and Helen Smith describe in Chapter 4, there is apparently little consensus over what a community mental health team is, let alone how they can function most effectively. Similarly, as discussed by Richard Ford and Edana Minghella in Chapter 6, few studies have examined and defined users' agendas in research nor taken this into account in providing interventions or measuring outcome.

Notwithstanding these problems, of the models proposed, it is perhaps the 'enlightenment' model that best – although not entirely satisfactorily – describes the situation in relation to people who have serious mental health problems, whereby 'it is not the findings of a single study nor even of a body of related studies that directly affect policy. Rather it is the concepts and theoretical perspectives that social science research has engendered that permeate the policy-making process' (Weiss, 1986). Moreover, local service providers now have an opportunity to add their voice to the fray. As Trusts evolve their own research and development plans in line with the Culyer Report (Department of Health, 1994) hopefully research and development will become more focused on problems in the real (not ideal) world.

## IMPLEMENTATION: POLICY AND RESEARCH IN PRACTICE

When the complexities of the relationship between policy, practice and research are considered it is not surprising that the implementation of policy and research in the practice arena is problematic. Although the flow of guidance from the Department of Health/NHS Executive is considerable (see Box 1.1), neither this, nor the more specific recommendations that arise from multiple research projects in this area are having sufficient impact on service delivery. The recent review of inquiries into community care published by the Zito Trust makes salutary reading and provides evidence of the tragic results of inadequate services. For example, recent data from the National Census of Community Mental Health Nurses suggest that people with serious mental health problems are still not being targeted by the largest professional group that work in secondary services (Brooker and White, 1997). Questions therefore arise over how best to ensure that policy and research are implemented.

The adequacy of educational strategies to promote the implementation of evidence has been reviewed in Chapter 13. Although recent policy has attempted to highlight the, as yet largely theoretical, benefits of multiprofessional training, there is little evidence that such training can work or is more effective than other, unidisciplinary models currently in operation. In a review of 102 trials of interventions to improve professional practice, Oxman *et al.* (1995) conclude that a multifaceted approach is most effective in promoting new ways of working. In the area of serious mental health problems this might include far more emphasis on effective interventions in pre-registration and undergraduate training of all health care professionals coupled with more systematic post-registration/graduate training. In Sheffield the NHS Trust providing mental health services has developed a 'breadth and depth' strategy in an attempt to improve services in line with available evidence. This involves the provision of brief practical training in psychosocial interventions and service organisation issues for multidisciplinary practitioners working in a variety of different voluntary, local authority and health service settings to benefit a total of 75 staff over three years; funding six places per year (for three years) on a one-year postgraduate certificate in psychosocial interventions; and, funding three places on a postgraduate diploma/MSc level 'trainers' course in organisational, teaching and clinical skills for working with people who have serious mental health problems. It is hoped that by providing multidisciplinary training, and advanced training for senior clinicians in the service, skills and knowledge will be implemented, diffused within the service and supported within multidisciplinary teams. Since the School of Nursing has funded a lecturer to be trained to MSc level, it is also hoped that this evidence will permeate pre-registration nurse training. This is just one approach and its success is unclear as evaluation of the project is far from complete. However, for this type of initiative to be developed, implemented and evaluated adequately costs are involved and there needs to be commitment at all levels: by practitioners, managers, commissioners and regional education and development groups.

*CONCLUSION*

This book has attempted to draw together evidence for good practice in commissioning, planning and providing services for people who have serious mental health problems and to assess the overall contribution made by policy and research to this process. Generally, a hopeful picture has been presented; much has been achieved in recent years, and there are now clear indications of how effective services might be developed. However, the picture is still far from complete and in Box 14.3 a number of remaining key issues are outlined for key stakeholders. Although each of the contributors has addressed a specific topic area in their chapter, inevitably there have been areas of overlap; additionally common themes have arisen throughout the text. Box 14.3 can, of course, be read in a number of ways. Thus, there is a range of issues for users of services that require attention which include, for example, the identification of user-defined outcomes, further involvement in the planning and provision of services and meaningful involvement in multidisciplinary training programmes. Alternatively the book has identified a series of issues with implications for clinical practice, examples here include 'new' interventions (and the associated training requirements), unresolved conflicts about the targeting of specific client groups and the impact of multidisciplinary team working on the effective delivery of care. Ultimately the delivery of high quality community-based services for people with serious mental health problems will not depend solely on the individual efforts of researchers, purchasers, managers, policy-makers, users or clinicians but on a concerted team effort by all these players. It is to truly multidisciplinary team working that we should all aspire.

**Box 14.3** Main issues for key stakeholders

| | Department of Health/Regional Office | Regional Educational Development Group | Commissioners | Providers | Teams/Practitioners | Users |
|---|---|---|---|---|---|---|
| Research | • Reappraisal of research priorities as major commissioner to develop implementation and user perspective <br> • Workforce capacity strategy <br> • Strategic context | • Evaluation of outcome of strategy | • Evidence-based commissioning <br> • Quality specifications <br> • Audit <br> • Commissioning identified outcomes | • Culyer <br>  – identification of research skills <br>  – local evaluation <br>  – multidisciplinary research capacity | • Implementation/Development <br> • Responsibilities and role to be specified in contracts and through staff appraisal <br> • Membership of R&D project teams | • Identification of user-defined outcomes <br> • Role in routine audit (users' satisfaction) <br> • Membership of R&D project groups |
| Practice | • Policy context, e.g. *Health of the Nation* targets <br> • Serious mental illness versus GP fundholding <br> • Supervised discharge <br> • Clinical effectiveness | • Community mental health teams <br> • Varying roles of team members | • *Health of the Nation* targets <br> • Conflicts between policy priority, e.g. SMI and GP commissioning power <br> • Audit: outcomes, e.g. HoNOS <br> • Innovation, e.g. early intervention <br> • Costs of services | • Balancing competing priorities <br> • Principles of service provision <br> • Types of contract <br> • New interventions, e.g. drugs, psychological intervention <br> • GP fundholders | • Systems for clinical supervision <br> • Audit outcomes <br> • Difficult to engage users <br> • Team-working | • Involvement in provision and planning of services <br> • Definition of 'user' constantly expanding |
| Training | • National strategy (in light of national review) | • Multidisciplinary <br> • Clinical effectiveness <br> • Addressing policy concerns, e.g. SMI and primary health care <br> • Lack of evaluation of different models | • More specifically in contracts <br> • Funding for training <br> • For particular outcomes | • Development issues <br> • Outcomes and contracting <br> • Local consortia/REDG <br> • Responsive providers <br> • Skilled providers | • Resource issues, i.e. contract requirements and time needed <br> • Access to expert supervision <br> • Multidisciplinary versus professional agendas <br> • Fidelity in service settings | • Identify and resource training needs of users <br> • Involvement as trainers for m-d groups |

*REFERENCES*    Borrill, C.S., Wall, T.D., West, M.A. *et al.* (1996), *Mental Health of the Workforce in NHS Trusts*. Phase 1. Final Report. Institute of Work Psychology, University of Sheffield and Department of Psychology, University of Leeds.

Brooker, C. and White, E. (1998), The fourth national quinquennial census of community mental health nursing: Final Report to the Department of Health.

Brooker, C., Molyneux, P. and Repper, J. (1998), Auditing Clinical Outcome and Staff Morale in a Rehabilitation Team for People with Serious Mental Health Problems. *Journal of Advanced Nursing*, in press.

Brooker, C., Repper, J. and Booth, A. (1996), The effectiveness of community mental health nursing: a review. *Journal of Clinical Effectiveness*, 1(2), 44–49.

Bulmer, M. (1986), The policy process and the place in it of social research. In: Bulmer, M. (Ed) *Social Science and Social Policy*. London: Allen and Unwin.

Department of Health (1989a), *Working for Patients*, CMND 555. London: HMSO.

Department of Health (1989b), *Caring for People*, CMND 849. London: HMSO.

Department of Health (1991), *Health of the Nation*, CMND 1532. London: HMSO.

Department of Health (1994), Taskforce on R&D in the NHS (Culyer-Chair) *Supporting Research and Development in the NHS*. London: HMSO.

Department of Health (1995), *Building Bridges*. A guide to arrangements for inter-agency working for the care and protection of severely mentally ill people. London: HMSO.

Department of Health (1995), *Critical Reviews Advisory Group: Schizophrenia*. London: HMSO.

Department of Health/Social Services Inspectorate (1993), *Health of the Nation Key Area Handbook: Mental Illness*. London: Department of Health.

Ford, R., Beadsmoore, A., Ryan, P., Repper, J., Craig, T. and Muijen, M. (1995), Providing the safety net: case management for people with a serious mental illness. *Journal of Mental Health*, 1, 91–99.

Oxman, A.D., Thomson, M.A., Haynes, R.B., Davis, D.A. (1995), *No magic bullets: a systematic review of 102 trials of interventions to help health care professionals deliver services more effectively and efficiently*. Report prepared for the North East Thames Regional Health Authority R&D Programme, London.

Perkins, R. and Repper, J. (1998), *Choice or Control? Dilemmas in community mental health practice*. Oxford: Radcliffe Medical Press.

Repper, J. and Brooker, C. (1996), Public attitudes to mental health facilities in the community. *Journal of Health and Social Care in the Community*, 4, 290.

Repper, J. and Brooker, C. (1998), Difficulties in the measurement of outcome in people who have serious mental health problems. *Journal of Advanced Nursing*, (in press).

Repper, J., Sayce, L., Strong, S., Wilmott, L. and Haines, M. (1997), *Tall stories from the backyard*. A national survey of opposition to community mental health facilities. London: MIND Publications.

Royal College of Psychiatrists (1995), Clinical Standards Advisory Group: Schizophrenia. London: Royal College of Psychiatrists.

Weiss, C. (1986), The many meanings of research utilisation. In: Bulmer, M. (Ed) *Social Science and Social Policy.* London: Allen and Unwin.

# Index